THE VET AT NOAH'S ARK

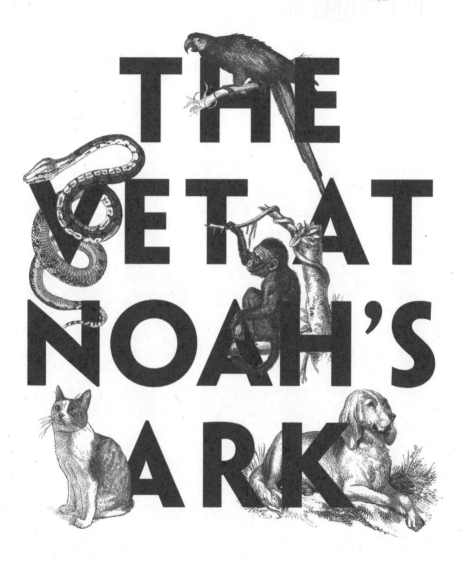

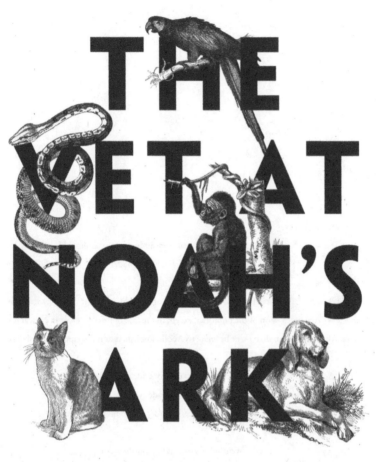

THE VET AT NOAH'S ARK

STORIES OF SURVIVAL FROM AN INNER-CITY ANIMAL HOSPITAL

DR. DOUG MADER

FOREWORD BY DR. KEVIN T. FITZGERALD

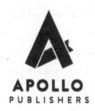

APOLLO
PUBLISHERS

*This book is dedicated with eternal love to Wok
and to all the Woks in everybody's lives.*

CONTENTS

FOREWORD

By Dr. Kevin T. Fitzgerald

In the early 1980s veterinarian Leo K. Bustad coined the term "human-animal bond." The American Veterinary Medical Association defines this as the "mutually beneficial and dynamic relationship between people and animals influenced by behaviors essential to the health and well-being of both."

Since *All Creatures Great and Small* was first published in 1972, a host of animal writers have tried to re-create the special magic and charm of James Herriot's book. Very few have succeeded. A large part of the appeal of the Herriot books was just how accurately they captured both the quaint nature of the English countryside and the state of veterinary medicine at the time. Readers got to accompany a country veterinarian on his daily rounds and in doing so met an enchanting group of people and animals.

In *The Vet at Noah's Ark*, you get to ride shotgun with a modern clinician, the remarkable Dr. Doug Mader, as he meets his patients and their families. Human beings have been given three gifts: the wondrous biodiversity of our world, our intellect, and our empathy. I have known Dr. Mader for over thirty years, and he is one of my favorite people because he has so much respect for our world's biodiversity, has an enviable intellect, and has empathy flow from every cell of his body.

In the following pages you will meet an unforgettable cast of characters, both animal and human, and watch as Dr. Mader treats them all with
affection, respect, and love. He is the embodiment of "the bond." You will
also get to play "armchair veterinarian" and make your diagnosis as each
case unfolds. In fact, this book is almost a primer in how to work up a case.
Best of all, in these stories you will get to meet Dr. Mader and see him where
he is undoubtedly most at home, with his patients.

To consider Dr. Mader just a veterinarian would be like considering
Muhammad Ali to be just a fighter. Dr. Mader has become world-renowned
through his iconic textbooks, his groundbreaking work with sea turtles,
and his animal adventures to the Arctic and Antarctica, and he has earned
his well-deserved reputation as clinician, teacher, and conservationist.
There are some ten million other forms of life on Earth, and Dr. Mader
has spent his life treating and studying a large number of them. Of course,
veterinarians love animals, but the best veterinarians love people as well.
Doug Mader's understanding and love of all life come through in this solid
read. Have fun with this book.

Dr. Kevin T. Fitzgerald
Animal Planet's *Emergency Vets* and *E-Vet Interns*
Staff Veterinarian
VCA Alameda East Veterinary Hospital

Preface

Fortunately for my patient I had recently attended a national medical conference. While there I'd visited a surgical instrument vendor and purchased the highly specialized equipment that allowed me to perform the delicate surgery through which I was currently sweating.

"Dab!" I commanded, but it came out more of a plea than an order. Stacey, one of my surgical nurses, carefully reached around my hunched shoulders and blotted the sweat from my brow, cautious not to dislodge the magnifying headset I was wearing to help me better view the minuscule parts of my Lilliputian patient.

No heart monitors or ECG units worked on such diminutive creatures, so monitoring the anesthesia was always a difficult and challenging task. You hear doctors joke, "The surgery was a success, but unfortunately the patient died." I never found that funny.

It's not uncommon for a patient to lose a small amount of blood during a surgery. Blood transfusions are commonplace in most human procedures, and rarely a problem. However, when your patient weighs barely over an ounce, losing even a few drops of blood can spell disaster.

A light veil of blue smoke wafted up from the tiny incision, forming an ominous, ever-changing ghost dancing over my patient as I used an electronic scalpel to cut through the paper-thin skin. The "blade," which is actually a radio current that cuts and coagulates the tissue, results in a minimal loss of precious blood. Thankfully, the cutting was done, and the procedure was halfway completed.

"Dr. Mader," a voice called into the surgical room. I had a steadfast rule that people were not allowed to enter the surgical suite while an operation was in progress.

"What?" I replied, with some irritation.

"We're running out of food for the ward patients." Leanne was new. She wanted badly to impress me, and I could hardly get mad at her for her compassion, but this really was not the time to be discussing supplies.

"It'll have to wait, Leanne. I'm a little busy right now."

"What an idiot!" Stacey smirked.

"C'mon, Stace," I replied. "Remember when you were just starting out and all enthusiastic." I reached for a sterile cotton-tipped swab and dabbed up a dollop of blood just as it started to ooze from the quarter-inch incision. Then, using an iris forceps—a miniature replica of common tweezers that has tiny teeth—I aligned the sides of the wound in order to suture it closed.

"Yeah, I suppose," she mumbled, turning back toward the counter where she picked up and opened a pack of surgical thread as fine as a human hair. She dropped it onto my tray, being careful not to contaminate any of the instruments. Stacey was a bit rough around the edges. She was one of the ex-cons whom I had working for me over the years. Most came and went, but Stacey stayed. For the sake of my patients, I was glad she did. She was competent, smart, and always one step ahead, which made my life in the operating room much easier.

The suture was black, the same color as my patient's pelage, making it rather difficult to see, even under the harsh surgical lights.

"Stace—" I started to speak.

"Yeah, yeah." She reached over and adjusted the focus on my headset.

The binocular lenses allowed me to see even the tiniest thread.

"When are you going to be finished?" Leanne's voice pierced through the partially opened surgical suite door, interrupting my concentration.

"Get outa here!" Stacey yelled. "And don't open that door!"

"Hey, you two!" I interjected. There's nothing like playing surgeon and housemother at the same time. Then, to Leanne, "I'll be finished in about ten minutes. Whatever you need will just have to wait."

"She's clueless." Stacey laughed again.

I returned to my task, eager to finish the procedure and wake up my patient. Amputating an ear does not rank as an overly difficult procedure in most cases, but then again, Mickey was not like most of my patients.

I had first met Mickey the mouse about one month earlier. He had come in with his family, Mrs. Davenport and her two children, Donnie and Leslie, ages six and eight, respectively.

It was not uncommon for people to bring such unusual pets to see me. I had established a reputation as an "exotics expert," "exotic" generally referring to any animal that is not a dog or a cat. Since most veterinary schools teach only "domestic" animal medicine—meaning, dog, cat, horse, cow, and other farm animals—most veterinarians have neither the training nor the desire to treat nontraditional pets such as mice, birds, reptiles, and the like. In fact, I had such an unusual client-pet constituency that people would often hang out in our reception area just to see what would walk, crawl, slither, or fly in for a doctor's visit.

Mickey had been scratching nonstop for almost a week, little Leslie had dutifully reported. She got the creature from a school classroom project where students were encouraged to take pets home and learn how to care for them.

At our first encounter Mrs. Davenport had expressed concern over money. She wanted to help Mickey but couldn't afford a large vet bill. I have always been a sucker for schoolchildren and animals. I believe that pets are an integral part of a child's life. Not only is the human-animal bond important, but the relationship also teaches a child important lessons in responsibility, finances, and, most of all, life and death.

I did not want to give away my services, as that would defeat the purpose of teaching the value of financial responsibility. Children have to understand that owning a pet means caring for it in health and in sickness. That means paying for the pet's care when it falls ill.

At the same time, I did not have the heart to let any animal suffer. What kind of impression would that make on young children? "Veterinarians don't really care about the animals. They're only in it for the money." Unfortunately, that's a common misconception among many pet owners when they receive their bill.

"I'll work with you," I had told Mrs. Davenport. The assurance that I would be flexible usually assuaged the concerns of clients who asked for discounts.

Mickey had a severe mite infestation, not an uncommon problem in mice. These cases are usually treated by giving the patient a medication that kills the mites, and within a couple of weeks the problem resolves.

Unfortunately for Mickey, after his first treatment he had developed an allergic reaction to the mites as they were dying under the skin. This was not an unheard-of complication, and as soon as the problem was identified, I started him on medications to soothe the itchy skin. I also started him on antibiotics because he had been scratching so badly that he had severely damaged his skin, leaving deep cuts and lacerations that culminated in a nasty infection on the side of his face. His little whiskers were covered with dried blood.

Mrs. Davenport had taught Leslie how to administer the medication twice a day, and the little girl had assured me, with tears in her eyes, that Mickey had taken every treatment. Nonetheless, he had come back a third time, even worse off than before. Mickey had been scratching so badly that he had actually scratched off the majority of his right ear. It was only hanging on by a thread of tissue, attached at the base. The rest of the ear had become necrotic, or dead, from the damaged blood supply caused by the incessant scratching.

Why pet owners tend to wait until it's too late is one thing that I always have difficulty understanding. A person whose ear is about to fall off will usually go to the doctor right away, but for some reason people with pets often wait. If I had been able to treat Mickey's ear when it was first torn, I could have saved it. Unfortunately, it was too far gone by the time I saw him, and the best I could do was amputate the remaining portion and sew up the damaged skin to prevent the infection from spreading.

These charity cases are never easy. If I had charged Mickey's mom every time she came in, the fee would have been several hundred dollars. But by offering to "work with" Mrs. Davenport, I had painted myself into a corner. I couldn't just decide to pull out in the middle of Mickey's treatments and say, "Gee, I'm really sorry Mrs. Davenport, Donnie, and Leslie, but I can't afford to continue. I think it's time to let Mickey die."

I finished placing the last suture in the side of Mickey's skin. His fur had been shaved over the right side of his face, giving him a punk rock look. With the half-shaved head, black fur on one side, white-and-gray skin on the bald side, a missing ear, and sutures, he would fit right in on the streets of Hollywood.

"That looks great," Stacey announced as I removed the little facemask that had been used to deliver the anesthetic gas Mickey had been breathing during surgery. She was good at saying the right thing, whether she meant it or not. Stacey could be hard to read.

Mickey took a big gasp, coughing out the last of the anesthetic gas as he began to recover from the amputation. Surgery is painful, and yes, mice feel pain.

"Let's get him some torb," I said to Stacey as I stroked Mickey's fur. "Torb" was short for butorphanol, a painkiller.

"I'm on it." Stacey knew the dosages and did not need to be told. I considered her my Swiss Army knife: she could do it all. She took out the bottle of pain medication and started withdrawing the liquid with a micro-syringe for our tiny patient.

At first I was concerned about having Stacey around the hospital. In her younger days she had been busted for cocaine after she bought from an undercover narcotics agent. Somehow, and I never learned the details, she got off with minimal time served. Her parents weren't wealthy, but they came up with the money to get her into drug rehab. She got started in a work program as part of her probation, and that's how she came into my life.

I hired her as a kennel helper, a menial job that involved cleaning cages, feeding the patients, washing the dogs and cats, and doing whatever other thankless jobs needed to be done. A housekeeping position was a safe place to start new staff, as it involved little responsibility and any mistakes were rarely life-threatening for the patients.

Stacey was a quick study. She frequently took books home to read at night, and she always kept copious notes. So now, a year and a half after taking a chance with her, I was decidedly better off for having her as an animal nurse. I watched without worry as she handled drugs that not only had abuse potential but a street value worth hundreds of dollars. Stacey had come a long way. I smiled an inward smile at the whole scenario and the small role that I had played in it.

Mickey was standing and starting to self-groom. He would hold up his little front feet, lick his paws, and then brush them over his face, pausing only to lick the paws once again, then start the whole process over. That was a great sign. Mickey was going to do just fine.

"Thanks, Stace," I said as she was disposing the used syringe and needle in a bright red biohazard container. I noticed that she had to jostle the canister to get the syringe to fit inside. It was just about full. Time to replace it. I would have to pay a fee to have these "biohazards" properly disposed. We couldn't just toss the full container in the trash. It cost the hospital about $500 a month to have a service come and collect the containers and replace them with empty receptacles.

I pondered what I was going to charge Mrs. Davenport and her children for Mickey's surgery. I scanned the surgery room. I had used an anesthetic machine that costs over $5,000. The anesthetic gas, the same type used in human hospitals, goes for about $500 per fifteen minutes when used in people. Mickey's surgery took about twenty minutes. The binocular headset that I was wearing to magnify the small surgery area on the side of Mickey's head cost about $1,750. The surgery pack, with the delicate instruments that I had just purchased, cost about $2,000. Cleaning and re-sterilizing the surgery instruments, $75. Consumables, such as suture material, gauze, scrubs, surgical drapes, and other miscellaneous items, $45 or more.

Stacey's salary? My time? We had just successfully anesthetized a mouse and amputated its ear. That requires a bit of skill that not all veterinarians have. What was it worth?

Not to mention the postoperative recovery time still to come, the salary of a technician to monitor the post-op patient, cage space, food and water, and a prescription of antibiotics for when Mickey went home. And the follow-up visit—Mickey would have to come back for at least one recheck and suture removal.

As I said, I'm a sucker for schoolchildren and animals. "Charge Mrs. Davenport seventy-five dollars, Stace." I handed her the patient's chart. She paused just before grabbing the manila folder, looking at me quizzically.

"That's for everything," I responded, letting go of the medical record so that she would have to grab it.

"Can I talk to you now, Dr. Mader?" Leanne's nails-on-chalkboard voice etched into the operatory.

"What, Leanne?" I turned. Stacey laughed as she gently cupped the alert Mickey in her palms, lifting him off the surgical table.

"We have no mice left to feed to the snakes. Can I have ten bucks to go get some?"

Finding Noah's Ark

Noah's Ark Veterinary Hospital, or NAVH, had not always carried that name. When it opened some eighty years before, it had been known to everybody in town simply as Doc Brown's Vet Hospital, the only place around to take your sick pet. Over the years it had changed hands only three times, my partner and I being the fourth owners. After Doc Brown the name was changed to All City Pet Hospital, then, with the last owner, All City Dog and Cat Hospital.

No matter what you called it, NAVH had the distinction of being the oldest animal hospital in the city. To some, it was still ol' Doc Brown's place. Believe it or not, there were still a scant few active clients who had taken their pets to Doc Brown when they were little children. It did not matter that the art and science of veterinary medicine had advanced fantastically since Doc Brown's passing. To those original clients, there would never be an equal to the old practitioner.

My friend William—Willy, as he liked to be called—and I had been looking to buy a veterinary practice of our own for over a year. I had recently completed a residency program in primate, zoo, and laboratory animal medicine, along with an additional two years of training postgraduation from regular veterinary school, and was currently working as a university veterinarian in Northern California. Willy had received his DVM, or Doctor of Veterinary Medicine degree, several years earlier and was working for another veterinarian in Southern California.

We were living at opposite ends of the state and made frequent calls to each other to lament the frustrations of working for someone else, constantly commiserating about how we would do things differently if we had our own hospital. It didn't take long to realize that we had similar interests and goals, and we ultimately decided to form a business partnership and start our own veterinary hospital.

While we had similar interests, we had rather opposite skill sets. Willy had been a veterinarian for several years and truly loved working with pets, but his prime interest was in business management. While working as a small animal doctor he had also attended night school and received his MBA. I had less interest in the business side than in building the medical portion of the practice. I wanted to be able to offer academic-level health services in a private setting.

My interest in medicine started when I was in middle school. At first I wanted to become a people doctor. That all changed when my sister got a horse. It didn't take long to realize that a lot of the cute girls hung out around the stables, many of them crooning over the sinewy blacksmith who came to shoe their horses. I figured I could be that guy, so I took all of my hard-earned paperboy money and moved away at age fifteen to attend farrier college. I quickly fell in love with my new passion as a horseshoer—not because of all the pretty cowgirls but because I was able to make a real difference to the animals. I soon became friends with the local equine veterinarian and, working side by side, was able to design and create custom horseshoes that would make a lame horse walk normally again. I worked my way through high school, college, and graduate school as a blacksmith.

Watching the equine veterinarian work his magic, I knew that I didn't just have to limit myself to hooves. My original interest in human medicine had morphed to horse medicine. I planned on smithing through veterinary school because I could do it part-time and still make enough to pay tuition.

That all came to an end thanks to an underage drunk driver. When I was in graduate school, a high school kid lost control while drag racing his friend and rear-ended my car, sending me and my passenger into a fiery roll down the highway. After multiple surgeries and a year plus of rehab, I never had the strength or confidence to return to horse work. I could no longer handle the constant physical trauma of struggling with more than one thousand pounds of muscle. Wanting to avoid another injury, I changed paths and pursued exotic animal medicine.

◆ ◆ ◆

Buying a veterinary hospital is not like buying a used car. There are no lots where you can go and test-drive several hospitals, ultimately deciding what and where you want to start a business.

The classified ads in the back of the scientific veterinary journals listed veterinary hospitals for sale, grouping them by geographic location. We had mutually decided to pick a hospital in the southern part of the state, preferably near the beach, since we both had a passion for the water. As such, we set boundaries from San Diego north to Santa Barbara.

Over the months we called, wrote letters, and visited dozens of veterinary hospitals. Some were too small, some were too far inland, some were too expensive, some were outdated and in bad parts of town. When you are in the market for a used item, you don't have the latitude to be choosy. It seemed that every hospital that we evaluated had at least one major flaw.

One place had them all.

Imagine our enthusiasm when we came across the following advertisement in the classifieds of one of the premier veterinary journals:

Small Animal and Exotic Veterinary Practice. Excellent coastal
location; just blocks from the beach. Great clients. Well equipped.
Owner ready to retire!

Wow! That had our names written all over it. I flew down from Northern
California as soon as I could get a weekend off, and Willy and I made an
appointment to visit the practice.

Once we got there, it seemed hardly worth the price of the plane ticket.
The hospital was in a leased building, smack in the middle of a bad section of
town, on a street infamously nicknamed the California Corridor. California
Street, a busy thoroughfare in front of the building, essentially split the city.
To longtime residents, the "Corridor" was not a place to go, day or night.
Several street gangs had been battling for turf along the Corridor for the
last few years, and the street—specifically the portion that started just one
block west of the hospital—had been the site of much bloodshed.

The building itself had no off-street parking. Clients had to park
curbside on the front or side of the orange-and-brown two-story building.
The combination of Southern California sun, salty air, and old age had left
the facility looking much like a badly sun-bleached pumpkin. The windows
were cracked, the stucco chipped, and the paint that hadn't yet peeled was
scarred with graffiti. Two planters full of trash and replete with dry rot
leaned under graffiti-etched plate glass windows bordering the entrance.

Next door was a motorcycle repair shop, a strip bar called the China
Girl, and a furniture reupholstering sweatshop staffed by undocumented
immigrants. Across the street was a decrepit fast-food restaurant, and
immediately adjacent, a vacant concrete shell, once home to a lumberyard
that now served as partial shelter for the city's homeless and a hideaway for
gang members on the lam.

Did Willy and I really need to waste our time looking inside? We were
also concerned about leaving Willy's car unattended.

But curiosity won out. After all, I had flown all the way south just to have a look. It had sounded so good in the journal. Everybody knows that the best restaurants are always in the worst part of town. Perhaps it was similar for veterinary hospitals.

As soon as we entered the building we were greeted with the stench of animal urine, likely from the brown carpets saturated with years of bodily fluids. At least the brown hid the stains. To enhance the depressing effect, the carpets were accented by dark, fake wood paneling and highlighted with water-stained cork ceilings.

In the front corner of the waiting room two doves cooed in an old wrought iron cage, hastily crafted in Mexico eons before, no doubt laced with lead-based paint. A radio crackled an unintelligible mumble from somewhere behind the receptionist's desk.

"Do you have dogs or cats?" asked the jump-suited teenager, chewing her gum as she spoke.

"Excuse me?" I asked, trying to hold my breath.

"If you have dogs you can stay here. Cats and other critters, you have to go in the other door." She flicked her head toward the far side of the building.

I explained that we were there to see the practice, that we were interested in potentially buying the place.

"Cool. It's about time someone took a look at it. He's been trying to sell it for years." She smiled and sashayed out of sight.

A little voice in my head kept repeating *Leave, leave, leave.* We thought about having a seat but were convinced otherwise by a look at the bench covered by hair, fur, and an unidentified dry liquid residue.

The practice manager appeared a few minutes later. All businesslike, she shoved several papers into our hands, explained that this was the premier veterinary hospital in the city, that it had been there longer than any other veterinary establishment, and that it actually grossed much more than the financial papers stated—the owner had a great accountant, and he was able to "bury the fat" so that even the best IRS auditor could never find it.

Leave, go now, run . . . the voice in my head continued, but I ignored it.

The manager gave us the grand tour. The building was old. Little had been done to maintain it since the owner had decided to sell, and he did not want to put any more money into a building that was already, in his opinion, in excellent condition. A stairwell to the second floor bisected the front half of the building, separating the client waiting rooms into two separate areas, hence the dog and cat sides. The inside was designed like a big U, mandating that staff trek from side to side in order to attend to the needs of both dog and cat clients. A scarred asbestos tile floor started where the carpet ended, also accented with dark wood panels and brown trim. Everywhere you turned was another door, and there were only a few windows, effectively chopping the place up into little cubicles, and with minimal natural light, the place felt like a dungeon.

There were ample cages, albeit most were old painted wood—brown, of course. The chain-link dog runs were stitched together with hay baling wire, just waiting for some dog to get its head caught in the large gaps.

The biggest shock was in the surgery area. The room was so narrow that there was barely enough space for one person and the surgery table. An antiquated gas anesthesia machine collected dust on the far side of the soiled surgical table. Its hoses were cracked, and the oxygen canister registered "empty."

We had seen enough. Surgery had always been a passion of mine. How could I ever work in such conditions? We thanked the practice manager and excused ourselves before the owner had a chance to introduce himself.

"Ya gonna buy it?" the young blond asked between bubbles as we scurried past on our way to the door.

◆ ◆ ◆

When push came to shove, the simple truth was we couldn't afford anything else. We took a chance that the neighborhood would improve, and we had faith in our own abilities to make it work. And so Noah's Ark Veterinary Hospital was born.

Everybody thought we were crazy. We wanted to prove everybody wrong.

Had we only known.

AUGUST

The Karens

I had four more days left to submit my application for the American Board of Veterinary Practitioners—Companion Animal Practice specialty examination. I stared at the calendar on my desk and fretted that I would not have time to get it finished.

Willy, my partner, was still out of town on his annual vacation. He liked to travel and opted to take six weeks off in the middle of each summer—our busiest time of the year. I'd been meaning to talk with him about that, but I just never seemed to have the time.

Two new veterinary students were starting their summer externships that day. Externships are university-approved out-rotations where fourth-year students get to experience life in the real world under the supervision of a recognized expert in a particular discipline—in my case, exotic animal medicine. These two just happened to be from my alma mater, UC Davis.

Our practice had grown since we bought it. We purchased the building and expanded upstairs. In addition, we had taken the practice from a one-doctor hospital to one having four full-time veterinarians. Noah's Ark Veterinary Hospital had earned a reputation as being one of the top veterinary hospitals for exotic animals in the United States, and students from veterinary schools all across the nation vied for the opportunity to spend four weeks externing with us.

Our daily protocol called for me, associate doctors Debra and Cliff, head technician Stacey, and the students to meet in the conference room for morning rounds. Since this was the first day for the two new students and we had to explain the hospital protocols, rounds took a little longer than usual.

I had a long list of surgical procedures on my schedule for the morning. Fred, my other surgery technician, was excellent. Like Stacey, he was another of our ex-cons. Also I was glad to have him, just like I was glad to have Stacey. He could anesthetize a dog one minute, a hummingbird the next, and a cougar the next.

The associate doctors saw most of the dogs and cats, but all the doctors would examine exotics if asked. Being the chief of staff, I was responsible for overseeing all cases, and that's what morning rounds were for: to review every case, every day.

Each doctor had cases assigned, and each student had daily tasks laid out on the table. Coincidentally, both of our new students were named Karen. So naturally we immediately nicknamed them Karen 1 and Karen 2. The general rule was that each student had to shadow their assigned doctor, going into examination rooms, helping with diagnostics, and assisting with treatments and surgery.

The largest, and hardest, part of a veterinarian's job is interacting with the pet's owners, a skill not well taught in veterinary school. We have to be able to effectively communicate with scared, emotional, stressed, and oftentimes financially strapped owners and entreat them to allow us to take care of their pet. We also have to be able to handle the guilt that comes with seeing pets suffer when their owners won't spend the money to attend to their pet's medical needs and also not allow them to make us feel it's our fault their animal is suffering.

I not only had to be a veterinarian and educator (of students, staff, and pet owners) but also a businessman, manager, and counselor, dealing with all the problems of operating a hospital and overseeing its staff members. As rounds wrapped up, Lori, our newest receptionist, approached me with a clipboard full of messages:

"Mrs. Peterson is on the phone and wants to know if she can get a refill for Potsie's skin meds." *Has it been more than six months since her last visit? No? Then you know the rules; she has to make an appointment.*

"The washing machine is broken, and we don't have any clean towels for the baths." *When did it break? Yesterday? Why did you wait until today to tell me?*

"Catherine Defield called. She's really pissed because her dog chewed out all the stitches from its surgery last Monday, and she wants you to come to her house to replace them for free."

"The guy from the gas company left a note. You can't get your permit, and they are going to disconnect the gas line unless you call them back by noon." *What time is it now? 8:30? When did he come in? Yesterday you say? Oh, you forgot to tell me . . .*

Somehow, I had to concentrate through all of this.

"Oh, yeah," Lori added as she was about to leave. "Some doctor called. He said not to forget that your application for the boards is due next Monday!"

Just like human medicine, veterinary medicine has progressed to the way of the specialist. In human medicine, if you have a sneeze, you go to the general practitioner. If you have something more serious, you get referred to a specialist. It is malpractice for a doctor not to refer a patient to someone with better, more advanced training, if one is available.

The same trend has occurred in veterinary medicine. Back in good old Doc Brown's time, he did everything. If the dog had a sneeze, he took care of it. If the cat had a broken bone, he put on the cast. In the terrible event that your pet had cancer, he was the one who put it to sleep.

No longer. Now there were just about as many veterinary specialty categories as there were human medical specialty categories. There were veterinary surgeons, ophthalmologists for eye problems, oncologists for cancer treatment, theriogenologists for reproductive matters, and many, many more.

That said, there were no specialty categories for exotic pets. Zoo veterinarians had their own specialty category, as did laboratory animal veterinarians. But there was no specialty category for vets dealing with exotic pets like bunnies, birds, snakes, ferrets, or fish.

Although my residency—an additional two years of training that I took after I graduated from veterinary school—covered both zoo and laboratory animals, and I was qualified to take either of these specialty boards, they did not have direct relevance to what I was currently doing.

Board certification is not necessary if you are a general practitioner. In fact, of the one hundred thousand-plus veterinarians licensed in the United States, only about one tenth have some type of board certification. Most of these are in university settings or large specialty practices.

For me, I felt board certification was necessary. Not that my clients would care. In fact, the vast majority of them, if I added some extra credentials after my name, would just think it was an excuse to charge more. They did not seem to understand that it meant that I had an additional level of training and knowledge and could provide more advanced care for their pet.

The most important reason that I wanted to get board certified was not for the clients but for me. I like to stay on top of things, and I always want to know as much as I can about any subject. If I wanted to pass the specialty boards I would have to know everything better than all those I was educating. Getting "boarded" would also add to my credibility as a teacher and writer among my professional peers.

Most veterinary schools do not consider exotic pet medicine important and devote very little time to educating students how to care for a guinea pig, fix a sick snake, or heal an ill bird. One way that I could personally correct this academic shortcoming is to teach exotic pet medicine at the same level as teaching for dogs and cats in the schools, doing it right here in my own hospital with the students who came to learn from me.

Although there were no exotic pet specialty boards, I was determined to become board certified in some discipline. The American Board of Veterinary Practitioners offered a specialization in "Companion Animal Practice," which covered all aspects of veterinary practice in dogs and cats and included other pets considered to be companion animals, such as birds, rabbits, and other non-domestic species.

There are strict guidelines and qualifications that must be met before a veterinarian can even apply to take a specialty board examination. In essence, you have to pre-apply to see if you are qualified to actually sit for the exam.

I was still at that stage. I had to submit a list of my qualifications and credentials establishing that I had completed a postgraduate residency training. I had also been in practice for over six years and had published many scientific articles. So I figured it would not be a problem for my application to be accepted. The entire process, from start to finish, takes one year. I was reasonably confident that I would be sitting for the exam next summer. I just needed to find the time to get my application finished.

• • •

I have been blessed (or cursed, depending on your perspective) with the need for little sleep, usually getting by on about four hours a night, and I had been up late the previous night finishing my application. I arrived at work early and was sitting at the table in the conference room reviewing my paperwork when the two Karens showed up at 7:45 for morning rounds. One was bright and happy, the other bedraggled with dark circles under her eyes.

"I can't believe you didn't hear anything!" Karen 2 exclaimed as they each selected a chair around the round oak table. She was clearly distraught.

"I didn't hear a thing." Karen 1 smiled, shaking her head back and forth.

The hospital had two apartments upstairs. Our night technician lived in one, so that there would be an employee here 24/7 watching the patients, and the externs shared the second one.

"What are you talking about?" I looked up, curious.

"There was a drive-by shooting last night," Karen 2 exclaimed, "right outside our window!"

"She's dreaming," Karen 1 laughed. "I didn't hear anything."

"Dreaming, my ass!" Karen 2 jabbed. "Ya wanna go look for bullet holes?"

"Unfortunately, it happens all the time," I said, trying to de-emphasize the event. The sad fact was, it really did happen all too frequently.

While the students were quibbling, I gathered the voluminous paperwork for my application and stuffed it into an overnight envelope. To this collection, I added a $200 check for the filing fee. If my credentials were accepted to take the test, then I had to pay an additional $400 for the test.

"Excuse me a second," I said to no one in particular. The associates had not arrived yet. I got up and left the table and took the package to the reception area where Lisa, my office manager, was busy checking in a client.

"Could you please overnight this for me? It's the application for my boards. It has to be there by Monday." The client was listening as I handed the large, heavy envelope to Lisa.

"What's that? What are the 'boards'?" the client queried.

I was proud of what I was about to attempt, so I rattled off all that was involved in getting this veterinary specialty designation, winding up with the observation: "Very few veterinarians are board certified."

The client's response: "Does that mean you are going to increase your prices?"

◆ ◆ ◆

That night, my usual abbreviated sleep was even less satisfying than I had hoped. I dreamed about applications, big envelopes, and missing deadlines. When the alarm rudely screamed at 5:30 a.m., my first thought was that there must be a fire. I spun out of bed in a huff, heart racing, and out of breath.

I stood up, my heart still pounding and my body sweaty from a lack of good sleep. Sidney, my cat, was snoozing on the foot of the bed. I covered him with the blanket and headed off to a cold shower.

Ellen had yet to get home. My wife was an intensive-care nurse at the local trauma center and worked the graveyard shift, which meant that she was usually getting in just before or shortly after I was leaving for work. The opposite was the case at the end of the day.

I hated her graveyard shifts. Aside from the fact that we worked polar opposite schedules, and I rarely got to spend time with her, all the kooks surfaced in the dark hours of the night: the drunks, the crazies, the gangbangers. She had to deal with bad stuff on a regular basis. I liked to be around when she got home in case she needed someone to listen to her vent.

After breakfast I had a few minutes to kill before leaving for work, so I went into the backyard and picked some fresh flowers for the table. Dewe and Traci, my tortoises, like Sidney, were still asleep in their burrows under the rosebushes. It must be nice to actually sleep in on a Saturday morning. I left a love note next to the flowers and headed out for work.

On the way in, passing through an intersection, I saw a hand frantically waving from an approaching car. Instinctively I waved back. It was Ellen.

A married couple living separate lives.

◆ ◆ ◆

Karen times two were already waiting for me in the conference room when I arrived for rounds that morning. Stacey had a stack of about twenty charts piled up on the table and was feeding them to Cliff. His shirt was not pressed, his tie wrinkled. As usual, his hair looked as if it had not been washed in several days.

"What do we have on tap?"

"Mostly the usual stuff," Karen 1 responded. I was amazed how rapidly and comfortably she seemed to fit in with the way we did things at NAVH. She was the type of student whom I would love to hire as a staff veterinarian once she graduated.

"Like?"

"You know." She ran a pen down a patient list that Stacey had attached to a clipboard. "Another parvo dog, a renal case, a whole bunch of sick birds and lizards, and a vomiting basset."

The basset was new. "When did the basset come in?"

"Last night on emergency," Cliff piped in. "I was here most of the night with it." That explained his appearance.

"What happened?"

"Nothin' big," Cliff responded nonchalantly.

"Not to be nosy, but do you mind filling me in on the case?"

"Oh, yeah." He pushed some manila charts around on the table, ultimately selecting the basset's chart. "Barney the basset came in last night about 9:30 with intractable vomiting. I NPO'd him and started him on some metoclopramide."

"And?" NPO stood for *nil per os* (nothing by mouth)—no food or water, a common course of action for a patient with severe vomiting. Metoclopramide is a drug that is used to stop vomiting, often used in chemotherapy patients. Not a bad therapeutic plan, but more needed to be done, like finding out why Barney was vomiting in the first place.

"And what?" Cliff asked.

"And is that all?" His brevity disappointed me. We had set ourselves up as a teaching hospital, so it was particularly important to come up with a thorough medical workup. I realize that on late-night emergencies it's easy to get tired. All you feel like doing is stabilizing the patient and doing a more thorough workup the next morning.

"How is Barney this morning?" Cliff questioned Stacey defiantly.

"Fine." She looked back and forth between Cliff and me. She could tell there was some tension. "Hasn't puked since I've been here."

"It's 'vomit' or 'regurgitation,' Stacey, not puke," I corrected, trying to maintain a professional decorum, if only to set an example for the students. "No surprise the dog hasn't vomited. You've given him nothing to eat or drink, his alimentary tract is empty, and on top of that, he's on an anti-vomiting drug!"

"I was going to start him on some cottage cheese and rice this morning," Cliff offered. All fine and good, but we still had not gotten to the root of why Barney was here.

"Karen," I said to Karen 2. I had a tendency to address my questions to Karen 1, since she was so quick with her suggestions. But I did not want to play favorites. "How would you have worked up this patient?"

"Well," she paused, "I would have done what Dr. Nordic did," she said rather sheepishly, then gazed down at her notes, avoiding eye contact with anyone. "Except," she continued, "that I would have probably put him on fluids."

Now we were getting somewhere. At least Karen was addressing a major concern for a vomiting patient. Any vomiting patient, human or animal, is losing fluids and electrolytes. "Good point," I said, complimenting the quiet Karen. "What kind of fluid? How and how much?"

"Well," she said, looking momentarily at Cliff, as if apologizing for suggesting something that he hadn't done, "it really depends on whether or not it's stomach vomiting or lower GI."

"Why?" I was surprised she was being so thorough.

"If it's stomach vomiting," she started, "it means that Barney is losing hydrochloric acid, and we will need to replace his fluid loss with sodium chloride. If it's lower GI vomiting, we may need to use lactated Ringer's and monitor him for acidosis."

"How can you tell the difference?" Everybody was listening. This was perhaps the first time since Karen 2 had been here that she was on center stage.

"I think you can just test the pH of the vomit?" she answered hesitantly.

"Absolutely, and it's an easy thing to do."

"Just dip some litmus paper in it," piped in Cliff, as if he did it all the time. "If it's acid, it's from the stomach, and if it's basic, it's intestinal."

"Like you knew that!" Stacey sneered.

"Of course I know that. I just said it, didn't I?" he shot back at Stacey.

"Then why didn't you do it, idiot?"

"Hey!" What was with everyone this morning? They were quibbling like a bunch of schoolkids. I was pleased to find out that Karen had been listening all this time, not just being quiet and unresponsive.

"Okay, but we're still not finished." I turned to Karen 2. "What is your differential for vomiting in a—"

"Four-year-old dog," Stacey said, finishing my sentence.

"Yeah," I said, looking at Stacey, "a four-year-old dog?" I swear Stacey could read my mind. A "differential" is a list of possible causes for a condition. It is imperative to make a differential list for any medical problem so that you can then formulate a plan to try to figure out the cause.

"I would worry about a foreign body, gastroenteritis, either bacterial or viral, and intussusception initially. Toxins, metabolic disturbances, and head trauma should also be considered," Karen 2 responded without hesitation. She had clearly thought this through. I was really impressed with her clinical acumen.

"Is there any history that would suggest any of the above?" I asked. A foreign body is anything that the patient may have eaten that could be stuck in its intestinal tract, a common problem in dogs that like to raid garbage cans. Intussusception refers to an unusual condition where the animal's intestine swallows itself. If not caught in time, it can be deadly.

"There was no history of trauma, and the owner stated that Barney never eats out of the garbage," Karen 2 offered. Her hair was pulled back in two braids over each ear and held in the back of her head by a green turtle clip.

"So what would we do for Barney now?"

"Apparently the owner does not have a lot of money. He's a truck driver and does not even live in town. He was already complaining about the cost of the emergency visit," Karen 1 volunteered.

"That's why I didn't do anything else," Cliff interjected defensively.

"Did you document the owner's money concerns in the record?" I asked in general terms, to avoid direct criticism of Cliff.

"Of course not!" Stacey smirked.

"I was going to do it this morning at rounds. I was tired last night. It was late!" Cliff grabbed the record and clicked his ballpoint pen with dramatic flair.

"Dr. Nordic, you *must* document client communications. What if you died on the way home last night? We'd have no idea what happened."

"We should be so lucky!" Stacey chided.

"Okay! That's enough!" I made a T signal with my hands. "Stacey, don't you have something productive you can do?"

She looked around at everybody. "I'm sure I can find something," she said as she stomped out of the conference room.

"Dr. Nordic, I want you to call Barney's dad and see if you can get permission to get some blood work and an X-ray.

"I'll be glad to do it," Karen 2 chimed in. "If that's okay? He has that funny frog nickname—Toad!"

"Sure, but first please review what you are planning on saying with Dr. Nordic."

We finished rounds without too many more distractions. It appeared to be shaping up as a rather routine day, even after a rocky start. Typically, at the end of rounds, we discussed nonmedical issues such as meetings, events, and the like.

"Remember, tonight is volleyball and pizza!" I announced as everybody was gathering their charts. During the summer months we would close the doors a half hour early on Wednesday evenings and head to the beach. We would play until dark, then head over to one of the local pizza joints for food, drinks, video games, and pool, all paid for by the hospital.

The remainder of the day, after morning rounds, was relatively uneventful. Karen 2 was unable to get in touch with Barney's owner, who I had by now learned went by his CB radio handle, "Toad." I decided to take the X-rays anyway, since we needed to know what was happening. I figured that if the owner couldn't pay for them, I would eat the cost.

Not surprisingly, the X-ray showed a large bone stuck in Barney's stomach. I could take an X-ray without the owner's permission, but I could not do surgery without permission. It was imperative that we get in touch with him ASAP.

Thank God it was Wednesday. After a long, stressful day we all needed some brainless fun time.

Of all the negatives that come with living in Southern California, the weather is certainly not one of them. Typically mild all year around, this night was no exception. We were able to get to the beach shortly after 7:00 p.m. and found an empty volleyball net right on the water, not too far from the main road. We played hard, but without any real competition or skill. Karen 1 was excellent, not surprisingly, as she did everything well. Karen 2 did her best to just hit the ball in the direction of the net. Her attempts were met with much teasing and laughter, but to her credit she did not hold back.

As the sun set, it changed like a chameleon from yellow to orange to red to salmon while it passed through the layers of jet exhaust, car pollution, and oil refinery waste typical of Southern California smog. We played until we could no longer see the white ball, the sand was beginning to cool, and our stomachs were screaming for food.

Since it was a midweek night, we had no problem getting a couple of large tables together. Shortly after the food came and we were all gorging ourselves with pepperoni and sausage, Karen 2 suddenly dropped her slice and shouted, "That's him!"

She pointed across the bar. Everybody turned.

"That's who?" I asked, looking across the crowd. The music was blaring, and waitresses in short shorts were scampering around hoisting large, round trays heavily laden with food and drinks.

"Toad!" She pointed feverishly. "Right there!"

• • •

Toad, Barney's owner, had been unreachable the previous day because he had contracted an extra day-haul with his truck in order to get some money to pay for Barney's veterinary bills. He did not realize that his basset was so sick, and by the time he was back in town, he figured we were closed, so he hadn't tried to call.

Toad, who looked to be in his fifties, had been a trucker since he was seventeen. He stood about five feet ten inches tall and weighed somewhere in the neighborhood of 250 pounds. He had male-pattern baldness, which I didn't notice until he took off his sweat-stained PENNZOIL cap to wipe his brow. His teeth were tarnished a tobacco yellow under a flat nose, and his puffy cheeks and head blended into his shoulders without the benefit of a neck, giving his face a pumpkin-like appearance. He had found Barney as a puppy at a truck stop in Arizona, and the dog had been his driving companion ever since.

I explained Barney's condition to Toad and asked that he come to the hospital the following morning to visit his pet and review the X-rays. Unfortunately, he said, he had to leave again early in the morning to take a load to Sacramento. If he left before dawn he'd be back in Southern California by the end of the day. That way he'd have even more money to help with Barney's care. The cost did not matter. He would do whatever he had to do to ensure only the best care for his best friend. It was obvious how much Barney meant to him.

Needless to say, Barney was once again the main focus of attention at morning rounds. Removing a bone from the stomach is not a difficult surgery. Since Karen 2 had been the student most involved with this case, I asked her to scrub in on the surgery with me.

"Interesting," I remarked after we finished removing the bone from Barney's stomach, "considering the comments at morning rounds two days ago, that we found a bone in a dog that the owner stated, so emphatically, never gets into the garbage."

"Yeah," she answered, "I guess it goes to show that you can't believe everything that a client tells you."

I began to remove my surgical gloves. "Get a plastic bag and seal the bone inside so that we can show Barney's dad. And Karen, I'd like you to write up the surgical report for the record. Please let me see it so that I can proof and sign it before you put it in the chart."

"No problem."

I could tell Karen 2 was really enjoying this. "And one more thing, Karen," I said with a smile. "You did an excellent job."

• • •

Toad came in late that night after his haul to pay Barney a visit and leave a few hundred dollars toward his balance. Although still groggy from the pain medication, Barney wagged his tail feverishly when he saw his dad. It was a pleasure watching the two of them together. Karen 2 had also bonded with Toad and his dog. When things went well, I liked to let the students do the majority of the client communication. It teaches them the interpersonal skills necessary to be a good doctor, and it reinforces the human-pet bond and the commitment that we, as veterinarians, do our best to prolong it.

On my way back from lunch I noticed new graffiti on the side of our building. Although some graffiti was actually quite artistic, this was just a hastily penned tag. WS was scribbled gang style, block letters, sharp corners to each one, about three feet tall, with black spray paint. WS was the tag for the West Siders, a local neighborhood gang that was constantly battling for turf with the ES, or "East Siders." Our street, and about two to three blocks on either side, was right between their territories. Consequently, we were frequent targets of the graffiti wars.

As I looked at the offensive, scratchy-looking letters, I noticed three bullet holes in the stucco wall. Karen 2 must have been right about the drive-by.

• • •

When Barney came in for his suture removal, he was mostly doing well, but a small area of the incision looked red, possibly indicating the beginning of a brewing infection. Karen 2 asked me if it would be appropriate to give him an injection of antibiotics. I agreed it was a good idea and let her pick the drug with my approval. She was happy with my letting her do the decision-making and even happier with the progress of her patient.

Peter, one of our part-time pre-veterinary students, was scheduled to work all day. I always liked it when he was working. Most pre-veterinary students had something to prove. They felt that they had to demonstrate their worth, wanting to garner the coveted letter of recommendation that they could use for their application to veterinary school. With some exceptions, most pre-veterinary students were excellent workers and very dedicated.

Peter was an extraordinary student. He was very bright, enthusiastic, and pleasant. His only vice, if I had to pick something, was his lack of concentration when a certain co-employee was around. Peter was terminally infatuated with Leanne, our kennel helper. Peter was tall, clean-cut, well educated, and religious, and he came from an upper-middle-class family. Leanne was the total opposite: she was a high school dropout (by choice—she often declared that she already knew all that she needed to know to get by), lived with several guys, wore tattered jeans and a braless T-shirt when she was not working, and lived for rock and roll. She was also absolutely cover-model beautiful.

From my perspective, they had nothing in common. But Peter would dribble and turn to mush whenever Leanne was around. I had a talk with him about his infatuation and how it interfered with his job performance, and he promised that he would make an effort not to let it get out of control.

With the morning's procedures and appointments finished, and it being such a beautiful day, I offered to take the Karens to a café by the beach for lunch. Arriving back at the clinic afterward, we were all smiles. This was the quintessential Southern California day for a visiting student. Good medicine in the morning, a great lunch at the beach, and a full schedule of challenging patients in the afternoon.

As soon as I stepped in the front door I saw my first patient. Mrs. Davenport, her two children, Donnie and Leslie, and of course, Mickey the mouse, on Donnie's lap in a clear plastic transport cage with a blue-and-pink top. As soon as they saw me, the young children started to jump up and down. "Dr. Mader, Dr. Mader!" they shouted.

If it weren't so wonderful to see them, it would have been embarrassing. Donnie ran over to me carrying Mickey, proud and excited to show me his little friend, its ear all healed. The poor little mouse bounced around inside the plastic cage like a pinball as his master bounded over.

"You fixed him!" Donnie proclaimed.

"We all fixed him." I squatted down to be at eye level with my little friend. "I could not have done it without your help." I carefully took Mickey from little Donnie and held the cage up so that I could look at my patient. The surgery incision from his ear amputation had healed, and fur was starting to regrow. I also noticed that there was no evidence of mites or the severe scratching that had caused the original problem. Needless to say, I was delighted with his recovery.

"Dr. Mader," Mrs. Davenport said, pausing as she looked affectionately at her children, "we want to thank you so much for all you did." She smiled, took my hand, and lowered her voice. "And I really appreciate your most generous discounts. We couldn't have helped Mickey if it wasn't for you."

"I am so glad that I was able to help," I said my hand slipping out of her palm as I stood. "Just let me take Mickey to the treatment area and have his stitches taken out."

I often take the sutures out of a patient while the owners watch. It is sort of a ritualized "final act" to signify the resolution of the medical problem. But in this case it had been over two weeks since Mickey's surgery, and the sutures were starting to get embedded into the skin. Also, a new growth of fur made it hard to see the tiny knots. I decided to take Mickey into the back where I had better lights.

"Dr. Mader," Lisa said, intercepting me as I walked back toward the treatment area.

"Yeah?" I gave her a look.

"There's a doctor on the phone from a university who needs to ask you about some lizard thing."

"Okay," I said, handing the small cage to Lisa. "But could you please take Mickey back to Peter and have him take out Mickey's sutures?"

"No problem." Lisa took the patient and smiled at the little mouse inside. "Line three." She headed off with Mickey.

I took the call on the hallway phone. The afternoon was starting to get busy as the buzz of activity increased all around me. I was probably on the phone no more than five minutes when Leanne came up and stood in front of me. I looked up at her, but she did not say anything.

I turned my attention back to the caller and helped solve his problems, explaining the procedure he needed to follow to help his patient. After a few more minutes I looked up and noticed that Leanne was still standing there. I said goodbye and hung up.

"You need the phone?" I wondered why she hadn't just gone to one of the other fourteen phones in the hospital.

"No. Peter needs you." Leanne was expressionless.

All of a sudden I had a sinking feeling. I realized that I had not seen Mickey pass by me on his way back to his family. I quickened my pace, only to stop dead in my tracks as I turned the corner to the treatment room.

Peter was bent over the stainless steel table, cupping Mickey in his hands, performing mouth-to-mouth resuscitation on the little rodent. Maria, our kennel keeper, was crying, and Stacey, Karen 1, and Karen 2 were looking on in horror.

"What happened?" I asked, somewhat in shock. I looked at Leanne—why hadn't she interrupted me if there was an emergency?

"I was taking his stitches out"—Peter stopped his mouse CPR and looked up at me— "when he just stopped breathing!" His eyes were red and panicked, and he was choking back tears.

I took Mickey from Peter and gave him an emergency examination. I listened for his little heartbeat with my special neonatal stethoscope, but there was no sound.

"Stacey." I started to bark out an order.

"Right here." Stacey handed me an insulin syringe loaded with epinephrine. I gave her a momentary look, then took the syringe and focused all my attention back onto my patient.

With precision I inserted the delicate syringe needle through the skin and black fur on Mickey's chest and into his tiny heart. The clear plastic hub of the syringe immediately filled with dark purple blood, indicating that I was in the heart, but also indicating that things were really bad—blood from the heart should be bright red. I gently depressed the plunger, infusing the epinephrine directly into Mickey's vital organ.

Everyone was silent. The Karens watched intently. Stacey was busy making entries in Mickey's chart. I continued to administer CPR.

Mickey's thimble-sized chest heaved. I halted my CPR efforts and applied my stethoscope, listening for signs of a heartbeat. He squeaked a barely audible gasp, his tongue blue, eyes black with dilated pupils. Mickey, on his back, feet up in the air, rolled his short neck to the side and died.

"Don't you dare die on me!" I commanded my patient. I started aggressive CPR once again, rapidly compressing the little chest, alternately puffing mouse-sized breaths into him with my lips.

His body was limp.

He was dead.

Nobody said a word. Out of the corner of my eye I saw Peter usher Leanne out of the room. Maria turned away, tears flowing. Karen 2 whispered something to Karen 1. I stood there, in shock.

This was not happening. I waited for someone to tell me that Mickey was just faking it.

My head buzzed and pounded. Everything around me faded. Somehow I found myself looking down at an imaginary scene of chaos in the treatment room. I was in the center, leaning over the stainless steel table as a crowd of smiling faces stood all 360 degrees around me, pointing at the object on the table, laughing, and slapping each other on the back—it *was* a joke! This wasn't really Mickey! Leanne and Peter were just playing a bad joke on me: the mouse was a lookalike that they were planning to feed to the snakes. That must be it.

OK, everybody! The joke's over. You caught me. I really believed that this was Mickey. Bring the real Mickey out so that I can take him back to his family. You know, Mrs. Davenport, Leslie with her pigtails and pink dress, and Donnie, Mickey's best friend. The joke's over! They want to take Mickey home. Hey, why isn't everybody laughing?

My focus returned to the lifeless body lying motionless on the table. The little mouse's eyes were fixed, dilated black holes staring off into nowhere.

The lifeless body was missing an ear.

I looked up. Both Karens were watching me. The room was silent. Stacey reached out and picked up Mickey, wrapped him in a clean white tissue, and placed his body in a small cardboard box, the kind that we used as coffins for our small patients.

The ones that die.

I looked at the mouse nestled in the tissue bedding. It really was Mickey. This was not a joke. This was the cruel part of veterinary medicine. Losing a patient.

"Go take Mrs. Davenport and her children to the conference room," I whispered to Stacey. "Don't say anything other than to let her know I'll be right in to talk with her." I did not need to instruct Stacey. This was not her first walk of death, and, sadly, it would not be her last.

I wanted to find a dark hole and crawl inside. I wanted to go to sleep and wake up when this was all over. Where was my partner? Why couldn't he go talk to the Davenports? Maybe I could stall them until he got back from his ecotourism vacation. It was only three more weeks. I could tell them that Mickey needed more surgery.

I wanted to vomit.

I picked up my former patient. He looked so comfortable in the box, all cozy in the soft tissue. In my subconscious I was sure he was just sleeping and would wake when I brought him back to his owners.

But he was not asleep. Mickey was dead. He had been alive ten minutes before, healthy. He had recovered from six weeks of medical treatment and surgery. He was finally healed. No longer feeling any pain and discomfort from the mites and infections, he had started on his renewed life. Now, because of something we did, he was dead.

Now, I had to go try to explain this to his former family.

I looked around the room for a modicum of support. Some scintilla of hope that this would not be as difficult as I knew it would be. Everybody looked away. No one would look me in the eyes. Peter and Leanne were nowhere to be found.

Finally, Karen 2 spoke. "Dr. Mader, would you like me to go in there with you?"

I was genuinely touched. As much as I would have liked the support, this was something I needed to do alone. I knew that I should be using this as a teaching experience in learning how to handle such scenarios, but I just couldn't do it. I would meet with both Karens afterward and discuss what transpired.

"No thanks, Karen." I paused. "I think it would be best if we give the

Davenports some space. Those rooms get real small when there's bad news in the air." I looked down at Mickey, still looking peaceful in his cardboard coffin. "I'd better go do this now."

I have never cried over a patient, at least externally. Internally, I was all torn up. A half-hour earlier I had been loving my job, yet now I wished to be doing anything else. I had no plan as to what I was going to say. This was not something taught in school, not something you rehearsed.

I turned the corner to the conference room and saw the Davenports through the glass French door, waiting inside. The children were playing some game with a blue nylon dog leash that had been left behind by one of the employees, and Mrs. Davenport was just sitting there, staring blankly at the wall. Her expression suggested she knew something was wrong.

I handed Mickey, in his box, to Stacey, who was shadowing me down the hall.

What type of face should I wear as I entered the room? A smile? A frown?
I just walked in.

As soon as I entered the room the children started jumping up and down again, just as they had thirty-six minutes before, when I came back from lunch. That seemed like an eternity ago. Oh, how I wished I could rewind the clock.

I immediately squatted down to their level. Though they were just innocent children, both could see that I was not smiling. And where was Mickey?

I looked each child in the eyes, my expression somber. "I'm so sorry, Leslie and Donnie." I continued to look at the children. "Mickey passed away when we were removing his stiches."

"Can we see him?" Donnie spoke first. There was disbelief in his voice.
I looked toward their mother, and she silently nodded okay.

On some unspoken cue Stacey quietly slipped into the room and handed me the small coffin containing Mickey. I held it out in front of the children and slowly opened the lid, exposing the adorable little mouse, missing his ear, looking like he was comfortably asleep in his soft, white tissue bed.

But he wasn't sleeping. He was dead. We had killed him.

I watched their expressions as their eyes widened. Leslie covered her mouth with her hands and started to cry silent sobs, her chest heaving and mouth shaping little O's. Donnie looked to his mother for a clue as to what to do.

Once again I reached behind my back, retrieving a freshly laundered handkerchief from my hip pocket, handing it to the distraught little girl. Donnie stepped closer, attempting to look into the box. He reached out but suddenly paused. My hand was shaking, as was the cardboard box I was holding.

"It's okay, Donnie." Mrs. Davenport spoke to her son. "You can touch him."

Donnie lightly brushed his right index finger over the fur of the now cold little mouse. "Is he really *dead*?" Donnie looked at me, pausing between words. His eyes were moist, lips pale.

"Yes." I couldn't offer anything more.

"Why did he die?" Donnie continued to pet his friend, not looking at me anymore.

"He had a heart attack." I was not sure if he knew what that meant. "His little heart just stopped beating."

"Oh." Donnie pulled his hand away. He looked at his mother, expression changing in a microsecond. "Can we get another mouse?"

"Of course!" Mrs. Davenport said through silent tears. Her frown turned to a welcomed smile. "Of course you can."

"I get to name it this time!" Leslie shouted. Tears gone.

"No you don't!" Donnie threw his arms down, fists clenched. "You got to name the last one!"

Last one? Had they already forgotten Mickey's name?

I surreptitiously placed the box with Mickey's body on a shelf behind a book while the children were jabbering.

"Dr. Mader." Mrs. Davenport turned to me as she reached into a large paper bag sitting on the floor by her feet. The children were arguing loudly, the air charged with renewed energy. "The children and I wanted to give you this." She handed me a large, beautifully wrapped box. A shiny red ribbon adorned the top left corner.

I was mortified. Didn't Mrs. Davenport realize what had just happened? I had just killed her children's pet mouse! Now she was giving me a present? It did not make any sense. Could this be a bomb? I certainly felt as if I deserved one.

"Mrs. Davenport, I can't take this."

"Dr. Mader, please." She pushed the package into my hands. "You have tried so hard. Whatever happened to Mickey, I know that you did not do anything to harm him." She patted the back of my hand. "You are so kind."

I was not sure if I should open it or not. I felt so self-conscious. Suddenly Mickey's death was no longer the central issue. His little body was still hiding in the cardboard box resting out of sight on top of the bookshelf. Both children were watching me.

"Open it! Open it!" they cheered.

Without a word, I did what I was told. I was careful not to damage the pretty wrapping paper—Mickey and Minnie mouse characters riding a cartoon bicycle built for two. Inside was a colorful T-shirt with a Mickey Mouse design. Underneath the picture of Mickey's smiling face and large ears, written in a purple script, was "Dr. Mader—World's Greatest Veterinarian!"

◆ ◆ ◆

I could not sleep that night. I needed badly to talk to Ellen about what had happened with Mickey during the day, but unfortunately she had left for work by the time I got home. Instead, I took Wok, my chow chow, for a much-needed soul-searching walk.

We headed to the park a few blocks from my house. It was late. The hot midsummer day had morphed into an evening with a slight chill. The ocean fog was rolling in, and a layer of dew coated the grass. There were no other dogs or people around, so I let Wok off his leash so that he could gallivant across the playground, marking his territory with a quick lift of his fuzzy rear leg. Wok's fluffy, jet-black coat and black tongue were lost in the dark of the night. The only thing visible were the whites of his eyes and his big, sharp teeth. He had a formidable appearance, but on the inside, he was a wonderful, cuddly bear. No question, my best friend in the whole world. I could always count on him.

I found a graffiti-etched bench and sat, staring blankly into the night, while Wok continued his prowl. I couldn't help but compare Wok's prancing from bush to bush and tree to tree, marking each with his urine to denote his territory, with the gang members doing the same, but with spray paint.

It was not safe to stroll alone at night in this park. However, having Wok by my side was better than having a gun. People can't tell if you are carrying a weapon, but everybody can see a big dog, and strangers tended to give me a wide berth.

Wok finally finished staking out his territory and came over to join me on the bench. He gave me a loving look that only a dedicated dog can give, tongue lolling to the side, saliva dripping in little foamy beads to the bench, and smiling from ear to ear. He knew I was upset. I couldn't help but wonder what it would have been like if I had been little Donnie and Mickey had been Wok. I would have been devastated.

I told Wok all about Mickey and his family. I explained how Mickey had finally healed after all of his treatments and surgery, how he had come in for a simple suture removal and, in the process, had died. I told Wok about the present that Mrs. Davenport and her children had given me and that I was too ashamed to ever wear it.

Wok just listened to the whole story. He always listened to my problems, never criticized or passed judgment.

The next day, the Mickey issue would not go away. The entire staff, including both Karens, was buzzing about what had transpired.

In between clients I made it a point to meet with all involved and try to ferret out what had happened. After talking with Peter, Leanne, Maria, and Stacey, this is what I figured out:

It seems that Lisa had taken the cage with Mickey to Peter as she had been instructed. She even offered to help Peter take the sutures out, but Peter had declined, stating that he would get it done.

The first thing that Peter did was find Leanne, since he wanted her to help instead of Lisa. Leanne was and always had been a kennel helper, mostly doing laundry, cleaning cages, and bathing pets. She had not been trained in handling patients.

Peter loved to impress Leanne, and his favorite way to do so was to let her do "cool" things, like helping out with patient nursing, so he asked her to hold Mickey while he removed the little black stitches. Unfortunately, Mickey started to grow impatient and began to struggle during the process.

As Mickey tried to wriggle free from Leanne's grip, Leanne did the first thing any inexperienced handler would do: she tightened her hold on the little rodent. The tighter she held, the harder it was for the little mouse to breathe. As a result, he suffocated.

I had a long talk with both Peter and Leanne. Peter was genuinely crushed. I am sure that he cared about what had happened, but he also fretted that it might hurt his chances to get into veterinary school. I assured him it would not, providing that he accepted the responsibility for his actions and that he never allowed such poor judgment to influence his decisions again.

I also spoke with Leanne. As expected, her reaction was different. She said she felt "kinda bad" about what had happened, but she "was just tryin' to help," and if I had given her the proper training it never would have happened.

As a statement to the rest of the staff, I put both Peter and Leanne on probation for two weeks.

Peter accepted his punishment. Leanne complained that it wasn't fair.

I hoped that we could all move forward after the loss of Mickey. New cases awaited us, new challenges, and hopefully more satisfying results.

The morning was booked with surgeries. Especially good this morning was a surgery for the West Coast Turtle and Tortoise Club (WCTTC). The club, a nonprofit organization consisting of more than three thousand members from all over the western United States, was financially our hospital's number one client. Initially formed by a small group of turtle lovers who had shared interests, the group grew over the years in number and scope. It now held public turtle shows, published a first-class newsletter, and had sixteen different subchapters all over the state, each of which held monthly meetings.

The majority of the meetings and newsletter topics focused on different aspects of turtle care and husbandry, breeding, hatching reports, and general interest. On occasion they would have a veterinary- or health-oriented lecture at one of their meetings. That is how I became involved with them.

Willy and I had no sooner taken over NAVH when a woman representing herself as a senior member of the WCTTC made an appointment with me to examine a small tortoise with a broken jaw. The woman's name was Dorothy Shackleford, but everyone in the club called her Dottie. I figured she was in her late fifties or early sixties, but Dottie's age was difficult to gauge. Bony shoulders highlighted her gaunt stature with long arms that ended in birdlike fingers covered with silver rings. The nails, although polished with bright, ever-changing colors, were always stained brown from nicotine. Whenever you saw Dottie in public she was engulfed in a miasma of whitish smoke that circled in a halo around her silver-gray hair. Her gravelly voice signaled a life of smoking, the corners of her mouth permanently pursed from dangling a cigarette. Crow's-feet framed her squinty eyes like a permanent pair of spectacles.

Dottie immediately impressed upon me that she had been one of the founding members of the WCTTC. Furthermore, she made it abundantly clear that when it came to turtles, she had tried working with every veterinarian in Southern California, including old Doc Brown many years ago, but had yet to find any worth her time or money. She claimed to have more experience and knowledge than any vet.

Given that introduction, I had to ask: "Dottie, why are you here?"

"I can drive to Mexico and get whatever drug I need, but it's just so inconvenient." Dottie was much shorter than me and tended to step close when she spoke, looking up into my face, her cigarette breath forcing me back against the wall.

"So, Dottie," I said, trying to stay polite, "again, what do you need from me?"

"Obviously," Dottie stepped back, "I do not need a veterinarian. I already know what's wrong. I just need to find a source of medications closer than the border."

Of course, how stupid of me! That is why I went to school for all those years—so I could be a pusher for local turtles.

In fact, I was not all that surprised by Dottie's approach. It was true that special interest groups like the reptile clubs, the bird clubs, and, for that matter, many pet stores had better pet pharmacies than most veterinarians—at least here in Southern California. Most of these individuals or groups made the two-hour drive to Tijuana on a regular basis. If you happened to have a special prescription, perhaps one written by a Dr. Jackson or Dr. Franklin (i.e., a discreetly folded bill), you could even score narcotics if you knew where to ask. I knew something like this would happen soon enough, but I never expected it to be so blatant.

Thinking back on this encounter with Dottie, I realize that it was probably the most significant turning point of my career. You see, if Dottie liked you, she would tell everybody about you: what a talented veterinarian you were, how fair, and, most of all, that you were someone who could get medications at reduced cost.

I did my best to control my indignation and reluctantly donned my nice-doctor game face. As I began my examination of the little Hermann's tortoise, Dottie rattled on about how the turtle was not getting better even though she had been treating it for some three weeks. Just a few more antibiotic treatments, she assured me, were all it would take.

The first thing I noticed when I picked up the little turtle was how emaciated it was. Of greater significance and far overshadowing the weight issue was its jaw. Hanging down from the front of its face, under sunken, closed eyes, were the raw ends of the jawbone.

It had snapped off, on both sides, right in the middle between the cheek and the chin, forming a grotesque V flapping back and forth, dangling by mere shreds of damaged greenish-brown skin. The exposed bone protruded from each cheek like rusty tines on a broken fork. Its tongue, having been exposed to the air nonstop, had become a shriveled, brown-black dried-out piece of flesh.

The tortoise's legs and head dangled from its shell. He was too weak to retract them. The closer I examined the pitiable creature, the more my blood boiled. Dottie's voice prattled on like a bad radio talk show just inside my level of consciousness. This woman had veterinary drugs, had made a diagnosis, and was treating the patient. In legal terms, Dottie was practicing veterinary medicine without a license! If a veterinarian had done what Dottie had done to this turtle, it would have been malpractice.

I was furious. My mind raced as I tried to decide what to do. My gut reaction was to reach over the table, grab Dottie by the collar, and shake her—but that would not have helped the turtle. I can't stand to see animals suffer, and there was just no excuse for the condition of the animal I was holding in my hands.

I gently set the little tortoise back into the cardboard box in which it had arrived, giving its shell a gentle stroke with my fingers as I did. Stepping back from the table, I took a deep breath, centered myself, and gave Dottie the most penetrating look I could muster.

"Well," Dottie spoke first, "you can see why I need antibiotics, can't you?"

"Ms. Shackleford," I addressed her as I turned up the intensity of my glare. The next words that came out were critical. If I gave her the antibiotics she requested, I could preserve and possibly cement a future relationship with the WCTTC. And if I told her honestly what was on my mind, I might well alienate the club for good and end any chance of my ever caring for another turtle or tortoise in Southern California.

"Ms. Shackleford," I repeated, "this sick little tortoise does not need antibiotics. What this turtle needs is proper medical care."

"All he needs is a few more shots," Dottie interrupted.

"Proper, professional veterinary care," I persisted, increasing my volume. "If this patient had come to see me from another veterinarian's office I would be on the phone right now with the State Board of Veterinary Medicine, filing formal charges of malpractice." I did not give Dottie a chance to interrupt. "What I see here is gross negligence. In fact"—here I picked up the tortoise and turned the dangling jaw in her direction—"in my opinion, it's cruel to let any animal suffer like this!"

Dottie licked her lips, swallowed. "I've only had it for three weeks. It just needs a little more time—it *will* get better."

"No, Ms. Shackleford. This turtle will not get better without proper veterinary care. It has a compound, bilaterally broken jaw. The ends of the bone are dead from lack of blood supply. It is severely dehydrated and starving because it can't eat, and the last thing in the world you should do is put it on antibiotics."

Dottie was speechless. Her shoulders slumped, her mouth fell open, and she stepped back from the table and slouched against the wall for support. Her voluminous purse hung over her left shoulder by a thin fake leather strap. She looked down and fumbled aimlessly with the top zipper.

I can't remember ever coming down on a client the way I had just unloaded on Ms. Shackleford. I don't usually let my emotions dictate my interaction with clients. But as I looked down at the turtle, its broken jaw flipped back under its neck, its closed eyes sunken and matted with dried mucus that gave it a look of tears on a pained face, I knew that I had done the right thing. If Dottie had let this little turtle suffer so, there was no telling how many more had been or were being treated the same way.

Finally, somberly, Dottie looked up from her purse, reached over, and, picking up the Hermann's tortoise, handed it to me. "I guess I should leave it with you, huh?"

I was stunned. I had expected her to grab it, make some snide remarks, and storm out of the room.

"I'll do what I can," I said as I let her place the turtle in my open palms.

Unfortunately, but as expected, the turtle died the following day. Its prognosis was grave the moment it presented, but if an owner wants to try to save a pet, I feel that it is my duty to try everything I can. I called Dottie and informed her of the turtle's passing. She accepted the news with little emotion, stating as a matter of fact that she would send a check to my office to cover the bill.

I had just berated one of the icons of the WCTTC and failed to treat the first patient the group brought me. I was certain I would never hear from them again.

The next day a special delivery arrived at the receptionist's desk—a huge bouquet of beautiful flowers, accompanied by a large, heavy present and a greeting card, addressed to "Dr. Mader, turtle vet." The envelope had a smiling green turtle emblazoned on the rear flap.

Dear Dr. Mader,

I realize that we got off to a difficult start. Please accept these flowers and this book as a token of my appreciation for your efforts and a gift welcoming a future relationship. Both the WCTTC and I look forward to working with you, and especially, to learning from you in the years ahead.

Sincerely,

Dottie Shackleford and the WCTTC

Inside the gift wrap was a wonderful book called *Turtles of the World*.

◆ ◆ ◆

I said my perfunctory good mornings to the receptionist staff as I started my morning lap around the hospital before heading to the conference room. When I arrived in the treatment room I was alarmed to see the Karens, Peter, and Stacey huddling over a patient on the table. Off in the corner of the room, his face wrought with dread, stood Toad.

"What's going on?" I asked, scanning the scene. I nodded in Toad's direction. His eyes were uncharacteristically anxious, reddened.

"What's wrong with Barney?" I asked again, trying to peer through the mass of bodies surrounding the table. The old dog was prone, his eyes half shut. Not even a twitch from his usual happy tail.

"His skin is falling off," Toad stated, without emotion. His voice was calm, but I sensed an urgency that I had not heard since Barney first came in sick. It was obvious that Toad had not shaven. Pronounced shadows under his eyes darkened his rotund face. Despite the coolness in the treatment area, a patina of sweat dampened Toad's frowning forehead.

Clients are not trained in medical description. I have learned years ago not to take what they say too literally. What appears to them a catastrophic emergency is more often than not just a routine medical problem. In contrast, the true emergencies are often ignored until it's too late (like an eye that has popped out and the owner wants to wait to see if it will go back in on its own). So when Toad described Barney's skin as falling off, I was not convinced this was actually the case.

Curious and concerned, I stepped forward and my staff parted like the Red Sea. There before me lay our chubby basset. I was astonished to see that Toad's description was not far from the truth. As I got closer, Barney stood up, his long, sway back accented by his large, droopy jowls. He glanced up at me with pained, bloodshot eyes, obviously not wanting to move his head or turn his neck. "What's his temperature?" I asked no one in particular.

Karen 2, who had been Barney's primary caregiver all along, offered, "It's 105, even." Normal for a dog should be less than 102.5 degrees.

A band of skin about six inches wide around his midsection had turned completely black. It started at the top of Barney's back, just behind the shoulder blades, and circled his belly like one of those old, wide belts that men used to wear in the early '70s. At the very top of Barney's back, at the zenith of the black band, was a deep ulcer the size of a silver dollar. The skin was completely missing, exposing the raw, bloody muscle and sinew below. The edges around the crater were crusty and pasted with a yellow, sticky serum that matted Barney's tan fur into smelly, red-brown points like an inward crown of thorns.

To make matters worse, the blackened belt of skin encircling the midsection was hard, like beef jerky, and obviously painful to the touch. Where it came together on Barney's belly was a large fissure-like crack in lieu of a buckle, and from that dribbled a straw-colored, stringy fluid down onto the stainless steel table, forming a coagulating puddle of goo.

I had never seen this before, but I knew immediately what it was.

"What is it?" Karen 2 asked, sensing that I was finished with my assessment. Toad was hanging on my every word.

"Have you ever heard of toxic epidermal necrolysis, or TEN?"

All eyes flashed around the room, each hoping that someone else had the answer, and hoping even more that the answer would be a happy one. Finally, Karen 1 spoke. "Isn't that where the body has an idiosyncratic reaction to a medication?" I figured that Karen 1 would be the one who knew. She continued to impress me with her mind for facts.

"Yeah, it's really rare. Not an allergic reaction, like when a person reacts badly to penicillin. Nobody knows why this occurs, and it's much more violent than an allergic reaction—as is obvious here.

"What were we using, Karen?" I turned my attention to Karen 2, knowing that she had been treating Barney from the beginning and remembering that she had medicated Barney last week when he came in for what we took for a sore on his skin.

"Trimethoprim-sulfa." Her answer was tentative.

"Only that?" I asked, somewhat challenging.

"Yeah, that was all." She swallowed. I realized she might be feeling like she was the cause of all this.

"That is an excellent drug. I routinely use TMS for skin infections." I wanted everybody to know that Karen 2 was in no way responsible for Barney's condition, and I could see immediate relief in her expression.

"Did we"—I used the collective "we" so that everybody knew the administration of the medication was a team effort—"give Barney an injection of TMS, or did he just get pills?"

"An injection," Karen 2 said, stepping up to the table and pointing to the hole at the top of the belt, "right here."

"That makes sense." The ulcer Karen was pointing to was no doubt the start of the reaction. I have read that in severe cases of TEN some animals can literally slough off their entire skin the way a person might take off a full-length coat. Needless to say, such cases are almost always fatal.

"Toad," I looked up at Barney's concerned dad again, beckoning for him to approach.

"If he's gonna die, I don't want him to suffer." Toad wiped his nose with the back of his hand. "Just put him to sleep." His eyes welled up with tears.

I was not expecting that. Barney was Toad's traveling companion, his best friend. Toad took Barney everywhere. He loved that dog so much; it had to take an incredible amount of emotional self-control and selflessness to make such a statement. I have seen way too many owners not willing to accept humane euthanasia and have watched their beloved pets linger in terrible pain and suffering. But I was not ready to throw in the towel.

"Toad, I won't kid you. Barney is hurting right now. I am so sorry that he had this reaction to the medication." I was careful not to imply that it was something we had done wrong. Clients are often looking for any reason to blame the doctor when things don't go as planned, be it a veterinarian or a human physician.

"Like I said," Toad offered, his eyes welling up as I spoke, "I don't want him to suffer either." Toad reached a hand out and patted his friend on the head between his large, floppy ears. As he did Barney cringed and let out a yelp.

"Aw, man." Toad turned away and walked out of the room, wiping his eyes. Karen 2 followed him out of the room.

I stood there for a moment, thinking about Barney's options. I remembered that when a TEN reaction occurred, it usually was rapid, lasting for twenty-four hours or so. What skin was going to fall off would fall off during that critical period. If the patient lost all of its skin, it was certain death. If the skin loss was not complete, proper nursing care and skin grafting could save the day. Since the injection of TMS had been given almost five days earlier, I suspected that the skin reaction I was looking at was finished, and from this point on, no further damage need be expected. If I was right, I should be able to save Barney's life.

The rest of the day seemed to revolve around Barney. I continuously checked on him. The pain medications made him comfortable enough to curl up on a big, padded doggy bed. Stacey and Karen 2 wrapped a special bandage around him to protect his wounds.

By early evening most of the employees had gone home for the day. Greg, our night technician who lived in the apartment upstairs next to the students, had yet to check in. I looked over Barney's blood results while standing in front of his cage. He was soundly asleep and in the middle of some dog dream. His whiskers would twitch, all four feet would rhythmically flex, and he would emit an occasional whimper.

I couldn't help wonder what I would be feeling if it had been Wok in the cage. I knew I would have been devastated but that I would not give up. I decided that even if Toad could not afford the treatment Barney needed, I would donate it myself. I was not going to let Barney die.

◆ ◆ ◆

Ellen was not home that night, as usual. I took Wok for his evening walk to the park. We sat on the bench and I told him about Barney. I said that if he ever felt even the slightest bit ill he was to tell me right away.

The next morning, I arrived at work and uncustomarily walked right past everybody without my normal salutations, heading directly back to Barney's cage. "How's he doing?" Karen 2 was also up early and waiting when I arrived.

Barney was sitting up in his cage, ears flopping, face long, tail thumping on the cage bottom.

"Great!" Karen 2 answered, smiling. "I haven't changed his bandage yet. I thought you'd want to see it."

"Yes, thank you. That's good news." I opened the cage front and scratched Barney on his head, between his ears. His baggy eyes looked up at my hand, looking for food. "Did you feed him?"

"Not yet. I didn't know whether or not you wanted to anesthetize him this morning."

Karen 2 was thinking ahead. It was hard to believe that the two Karens had only a little over a week left of their externship. With good students, the time flies by; with mediocre ones, four weeks seems like an eternity.

We all gathered in the conference room for rounds. According to what I'd read the night before, as long as the TEN reaction had stopped, it should be possible to cut away the dead skin and replace it with skin grafts. The plan was to keep Barney for a few more days to get the infection under control and then I would attempt the surgical repair.

◆ ◆ ◆

Barney continued to do well that night. If his blood tests were normal, we would do his surgery the following morning.

The fourth Thursday of each month was always the monthly meeting for the Los Angeles Herpetological Society, or LAHS, the local club whose focus was reptiles and amphibians. The society meetings were held in the cafeteria of an intermediate school just on the fringe of the bad side of the city. The location was picked because it was next to the freeways, which was convenient for most of the members who had to drive in from out of town. But for us it meant driving directly through the inner slums, passing through the territory known for gangbangers and hookers. Most students considered it an adventure, although some were scared to death.

The two-hundred-plus avid amateur and professional herpetologists gathered together at the LAHS to discuss their favorite snakes, lizards, and turtles, compare breeding notes, talk about recent nature hikes, and discuss what animals each member had caught. In addition, a lot of the local breeders and pet stores brought animals or supplies to sell at display tables scattered around the periphery of the large hall. Meetings resembled a bazaar, with people milling around and tables covered with empty cages and live snakes, turtles, lizards, and mice (potential snake food). Occasionally, someone would have cookies or some other baked goods for sale for human consumption.

Every month the group had a guest speaker, usually a successful local breeder, a biology professor, or, at least a couple of times a year, me. I was not the featured speaker this month, but whenever I came to a meeting, people would always have questions about their pet's health. Not uncommonly, members would bring their sick animals to the meeting hoping to get a free exam. No sooner had we walked in the front door of the cafeteria than a horde of clients rushed up to great us with potential patients.

"Hey, Dr. Mader!" the first freebie hailed. "How ya doin'?" A young man with jet-black hair approached wearing a weathered leather jacket replete with zippers and chains dangling from the pockets. A silver loop pierced his right eyebrow, a silver stud ran through the left nostril, numerous studs, loops, and figurines pierced through each ear, and tribal tattoos covered the backs of each hand. Draped around his neck was a hefty, at least five-foot-long Nile monitor lizard.

"What's happening, Bean?" Bean worked at the largest reptile pet store in Southern California, was an excellent amateur herpetologist, and always kept his charges in the best of care. Inevitably he would have something to show me at these meetings, though there was rarely anything wrong.

"Lizzie's got respiratory or something. She ain't feeling too well lately."

Like "Monty" for pet pythons, "Lizzie" was probably one of the most common names for lizards. "'Respiratory' is the lay term for anything that causes a reptile to cough, sneeze, or wheeze," I explained to the two Karens. "It's a catchall diagnosis and doesn't mean much." Both students stepped forward to admire and examine the large saurian as Bean proudly showed it off.

"Bean, you know that there isn't anything I can do for you right here." I looked at him while I petted his lizard's large black-and-gold, diamond-shaped head. Lizzie's long, purple-black snake-like tongue flicked my wrist.

"I know, Doc. I was just hoping that you could prescribe me something."

"So you wouldn't have to spend money to come see me in my office?" Both Karens looked surprised I was so blunt.

"No, Doc, not that. I just didn't want to have to wait in case it was something serious."

"No worries, Bean." I used both hands to steady the large lizard's head and gently opened its mouth, exposing the four rows of large, razor-sharp teeth. There were in fact bubbles coming out of its windpipe when it hissed.

"See that?" I spoke to the Karens. They both leaned forward, almost standing on their tiptoes. Bean was a rather tall fellow, and I was holding the head up high.

"Yes," they responded, impressed. Just then a glob of thick yellow drool dripped out of the corner of the lizard's mouth and down the back of my hand.

"Sorry, Doc." Bean immediately wiped the saliva from my hand with his sleeve.

"No worries, Bean. Part of the job." I let go of the head and looked around for something to wipe off the rest of the slime. As if reading my mind, Karen 2 walked over to a table selling doughnuts and grabbed a handful of napkins.

"I'll tell you what, why don't you bring Lizzie into my office tomorrow afternoon and I'll have the students give him a free physical examination. We'll determine what he needs; then, all you have to pay for is the medication." I looked at the Karens for approval. They both smiled.

"Will that work for you?"

"Thank you, Dr. Mader! Very cool." He flashed a big smile and then quickly kissed Lizzie on the top of her shiny head. "I'll see you guys, ah, girls, and you, Dr. Mader, tomorrow! Thank you!"

I did not like giving away services gratis, but I kind of liked Bean. He was cool, and I could tell the students were really interested in the big lizard, the biggest they'd seen since starting three weeks ago.

◆ ◆ ◆

I arrived at work excited about Barney's surgery. If all went well, we would be able to save this wonderful dog's life. If not, then there was a good chance that Toad's best buddy would never go along on another ride in his big rig.

We got through morning rounds with efficiency. Barney's blood results came back normal. Karen 2 was excited because I told her that she could once again scrub in with me on Barney. By the time Karen and I finished rounds, Fred had already clipped the fur from Barney's entire trunk—from the back of his neck down to his chest, the top of both front legs, the entire torso, and all the way back to his hips and thighs.

After two hours of nonstop cutting and suturing, Barney was finished. By then he looked like a magician's assistant, cut in half and sewn back together, with the row of stitches giving the appearance of a zipper fastening the two halves of his long body.

The rest of the day went well. Barney slept off his post-surgical pain medications, and when he woke up he actually was feeling well enough to eat. Karen 2 stayed late at the hospital, waiting for Toad to come by and visit Barney after his day on the road.

According to Karen 2, Toad was pretty much in shock when he saw Barney's huge incision, even breaking down in silent tears. He managed to squeeze his short, stubby body partially into the cage with Barney and sat with him for over an hour. When Barney finally went to sleep, Toad took Karen 2 out for a burger. They had developed a real friendship. I wondered, with Toad's lonely life as a trucker, how often he got the chance to socialize with a young lady.

When I got home, I actually got to see Ellen. On Friday nights we play on a city softball league. Her coworkers at the hospital formed a coed team, and since I loved to play ball, they invited me to join the team. The best part was that it gave me a chance to spend time with my wife, even if it was with a large group. We played a competitive game but ended up losing in the last inning. It didn't matter—it was fun to get out and do something nonmedical.

◆ ◆ ◆

Euthanizing a pet has got to be one of the hardest things owners can do. I always try my best to help them with that difficult decision and to make the process as comfortable as possible. Every veterinarian in practice has at least one euthanasia horror story. One of the things that I have always done, especially for my really good clients, is to offer to come to their home to perform this sacred final passage. That way they don't have to load up their pet in the car, drive to the hospital, wait in the reception area to be called, be placed in an exam room, and then wait again for the doctor, a.k.a. the angel of death, to come in with the needle.

Daniel Benedict lived alone in a flat in one of the poorer parts of town, about two miles north of Noah's Ark along the corridor. He had a fourteen-year-old male black lab named Cuz that had been battling end-stage kidney disease for the past six months. Fourteen is old for a Labrador, and in reality,

Mr. Benedict had done an amazing job keeping him alive as long as he had.

Cuz, in his prime, was about 110 pounds. Though his disease had wasted him away, he was still a big-boned dog, and I was going to need help not only with administering the euthanasia but also carrying the large dog to the car when I was finished. I asked Fred to come along. Before we left, we gathered our supplies: medical gear, euthanasia solution, stretcher, blanket to cover the body, and plastic bags to protect the back of my SUV.

It was a typical August day—hot, hot, hot—and the thick brown smog created an inversion layer. When we arrived, Mr. Benedict was waiting for us at the front door. His place was small, sandwiched between two taller buildings so that what little breeze there was never reached his home. He did not have air conditioning, and even with windows open and several fans running, the temperature inside seemed well over the century mark.

He led us to a very small laundry room in the back of his home. There, between the appliances on a soiled comforter on the wood floor, lay Cuz. A lone, ivory-colored, half-melted candle flickered on top of the washing machine. The gray-faced dog was a skeleton of his once athletic self, so weak he could barely lift his head to greet us. The old dog was in kidney failure and constantly leaking urine onto the fetid blanket. The heat and the smell of smoke and body fluids combined with a lack of ventilation in the confined quarters made the laundry room unbearable.

"Is it possible to move him out to the living room, Mr. Benedict?" I didn't see how we could manage to work in the small space.

"Please, Doc, I'd prefer if we could do it here." He wiped a tear from his cheek. "This is where he has always slept. I'd like it to be his final resting place."

I was not here to debate. Things were tough. I looked at Fred. We'd make it work.

"Would you mind please turning on the light?" I looked up at a bare bulb hanging in the center of the ceiling.

"I'm sorry, Doc. It doesn't work." He nodded toward the dryer. "That's why I brought you the candle."

Black dog, dark room, dehydrated skin making the vein impossible to see. Again, I looked at Fred as we gathered the necessary items. I had to keep wiping the sweat from my eyes and hands onto my pants.

Finally, with grace and dignity, we were able to administer the euthanasia drug. Thankfully the dog passed peacefully, head resting on its owner's lap as it let out its final breath. I took a listen to its heart with my stethoscope to ensure that the life pump had stopped. No more suffering for the much-beloved Cuz.

"We'll give you a few moments." I had to step over the owner in the small space to get out of the room. Fred and I gathered our materials and went out to my SUV. The 100-plus temperature outside felt cool compared to the indoor oven. We both felt emotionally and physically drained.

I grabbed the large stretcher and a blanket and went back inside to retrieve the body. Fred and I carefully slid, then lifted the deceased pet from the cramped space between the washer and dryer. After Mr. Benedict gave Cuz a final kiss on the forehead, we covered the large dog with the blanket and carried it out and placed the body into the back of my car.

About a mile down the road I noticed a convenience store and pulled in. I was parched and needed something cold to drink. Even with the A/C in my car set on Arctic, we were both still pouring sweat.

As I pulled into the lot I noticed a man on the far side screaming and yelling at a driver in a parked car. One thing you learn in the inner city is to just ignore such drama. The need for a cold drink won out over any potential danger, so we went inside the store to grab some libations and get a respite from the heat.

The highly irritated man was still across the lot when we exited and deliberately did not look his way. Just as I was about to get into my SUV, the crazy noticed us and ran across the asphalt, jumping at Fred and yelling, "It's all your fault! You're the reason they're all dying!" He grabbed Fred by the collar and started shaking him violently, pushing him up against the side of my vehicle.

Instantly I ran around the front of my car and pushed the man away, screaming at Fred to "Get in the car, get in the car!"

Fred, clearly shaken, just stood there like a deer in the headlights. This seemed to irritate the man even more, and he continued to direct all of his rage at my stunned technician.

"You taunting me? You taunting me?" The man, wildly pointing a finger at Fred, was struggling to get past me. "I'm gonna kill you, muthafucka!"

The insane man was incensed, spittle flying about with each word, yellow eyes bulging out of his face. I had him by the shoulders and was able to parry him off every time he took a swing. Finally, I heard the door slam behind me, and I knew I had one chance to end this. I reached around the back of his head, grabbing him by his dreadlocks, and slammed his face into the rear side passenger window of my car.

"Unless you want to end up like this poor bastard," I yelled with all my might, pointing to the blanketed body in the back of my car, "get outa my face!"

The lunatic looked into the back of my SUV and saw the covered corpse, which, given its large size, could easily have been a human.

In an instant he froze. No struggling, no words. He just stared at the body. I could see the color drain from his face. Before I knew it, he turned and ran as fast as he could, until he vanished between the parked cars on the other side of the lot.

◆ ◆ ◆

"Did you see who's coming in this morning?" I directed my comments at Karen 2. It was the Karens' last day of their externship. They both had been fantastic and were going to be missed.

"Yep. Barney!" Karen 2 broadcast a big smile. She had really taken to the long dog and his owner, Toad. It had been a week since his major skin surgery, and it was time for suture removal.

"I'll let you take care of the procedure when he comes in, okay?"

"Great. Thanks!" She was obviously excited.

We finished rounds and proceeded to attend to the day's patient case-load. I was standing in the hall getting ready to enter a room when I saw Toad and Barney walk in the front door.

I paused for a moment, then decided to walk up to the reception area to say hi. Toad was all smiles, and Barney, tail wagging a million miles an hour, looked fantastic. His incision looked completely healed, and his fur was already starting to grow back.

This, I thought as I bent over and scratched Barney behind his huge, floppy ears, is why I do what I do.

Randy and the Sticky Buns

Since the hospital was closed on Labor Day, I got up early and took Wok to the shore before the crowds stormed the sand for the last hurrah of the summer. Wok loved the beach and water, and he loved to swim, unlike me. I may have grown up on an island and surfed as a young boy, but unlike the waters around the Florida Keys and Hawaii where I was raised, the Southern California water was *cold*. I'll man up and jump in for a dive if I'm wearing a thick wet suit, but I won't go swimming just for the fun of it.

Wok, on the other hand, would waltz into the water until he was in over his head, dog-paddle out past the breakers, swim parallel to the beach for a bit, then, when he was tired, bodysurf back in. Just like a kid.

After I took Wok home and bathed off all the sand and salt water, I picked up our new student from the airport. Randy was tall, well over six feet, and lanky. He spoke with a soft voice, and if it weren't for his prominent Adam's apple bobbing up and down, you often wouldn't know he was speaking. He seemed genuinely excited about the upcoming month.

Bart, one of my favorite clients, asked me to do a house call during my lunch hour the next day, so naturally I took Randy with me. Despite it being totally illegal, Bart kept a full-grown Galápagos tortoise, Bertha, in his backyard, and two medium-sized alligators in a custom cage in his garage, which had been remodeled to accommodate the large semiaquatic reptiles. The ceiling had been replaced by a panel of fluorescent, ultraviolet lights that mimicked the sun's natural rays. In summer Bart could leave the windows open, but even in Southern California, the winter nights could get down to the low 30s, so Bart lined the walls with several banks of heaters for the colder months. The windows were covered with security bars, much like in most homes in the inner city. These bars, however, were installed not to keep people out but the gators in.

Nothing was wrong with the reptiles. Bart was the perfect pet owner: he did not wait until there was a problem but had me check on his animals at least twice a year.

Randy and I got to his place just after noon. Bertha was easy to examine—she was over sixty years old and as tame as a puppy. She loved for us to scratch the top of her weathered, dark green shell and to rub the skin under her chin. She'd stand at perfect attention if you rubbed there, which allowed me to do a full exam.

I let Randy perform an examination on Bertha as well, and he was thrilled. He had brought along a small camera and got permission from Bart to take several photos, including him posing with the large reptile. Bart was okay with Randy taking the pictures, but under no uncertain terms was he allowed to let *anybody* know where they'd been taken.

The gators were not so cooperative. Fortunately, Bart was skilled at handling the beasts. He'd climb into their round pool, which essentially took up the entire two-car garage, then grab one by the tail and hang on until it stopped thrashing and spinning over. He would then jump on the back of its neck, pinning down its head and mouth. Once they were restrained, I'd take a roll of electrical tape and secure the chompers so that none of us would lose a hand.

We got through the examinations without any injuries but were soaked by the time we finished.

Bart lived several miles off the freeway, and we had to drive through some seedy parts of town to get back to NAVH. At one of the big intersections on the Pacific Coast Highway, traffic was snarled and halted in all directions. Suddenly I saw what looked like a person flying over the hood of a small truck several vehicles ahead of me, and immediately thereafter two others jumped over the same truck, obviously in pursuit. The first guy had a look of total panic on his face as he ran past our car, his torn T-shirt bloodied. Moments later the two pursuers, screaming and yelling and one carrying what looked like a baseball bat, ran by in the same direction. As soon as they passed, the cars ahead started to move. So did I, happy not to stick around for any encores. On the edge of the intersection, two low-rider-style cars pulled to the side, one partially on the curb, and several animated individuals congregating around the vehicles appeared to be arguing.

I looked over at Randy as we passed by. His face, stretched wide by a huge smile just a few minutes before at Bart's house, was now pallid and drawn.

"Welcome to the big city," I said with a smile.

◆ ◆ ◆

When I got home from work that night, after feeding Wok, I went for an evening run. I always wanted a dog that would run with me, but sadly Wok was not that dog. Wok was born with severe hip dysplasia. His hips were so bad that he needed to have a double hip replacement by the time he was two years old. I do not do hip replacement surgeries, but my colleague Dr. Elliott Roberts was one of the world's leading experts in dog joint replacements. Six months and two artificial hips later, Wok was back in the ocean swimming. He could walk, play, and run in the yard, but Elliott suggested that I not take him running with me because the prolonged exercise might damage the artificial implants. After I got back from my run, Wok was waiting for me at the front door, curly tail wagging full speed, leash in his mouth, ready for his evening walk to the park.

◆ ◆ ◆

Whenever Mr. Rockwell came in with his dogs it was more an event than an appointment. A former pro-football player, Mr. Lionel Rockwell towered six feet seven inches and weighed some 275 pounds of solid muscle. You would expect this hulking man to have Rottweilers, pit bulls, or some other similar macho hounds. Instead, he had seven Pomeranians—seven purse-sized, hyperactive, constantly yapping fuzz balls.

Mr. Rockwell had done very well for himself in football. He played for nine seasons before destroying his knee. However, unlike so many other young professional athletes who blew all of their money on extravagances only to find themselves penniless at the end of their playing careers, Mr. Rockwell invested in McDonald's restaurants—seven, in fact, just like the number of his dogs.

He drove a high-end Jaguar with the leather rear seat custom-replaced by a row of seven individualized cubicles, each with the name of a dog engraved on the brass plate over the top. Every stall was carpeted to match the upholstery of the Jaguar, and each had a small seat belt for its occupant. The dogs were trained to go to their specific spot when allowed into the car, and each waited patiently for Mr. Rockwell to properly strap them in safely before the ride.

We had no private parking lot, so clients had to park somewhere along the street, wherever they could find a place, and walk with their pets to the hospital. Whenever Mr. Rockwell arrived, he would call the office from his car phone so that at least two technicians could be out front waiting to help walk in the dogs.

It was time for his dogs to get their annual exams. Mr. Rockwell brought all the dogs in for their semiannual checkups. Seven dogs at a half-hour exam per dog was a full morning. Fortunately, after much bouncing and yapping, all the dogs checked out just fine. His veterinary bill was hefty, but that did not bother him, as he had left an open credit card on file and trusted us to charge him accurately. As he was leaving, he gave Lisa a fifty-dollar bill with the request to "Please treat the staff to a pizza lunch on me."

•••

I was extra busy because I had to interview a potential new veterinary assistant. Normally, Willy would handle the personnel stuff, since the management was more to his liking than mine (I preferred the medical side). However, this could not wait, as we were short-staffed; the animal care team was all putting in overtime hours, and the long days were taking their toll. So Lisa arranged for me to meet with the candidate over lunch.

Surgeries ran long, and the interviewee had to wait almost forty-five minutes. That meant that the interview was also cut short because of afternoon appointments. I walked back to the conference room where Lisa had Robert wait. He immediately stood up to greet me and extended his hand.

I have to admit, I was shocked by his appearance. He was wearing tattered jeans, unlaced high-tops, no socks, and a sleeveless shirt with a faded image of some type of devil on the front. His pale arms were covered with large black tattoos: crosses, knives, Gothic writing, a grim reaper, and headstones with names. The tattoos continued up onto his neck with more crosses, teardrops, some random numbers, barbed wire, and what looked like ravens.

Robert's facial bones were high and prominent over sunken cheeks, his lips thin, and, I am certain, carried a slight patina of black lipstick. His eyes were deep and dark and his ears festooned with dull, silver piercings. The jet-black hair was greased back and ended in a two-inch ducktail.

"I'm Robert." His grip was strong and confidant, as was his voice, though I had to wonder why someone would show up to an interview at a professional workplace dressed like a Halloween character.

"Dr. Mader. Please, have a seat." I motioned him toward a chair with a deliberately businesslike tone.

"Are you new to the area?" I wanted to break the ice, but I had trouble envisioning Robert interacting with clients, especially new ones. What kind of impression would he make on nervous owners when they saw all these signs of death and devil worship?

"Yes, sir, I just moved here from Hollywood." A polite response. I sensed a military upbringing.

"What brings you here?"

"I'm looking for a fresh start." He gave a barely perceptible squirm. As a veterinarian you learn to read body language. What people say is not always what they mean, but body language does not lie.

"Care to explain?" Time for the meat of the interview.

Over the next twenty minutes, Robert went on to tell me what had been happening in his personal life for the past year: homelessness, drugs, petty crime. It had been rough. One night a girl he had been dating OD'd. That was his wake-up call.

I took the time to listen and jot down notes. I needed to give Robert a fair chance in spite of my initial reaction to his appearance. I had learned my lesson with Dave, our wildlife volunteer and amateur magician. I had not wanted to like Dave when we first met during the British Petroleum oil spill in Huntington Beach a year ago, but, to my shame, Dave turned out to be a jewel.

When the oil tanker *American Trader* had ruptured its hull, spilling over four hundred thousand gallons of crude oil that washed up along the shores of the Southern California coast, Willy and I donated our veterinary expertise and hospital facilities to help treat injured wildlife. After the oil spill crisis was over, Dave showed up at our hospital offering to volunteer to help out with our community wildlife program. He came in on three separate occasions to drop off his résumé, but his appearance turned me off, so each time I told the receptionist to tell him we did not need extra help. I never took the few minutes needed to talk with him personally and thank him for all his hard work on the oil spill birds, or for coming by to offer help.

Months later, a perfect storm of staff problems, the flu knocking out half of our employees, and an avalanche of injured wildlife finally broke the camel's back. The overburdened staff and students just could not keep up with the proper care of our wildlife patients. If we were going to offer the service, we had to do it right or stop doing it altogether.

Reluctantly I had Lisa dig out Dave's résumé, and then I gave him a call. He was at the hospital thirty minutes later, and just minutes after that, he was cleaning cages and feeding possums, raccoons, ducks, and more. He'd been with us ever since.

Dave was gaunt with long, unkempt, grayish-brown hair, bushy eyebrows, a moustache, and a gold earring. He spoke softly, but only when addressed, and otherwise kept to himself. Dave, it turned out, was a Vietnam vet who had been blown up in the war and suffered many severe injuries, among them a skull fracture that warranted a metal plate in his head. He was on permanent government disability and could not take a paying job without losing his benefits. He lived a simple life, and his monthly income was enough to keep him comfortable. So he volunteered to help with the wildlife, which was one of his passions—the other being magic.

My myopia had nearly cost me a valuable relationship with Dave, and I did not want to make the same mistake with Robert. I had already decided before Robert finished telling me his story that I would offer him a job. There was something about him, something sincere, caring, honest—a doggedness under that demonic veneer. I'm not sure what it was, but I knew we could find a place for him at NAVH.

◆ ◆ ◆

I went into work early so I could be there when Willy made his big return, only to find him sitting at his desk going through a huge stack of mail when I arrived.

"I didn't expect to see you here this early. Welcome back!" I shook his hand and gave him a hug.

"It's good to be back!" He looked good, but he had lost some weight, grown a scraggly beard, and his hair was much longer, desperately in need of a cut. "My clock is twelve hours opposite yours. I've been awake since midnight!" He smiled, bags under his eyes.

"Well, glad to have you back. It's been a good month and a half. I'll fill you in over the next few days." I put my stuff under my desk.

"This was in my stack. It's for you." Willy handed me an official-looking envelope. The return address read "American Board of Veterinary Practitioners." The postal stamp was dated September 5, 1991.

The letter I had been waiting for, the one telling me whether or not I qualified to sit for the specialty boards, the letter that had been keeping me up at night, had been sitting on Willy's desk for the past eleven days!

• • •

Since Willy was back, I actually got my normal Tuesday afternoon off. With a sense of both excitement and angst, I drove south to see Dr. Elliott Roberts to give him in person the news that my credentials had been accepted to sit for the ABVP Specialty Boards in Companion Animal Practice. Elliott had always been my go-to guru on anything veterinary medicine, not to mention that he had taken care of Wok's hips when they were so bad. We had become friends as well as colleagues in the past couple of years, and when he found out that I was planning on sitting for the specialty boards he offered to be my official mentor.

As expected, Elliott was thrilled, though he also said he was not surprised. Before I knew it, I was walking out of his hospital with a stack of books in my arms that he wanted me to use as study guides for the exam.

The exam: two days, hundreds of questions, hundreds of slide images covering every subject from anemia to zinc toxicity, and anything and everything in between. I went home with my new library and started making my study plan. I had almost a year—eleven months, actually—to prepare for this test that would shape the rest of my career. I stopped at an office supply company on the way home and bought a large wall calendar, the type that shows the entire year in advance. I hung it up in my home office next to my desk and started listing the books I wanted to have read and by when. Elliott suggested that I start with certain subjects and then progress in a specific direction through the rest of the stack.

He emphasized that I should study the stuff that I found the most difficult first and leave the easy stuff until last. So for the next four hours I pored over the books and journals, and with great detail I assigned each to a particular month, week, even down to the day, when I wanted to have it read by. Not including the journals, there were thirteen textbooks that I needed to read, cover to cover, in the next eleven months. That equated to 1.2 books per month!

• • •

I had planned on taking the next day off, since I had worked the past six Saturdays in a row, but I needed to come in to work to get my camera and take pictures for some lectures I was preparing.

The hospital opened at 8:00 a.m. on Saturdays, but since I was not on the books to see appointments, I pulled in around 9:00. When I arrived, I was surprised to see the new veterinary assistant, Robert, laughing it up in the lobby with Pat Peters, one of our longtime clients.

Pat was quite a personality: a philosophy professor at the local university who was a "she," but a "she" who had a full beard and a deep baritone voice. She was small in stature, with dark, sun-weathered skin and hairy forearms—a self-professed "gender bender," as she liked to call it, who enjoyed experimenting with male/female hormones. She always wore baggy pants low on the hip and usually a dark, worn, and torn T-shirt over a braless chest. Her gray-accented brown hair, which never looked washed, was pulled back in a ponytail behind her head and tucked into the back of her shirt.

With her several pets, Pat was a frequent visitor to NAVH. She owned two scruffy dogs, a cat, a parrot, and a big fish tank. We had a large bulletin board that featured clients' photos along with their pets. Most pet owners were proud and willing to showcase their fur family on our VIP (Very

Important Pet) board. However, despite my frequent requests to take Pat's picture with one of her many critters, she steadfastly refused. I had even put out a $100 bounty to any staff member who could get a full-face photo of Pat with her beard. To date, nobody had been successful.

I guess it was no surprise that if anybody would accept Robert for his appearance, it would be Pat.

"Good morning," I greeted both of them. "I see you two have met."

"Oh my, Robert is wonderful!" Pat proclaimed. She turned to him and held one of his large tattooed hands firmly in both of hers. "I am so glad you have Robert on your staff." She turned back to me, still holding his hand. "I've always loved bringing or keeping my pets here when I am away. Now, I am even more pleased!" Robert was beaming.

"I couldn't agree more," I said as I patted Robert on his shoulder. "We are so thankful that he joined our team."

◆ ◆ ◆

"Where are your two hot babes, Dr. Mader?" Bean appeared like magic as soon as Randy and I entered the front door of the Los Angeles Herpetological Society meeting. Lizzie was draped around his neck in her usual repose, and he was wearing the same leather jacket as last month.

"Hello to you, too, Bean." I smiled back and turned to Randy. "I guess you just don't cut it."

"Noooooo! That's not what I meant. I'm sorry!" Bean turned toward Randy and, grabbing his hand, started pumping it before Randy could respond.

"No worries. I'm Randy," my new student whispered, smiling. Lizzie made a lazy lizard glance upward toward Randy's face, perfunctorily flicking its long tongue.

"My *babes*, my two veterinary students, finished up at the beginning of the month and had to go back to university."

"Oh, yeah. I forgot they were still students. They were so, you know . . ."

mature looking." Bean took Lizzie down from his shoulders and handed the large saurian to Randy. "Wanna hold her? She's cool." Randy had no choice but to take into his arms the large, black-and-gold, leathery lizard.

"The girls really did a great job fixing her up!" Bean was obviously excited, and I was glad to see him and his lizard doing so well. Clients like Bean were the best advertising that a veterinarian could ask for. Giving him the little price break really paid off.

On top of the normal monthly activities, the club was also hosting its annual bake sale. Proceeds were used to cover some of the costs of veterinary care for ill or abandoned reptiles before they could be re-homed. As the sick animals were usually brought to me, I naturally wanted to support the endeavor, so I escorted Randy to a large table covered with confections. Crawling amid the cookies, cakes, and breads was a fourteen-inch, shiny, blue-tongued skink. The long-bodied lizard, with its ridiculously short legs, half walked and half slithered among the munchables, stopping occasionally to take a lick of icing from one of the cupcakes.

Behind the table, handling the money, sat a young woman who had a four-foot-long red-tailed boa draped around her neck. She was alternately stroking it, handing out the food items, and collecting the money—all without washing her hands between transactions. All I could think of was the risk of salmonella bacteria from the reptiles contaminating the food. *How many people*, I wondered, *will eat some of these yummy sweets only to wake up in the middle of the night with a tumultuous case of diarrhea and projectile vomiting?*

"What can I get ya, Doc?" The snake lady smiled up from her chair, picking up one of the gooey confections with her bare hand and offering it to me. "These sticky cinnamon buns are reeaaal good."

In my mind's eye I pictured all the bacteria on her fingers glomming on to the large pastry. She wiped her sticky digits on her apron, then continued to stroke the boa.

"Oh my!" was all I could think of saying. I was dumbfounded. I did not want to be rude and refuse all the goodies, but I knew that there was no way I was going to eat *anything* I bought from this table. The skink looked at me and, as if on cue, licked its lips with its long, blue tongue.

"Why don't you just give a couple of those to Randy here." I stepped back, whipping out my wallet at the same time. I pulled out a Hamilton, handed it to the southern belle, and thanked her for all she was doing to help the sick reptiles.

"Thank yooouuu, Doc. Enjoyyy!" She had a lovely smile, accented by the large snake.

"Thanks," Randy softly responded for us both.

"I wouldn't eat that if I were you," I whispered as soon as we were out of earshot.

"Why?" He looked surprised and disappointed.

"Look." I nodded back in the direction of the food table at the lemon-frosted angel food cake. The skink was crawling up its side, leaving toe prints in the icing.

"Oh . . ." Randy dejectedly looked down at the sticky buns on the paper plate.

"Whadja get?" Bean and his lizard once again magically appeared.

"Some yummy sticky buns." I looked at Bean, big lizard hanging around his neck, inches from his face and mouth. "But after I bought them, Randy told me he was diabetic . . . and I don't do sugar after 7:00 p.m." I grabbed the plate from Randy's hand before he could say anything. "Would you like them?"

"Really?" Bean beamed one of his famous smiles. "Hell, yeah. Thanks, Doc!" Randy passed them over to the exuberant lizard lover. Problem solved.

The herp meeting went well and was a lot of fun. Randy enjoyed the event and learned a lot about the myriad reptiles and amphibians in the pet trade, what it takes to market a veterinary practice, and the intrinsic value of spending time with so many wonderful people who shared common interests.

All night I found myself thinking about the food and the reptiles and the risk of salmonella. As a health professional, I felt that it was my duty to say something to the club. I talked over my concerns with Wok when I got home from the meeting. I did not want to rain on the LAHS's parade and tell them that the club should stop having their bake sale. After all, they did it to raise money to help sick reptiles, and ultimately, that money would end up coming to me.

Wok had a great idea. He was always logical and practical. I called my physician friend, Dr. Kristin Sullivan, and asked her if she'd be interested in copresenting a lecture with me to the society on salmonella. I'd talk about salmonella in reptiles and amphibians, and she would talk about salmonella in people. Kristin was an R.D.—"Real Doctor," as veterinarians sarcastically refer to human physicians. She had brought her tortoise to me about a year before with a large bladder stone. Unfortunately, the surgery to remove the stone resulted in extensive damage to the internal organs, and though I tried my best to repair the tissues, the big tortoise died a few days later. Most pet owners would have blamed the doctor for not saving their pet, but Kristin had understood the risks of surgery, and although obviously sad, she was understanding when it passed away. Over time we developed a friendship that surpassed most others I have had in my life.

No surprise, Kristin was thrilled with the idea and was happy to help. I then called the president of the herp club and got on their guest speaker schedule for the following month.

◆ ◆ ◆

"You're gonna like the next one, Doc!" Lisa had a mischievous smile on her face as she handed me the chart. I glanced at Randy, who was shadowing me as usual.

I checked the entry in the medical chart, looking at the reason for the visit. "Health certificate for iguana moving to Australia." I showed the entry to Randy.

"That's not going to happen," I said, shaking my head. "Australia has extremely strict rules about imports."

I stepped into the room, a bit puzzled as soon as I entered.

"I'm Dr. Mader." I extended my hand in greeting to the portly woman standing in the corner next to the exam table. She was wearing a puffy down jacket, zipped up the front. "And this is Randy, my senior student."

"I understand you need a health certificate to take an iguana to Australia?" I did not see an iguana in the room.

"Not really." She shook my hand. "What I actually need is some tranquilizer for my iguana."

"I'm sorry. I'm confused." I looked at her.

"I'm aware you are not allowed to take iguanas or any reptiles into Australia. You don't need to tell me what I already know."

"Understood," I continued, bewildered.

"I know how I am going to get my ig into the country. I just need a sedative for the flight."

"I'm not trying or intending to argue with you, but you won't be allowed to bring your iguana into Australia," I said in a matter-of-fact voice. "Customs just won't allow it."

"Only if they find it." She was smug.

"And if they do, not only will they confiscate it, I know for a fact that they will kill it." "Euthanize" was too nice a word.

"They'll never find it." She smiled and started to unzip her puffy down jacket.

She removed the coat and placed it on the exam table.

"Check it if you want." She smiled and motioned in the direction of the discarded garment.

I nodded to Randy to take a look. He picked it up and felt up and down the material, checking the pockets and sleeves. Setting it down, he shook his head.

"See?"

"Okay?" I questioned. "So why do you need the tranquilizer? What's the magic here?"

"Again. They'll never find it. I just need to keep it quiet for the seventeen-hour flight."

The woman started to unbutton her long-sleeved, green-and-red-checkered flannel blouse. As she got to the last button, the shirt came off, and underneath was a heavily padded brassiere, supporting her ample bosom. The striptease continued as she reached behind her back, exposing fully haired armpits, unfastened the clasp, and proceeded to remove her bra. Well hidden and tucked high up beneath her breasts, stuffed length-wise into a silk stocking, was an approximately three-foot-long iguana.

"I·can guarantee that they'll never check here."

OCTOBER

Cheryl Knows Best

Cheryl Goldman, our October student, couldn't have been more different from Randy than a cat is from a dog. Cheryl was older than most students, in her mid- to late thirties. She had worked as an assistant manager in a grocery store and lived at home with her family after finishing college. Tragically, one evening about six years earlier, she had been riding in the car with her parents on icy roads during a winter snowstorm when they were hit by an out-of-control driver. Both of her parents were killed and Cheryl was badly injured, the glass from the windshield essentially scalping her right at the hairline.

A few years and several surgeries later, the insurance premiums, including those from auto and the parents' life insurance companies, had paid out several hundred thousand dollars. On top of that, it turned out that the driver who ran into their car was intoxicated. When the lawyers were done, Cheryl walked away with over $1 million in cash. Not that any amount of money would bring someone's parents back, but after a long, difficult convalescent period, the payout did allow her to follow her dream of becoming a veterinarian.

Her undergraduate grades were nowhere near what they needed to be for her to matriculate in the university in the state where she lived, so she applied to a private institution, and because she could pay cash, she was accepted with her less than stellar GPA.

Like Randy, Cheryl was reticent, but the similarities ended there. Randy was initially shy but outgoing and friendly if approached, and he had a magnetic personality. Everybody loved him, and the staff was genuinely saddened when his time at NAVH ended.

Cheryl, on the other hand, was both quiet and introverted. When asked a question, she usually answered with a simple "yes" or "no," nothing further. You had to pry her open, but if you pried too hard, she would clam up, so getting her to participate in morning rounds was almost painful.

Having lived through a horrific automobile accident myself, I could understand that she was having personal issues. I have had them myself, ever since my crash, and I did not lose my parents. That must have been horrible to deal with. I made it my mission to go out of my way with Cheryl during her month with us. I would do everything I could to try to get inside her cone of sadness.

Perhaps the most unusual thing about Cheryl when she arrived for her externship was that hidden in her luggage she had brought along her pet corn snake. Shortly after her arrival she asked one of the technicians if we had a cage she could borrow. We had several, and she could take her choice. She looked them all over and, after choosing one, put her snake it in and took it up to her student apartment.

◆ ◆ ◆

Lisa handed me the chart for my first client of the day. The first page contained the client information details. "PACKAGE," scribbled in pencil, in all caps, was written in the last name field. "THE" was written in the first name field.

Package, or perhaps I should formally say, Mr. The Package, had the reputation of being the go-to man in the Heights and Shore areas—the happening places for the yuppie rich and playful. Whatever recreational substance you needed, Package could get it. He had slicked-back jet-black hair and white-framed, mirrored wraparound sunglasses, and he sported a thumbnail-sized silver soul patch that glistened under his mid lower lip. A large diamond accented his left earlobe, and adding the final touch was a small diamond imbedded into the front of his left upper incisor. He always wore a silver satin blazer over a colorful silk, unbuttoned shirt, and skintight black leather pants. The highly polished, black cowboy boots came complete with silver tips. Hanging around his neck over a hairless chest, on a gold rope chain, was an ostentatious pendant that read "The Package."

You would expect a drug dealer like Package to have an unconventional pet—at least a hefty python or boa constrictor draped over his shoulders. Package's companion, however, was a pure white guinea pig, aptly named Powder. Powder had eerie pink eyes, and it too wore a thin gold chain around its short guinea pig neck.

Package had brought Powder in for its annual exam. He loved his geep, as guinea pigs are called for short. Whenever I'd see him hanging out down by the shore or in a restaurant, he'd have Powder cuddled in his arm, stroking its fur.

Package always treated me with respect, calling me "Doc" whenever he saw me. When it came time to pay his bill, he'd ostentatiously pull out a roll of $100 bills and pay in cash. The staff and receptionists thought he was the coolest dude on the planet. I wasn't impressed by his flashy persona, but it was not my place to judge, and all that really mattered to me was that he loved his pet.

Today was a good visit. Package liked it when the students were in. He even allowed Cheryl to do a physical exam on the geep after I did mine. All smiles from everybody involved. Powder passed his annual with flying colors, which was great news for a three-year-old guinea pig approaching upper middle age.

I explained the rather short life span of geeps to Package, and you could see the immediate concern on his face as his white cheeks scrunched up under his shades. "You tryin' to tell me that Powder ain't gonna live much longer, Doc?" He hugged the little rodent. Its pink eyes bugged out with the squeeze.

"No," I said, looking at the man—not the drug dealer but the concerned pet owner. "What I'm saying is that pets grow older so much faster than we do." I reached over and stroked the furry snowball. "I think, rather than bringing him in for annual exams at this point in his life, consider him a senior citizen, and bring him in every three to six months for regular checkups. That's all." I smiled.

He looked down at his charge, nervously rubbing its fur front to back, then back to front, over and over.

"I just can't bear the thought of losing him." I think I actually heard his voice crack.

"Listen, Powder is looking good. I suspect that with your care he is going to be around quite a while."

"Thanks, Doc." He smiled and looked up at me. "You're the best." He held out his free hand for me to give a pump. We did a manly thumb grasp, and he pulled me up close and whispered in my ear.

"And, if I can hook you up, with anything, it's on me." He stepped back.

"Thanks, Package. I'll keep that in mind." I looked over at Cheryl. Her confused look made it obvious that either she did not hear or did not understand his offer.

◆ ◆ ◆

The next day was particularly busy, but I was able to make it home about 8:00. After feeding Wok, Sidney, and the fish, I inhaled some pasta and then packed for an upcoming conference where I was to be speaking over the weekend. Since it was within driving distance, I had promised both Fred and Gene that I would take them with me.

I think the long days had finally started to catch up with me, because I was feeling a scratchy throat and a bit of a runny nose. All night long I was either freezing or dripping with sweat. I don't remember actually sleeping, but when the alarm went off it was like an explosion in my head. In order for us to get to the conference hotel in time for the opening reception, we had to leave the hospital by 6:00 a.m. I was soaked with perspiration, so I hopped in the shower while Wok and Sidney took the opportunity to get in a few more winks. By the time I left my house, my throat was on fire and I could barely say goodbye to my furry kids.

Fred and Gene were waiting on the curb in front of NAVH with their bags when I arrived. We tossed their stuff in the back and headed out to the already congested 405 freeway, just in time to hit the height of the morning rush-hour traffic as we traveled north through Los Angeles. We finally pulled into the hotel in Monterey just before five o'clock.

• • •

Between being unable to breathe and finding it hard to swallow, with my throat on fire and shivering from the chills or sweating like a horse—not to mention worrying about my presentations—I did not get a whole lot of sleep.

My three hours of lecture were the first of the morning. I rolled out of bed, exhausted, took a hot shower, put on my business suit, and headed out to the conference center without breakfast. On the way I stopped at the sundry shop in the lobby of the hotel for a cold Diet Coke and throat lozenges. What a taste sensation that was.

For the next three hours I lectured on turtles and tortoises. I taught veterinarians how to do an exam, sedate them, take a blood sample, get an X-ray, and even do surgery. Because of my involvement with the Herpetological Society and, especially, the West Coast Turtle and Tortoise Club, I had probably seen more of these shelled creatures than anyone in the country.

There were only three other veterinarians in the state who had experience with exotic pets, and as it happened, one was speaking about birds right after me. When I finished fielding questions from the audience, the next speaker stepped up to the podium to prepare for his presentation.

"Good morning, Dr. Woakes." I held up my hand in a casual wave but did not offer to shake his. "I'm fighting a nasty cold, so I don't want to shake your hand and spread my crud." I tried a smile.

Dr. Woakes briefly looked up and nodded disingenuously. The fact was, Dr. Ridley Woakes hated me.

He was trained in England, then moved to Los Angeles in the '80s, where he established his veterinary practice. Dr. Woakes despised the fact that I had started my hospital just a short way down the 405 freeway from his facility.

"I'm sorry. I'd like to stay for your presentations, but I'm not feeling so well. I am going to head back to my room and get some sleep." I pulled out a handkerchief and quickly wiped away a drip from my nose. "I'm sure that they will be excellent."

"No worries." He stepped back, as if not only avoiding my contagion but me. "Feel better," he added, feigning concern, and then turned his back to end the conversation.

I grabbed my stuff off the podium and headed out of the lecture room. As was typical, I was mobbed by attendees, generally the participants who were too shy to ask a question in front of a crowd or had some convoluted question that would have taken hours to resolve.

I have always figured that if a conference hired me to speak, I owed it to the attendees to stay as long as necessary to make sure all of their questions got answered. After about twenty minutes I was done. I was sweating like a pig, my collar was dripping wet, and my throat felt like it was going to swell so tight I would not be able to breathe or swallow. I really wanted to head directly to my room and fall flat onto the bed. But what the heck; I decided to slip quietly into the back of the room and listen to Dr. Woakes lecture on avian exams.

As soon as I did, I was mortified at what I heard.

"With all due respect to Dr. Mader, he is young and inexperienced. I totally disagree with him that you need to sedate a tortoise to get a blood sample from the vein in the neck. When you do that, you risk causing damage to the vessels, resulting in a *huge* hematoma," he said, holding up his fist next to his jugular vein on the side of his neck for emphasis, "and, can, well, potentially kill the patient." He opened his hand and made a slashing motion across his throat.

"It is so much easier to just grab one of the toes and cut the nail back until it bleeds. Then, you can just let the blood drip, drip, drip into a little tube." He smiled. "Simple!" He held his hands up over his head, palms open, as if celebrating a victory.

I wanted to scream. Really? Cut the toenail back until it bleeds? How would he like it if he went to the doctor for a blood test and the nurse cut back his fingernail until it bled? How inhumane was that?

It's probably a good thing I had no voice left, or I might just have yelled out. But common sense won out, and instead I stood quietly in the back of the room and listened to the rest of his talk.

After his lecture was over I waited for the audience to clear, then walked up to the podium. He was gathering his material, so I stood quietly in front of him until he looked up. "I decided to stay for your lecture."

He blanched. I stared him down for what seemed like an eternity. I guess I was hoping for an apology, but I knew that would never happen.

"I thought you were sick" was his only response.

"I didn't learn anything new about exotics, but I learned a whole lot about you." I turned and walked out.

• • •

After the tête-à-tête with Dr. Woakes, I retreated to my room to get some rest, but I was so livid I couldn't unwind. I went back downstairs to the coffee shop for a hot chocolate and then took a short walk along the docks outside the hotel and enjoyed watching the shorebirds and California sea lions in the harbor. The wildlife settled my restless soul, and when I finally made it back to my room, I crashed for about two hours. I felt guilty missing the afternoon lectures, but I needed to sleep more than I needed to learn about dog diarrhea and cat barf.

I awoke the next morning feeling a little more alive. The plan was to attend the morning lectures, then leave at noon for the drive back to Southern California. After showering and grabbing another Diet Coke, I sat in on the first lecture of the morning, "Avian Endoscopy" by Dr. Michael Taylor, an exotics animal professor from the University of Guelph in Canada.

I had never met Dr. Taylor before, but I had read many of his publications. He was about the same age as Dr. Woakes, sophisticated with dark, neatly coiffed hair, a pleasant Canadian accent, and dressed in a black pinstriped suit.

"Good morning!" He beamed across the early Sunday morning room of still sleepy veterinarians. "Thank you for getting up so early to come hear me speak. And, please pardon my accent, eh! Before I start talking about avian surgery, I would just like to make a few comments regarding some things I heard at yesterday's lectures." The room was silent.

"I don't know Dr. Mader, but I thought his lectures on tortoise medicine were excellent. I have been teaching exotics at the veterinary school for fifteen years, and I'll tell you that trying to get a blood sample from a shy tortoise, one that is completely tucked into its shell, is nearly impossible, eh.

"From now on, I'm going to give my tortoise patients a little sedative as Dr. Mader recommends, prior to getting a blood sample. Once they are relaxed, it is so much easier on us veterinarians and, more importantly, on the patient. I think taking a scared little tortoise, yanking its leg out from inside its shell, and then deliberately cutting off a toenail, destroying normal, healthy tissue, vessels, nerves, and, possibly bone, just to get a blood sample, is inhumane, borderline malpractice, and, in *my* opinion, should never be done, eh?"

The entire room erupted in applause.

◆ ◆ ◆

Stacey, Maria, Cliff, Willy, and Greg were all sitting at the conference table when I arrived at work. Greg was never at morning rounds. Cheryl, our student, was nowhere to be seen.

They all stared at me silently as I entered the conference room. "What's up?" I set my stuff down on the round table. "Why are you all here so early? Why the dour looks?"

"Her snake ate Greg's finches," proclaimed Cliff, tapping his pen on the table for emphasis. His head was cocked to the side. Nobody else spoke.

"What?" I was waiting for the punch line.

"The student, *your* student. Her fuckin' snake ate Greg's finches!"

Greg kept two gouldian finches in a round, hanging cage in his upstairs apartment, next to the student apartment. They were a gift from a client who was moving and could no longer keep the little birds. The gorgeous, multicolored finches were worth over $400 each and highly prized by collectors. More importantly, Greg had really bonded with the songbirds.

"What happened?" I pulled out the chair and sat down.

Greg now took the initiative: "She came to me Friday night and said that the cage we gave her was too small. I looked around our storeroom and offered her a few other cages that we had, but none were good enough." He was visibly shaken. "The next thing I knew she said, 'Just forget it,' and stormed back to her room. She didn't talk much all Saturday morning, and after we finished seeing appointments she just slipped back upstairs without saying anything to anyone."

"The funny thing," Greg continued, "was that when I came on duty Saturday night, I noticed that the original snake cage that we gave her was back in the storage room, but a larger bird cage was gone. I figured that she had just switched the glass terrarium out for the larger cage.

"But when I got back to my room Sunday morning, after finishing my shift, I did not hear the finches singing like they usually do when I walk in the room," Greg sniffled. "I looked over at their cage and did not see them. When I got up close and looked inside, I found her snake coiled up in the bottom, with an obviously swollen stomach!" He started to cry.

I rubbed my hands over my face, pressing on my temples with both palms to try to control my blood pressure.

"I am so sorry, Greg." What else could I say? "I know it is not the same, but I'll take responsibility for your finches."

"That's not the point!" Willy spoke up, obviously also very upset.

"I know." I looked at Greg. "Please don't think I don't value your bond with the birds."

"That's okay." Greg wiped away a tear. "But what are we going to do about her?" He was referring to Cheryl. "She deliberately put the snake in an inappropriate cage—a *bird* cage!"

"Obviously, it just crawled out between the bars," Cliff deadpanned. "She's so fuckin' stupid."

"That's enough, Cliff." I don't appreciate that type of talk, no matter how upset he was. "I'm sure she didn't do it on purpose." I stood up, leaving my stuff at the table.

"Well, this is a fine 'Welcome back.'" I looked at Stacey, "Where is Cheryl now?"

"No clue. She never came down this morning."

"We kinda had words yesterday when I found her snake," Greg stated.

"It was more of a screaming match is what I heard," Stacey interjected.

"Okay. Let me go talk with her." God, all I wanted was to go home and start the day over—or go back to Monterey and watch the pelicans, gulls, and sea lions.

◆ ◆ ◆

It was a good thing that the next day was my normal half day. I had originally planned on working all day to get caught up, but after the previous day's events with the student, I was emotionally drained.

I spent a couple of hours talking to her about what had happened. In short, she felt that the snake cage the staff had given her was too small for her snake, so she switched it out for a larger birdcage. Even though the birdcage had bars instead of glass, she did not think that the snake could get out. Saturday afternoon after work she had noticed that the snake was missing. She spent the rest of the day looking for it but decided not to tell anybody because she figured she would find it in her room before anyone would know that it went missing. She said she had no idea that Greg had finches in his room next door, or she would have told him.

She offered to replace the finches. Money was not an issue. I explained to her that replacing someone's lost pet, although it might be a gesture of good faith, was not absolution, nor was it a very sensitive thing to do.

After finishing my morning appointments, I slipped out the back door and went home. Since it was the middle of the day, Ellen was fast asleep. Wok was surprised to see me, so I had him go get his leash while I grabbed a large beach towel, and we headed out.

We drove down the coast past Huntington Beach, the surfer's paradise made famous in the '60s by the Beach Boys, to a largely unpopulated area of wetlands that had been set aside by the state as a wildlife sanctuary. We got out of my SUV and took a long walk down the sandy beach, watching the birds dart about, diving into the water, snatching tiny feeder fish from the surface, and flying off while others cawed and screamed as they tried to steal their catch.

I felt bad for Greg, for the loss of his finches, and also for Cheryl. Clearly she had serious emotional issues far more complicated than I could help her with. I hoped she was getting professional counseling. This latest incident surely did not help matters.

I watched Wok watching the world around him. He looked so content. I often wondered what it would be like to be an animal. *Did they worry about the stuff that I had to deal with every day? What was their biggest concern? Did they think about tomorrow?*

I knew one thing: I loved him more than anything.

• • •

Cheryl did not show herself until one afternoon a few days later. She was not missed, as none of the staff wanted anything to do with her. I tried to keep her close to my side, taking her with me into exams, helping with X-rays and the like, so she would not have to interface with the others.

One thing that Cheryl had made perfectly clear when she originally sent me her application for the externship was that she loved reptiles, specifically turtles and tortoises. On her first day I promised her that she would get lots of opportunities to see both.

I felt that today would be a "turnaround" day for her. First off, wildlife Dave was bringing in a western pond turtle that had been found injured on the side of the road. But more importantly, the WCTTC was bringing in two desert tortoises for surgery, one with a large bladder stone and the second with an egg impaction. Two very cool surgeries: in fact, surgeries I had lectured on extensively just that past weekend.

Cheryl did seem excited about the day ahead. It was probably the first time I had seen her smile since she arrived at the beginning of the month, and certainly since the events of the weekend. I asked Fred to let Cheryl assist him in getting the tortoises prepped for surgery. He whined about it, but after reminding him about the fun, expensive weekend that we just had in Monterey, he reluctantly agreed.

Cheryl questioned *everything* that Fred did. Not in an inquisitive way, but more like she was challenging his actions. I could tell that his patience was wearing thin. Once the first tortoise was anesthetized and on the surgery table, I scrubbed in and had Cheryl also scrub in alongside me. I took the bone saw from the instrument stand and was about to make my first cut through the shell.

"Why are you cutting there?" Cheryl asked.

"This is where we make our bone flap. There's a very limited space to make the window into the inside so we can access the bladder and remove the stone."

"Yeah, but why there?" Her tone was more critical than inquisitive.

I explained the anatomy of the shell, the anatomy of the heart and pelvic bones underneath that you could not see, the entry point to the bladder, and more. It felt like I was repeating my lecture from last Saturday.

"Why don't you start your cut here?" She pointed to the small area between the back legs.

"I could." I looked up at her. "But since I'm right-handed and I stand on the right side of the patient, it's more ergonomic for me to make my first incision here." I pointed to the area just behind the left shoulder.

"You're supposed to start between the hips." With her gloved finger she pointed again to the shell area between the back legs. The smallest sterile gloves that we had in stock did not fit her tiny hands, leaving about a quarter inch of wrinkled latex at the end of each digit.

"Just watch." I clenched my teeth; I told myself that this was going to be a good day for her. "It's important that a surgeon be comfortable when he or she operates."

Once inside the tortoise's belly, I pointed out the baseball-sized, spiked bladder stone to Cheryl.

"Are you going to take the bladder out, or are you going to cut up the stone into little pieces inside the coelomic cavity?" she asked.

Reasonable question, but I wondered why she did not just observe and learn. I gently lifted the bladder, containing the large, hard stone, out of the belly and rested the calculus on some saline-moistened gauze. It looked like a Kiwano melon, a roundish, hard yellow fruit covered with pointy spikes.

"Why don't you use stay sutures?" Cheryl's questions were becoming more pointed—and distracting.

"If the stone is small, or if the tortoise has a deep shell, I will use a stay suture to help hold the bladder." I looked at her. "Cheryl, I need to focus, so would you please try to hold your questions until after I finish?"

"How do you expect me to learn if I don't ask questions?"

"Questions are fine, Cheryl. But maybe just observe for now, and we can go over the surgery in detail when we are finished. I promise to address all your questions." I looked for a sign of agreement in her eyes.

"Go on," she answered without making eye contact.

I finished the procedure in silence. I asked her to stay with Fred until the patient recovered, but she said that she had something to do and walked out of the surgery suite. Fred gave me a look and shrugged. About forty-five minutes later, Fred had the second tortoise anesthetized, prepped, and on the table. I asked where Cheryl was, and he said that she was outside with Dave working on the pond turtle and did not want to watch this one. I thought this odd, especially for someone who claimed to love turtles and tortoises, but in a way I was glad she decided not to participate.

When I finished the surgery, Lisa told me that Dave was waiting to talk with me in the conference room.

"Hi, Dave." I smiled. "You got some magic for me?"

"No, but I wish I could make someone disappear." Dave looked pained. I knew immediately what was going to come next.

"What did she do?"

"I'm not a doctor. I'm not a vet student. Heck"—Dave really seemed upset—"as she pointed out, I'm not even a technician!" He leaned back in his chair. "I'm just a loser ex-Nam grunt."

I did not like to hear him so upset. I sat down next to him. I also did not want to stand above him while he was talking.

"But *I do know wildlife*!" His voice cracked. "Is she some type of super brain or something? I'm not trying to make trouble. I know that I'm just a volunteer, and she's supposed to be the one here learning."

"What happened, Dave? Please tell me." I leaned forward.

Dave went on for the next twenty minutes about Cheryl's telling him what to do with the turtle, how to feed it, how to house it, how to treat it, and on and on. He told me that she criticized everything he did.

"I'll talk to her, Dave." I patted him on the shoulder as I stood. "I'm really sorry if she upset you."

"I feel bad for bringing this up. I only just want to help." His eyes were bloodshot, and he was squinting, and I could tell he was getting one of his migraines.

"You did nothing wrong, Dave. All of us appreciate what you do." I gestured toward the door. "Why don't you go home and get some rest. You look like you've got a headache coming on."

◆ ◆ ◆

By the next day, both of my tortoise patients were active and already eating. I was surprised, or maybe not, that Cheryl was not in the treatment room when I arrived. I expected to see her working on the animals she claimed were her favorites.

"Where's Cheryl?" Maria was cleaning one of the cages, and the only employee within earshot.

"Out back." She nodded her head toward the wildlife area. I could detect a barely perceptible eye roll.

"What's up?"

"She don't like you."

"Oh?" I put the bladder surgery tortoise back in its cage. "Care to elaborate?"

"Nutin' to elaborate," Maria said flatly and then went back to cleaning. She stuck her head and shoulders deep into the cage to avoid me.

I walked over to her and opened the cage door so I could lean in next to her. "Don't poke a bear and expect to walk away."

Maria stopped scrubbing and looked at me. "She said that you don't know what you're doing. That's why she didn't want to scrub in with you on the second surgery."

Ugh! I'd expect something like that from Dr. Woakes, but a student? It didn't seem appropriate for her to go around telling my staff that I didn't know my stuff.

"Did she happen to say why?"

"She said you were doing the surgery all wrong. Said there's no reason for her to watch you do surgery if there was nothin' she could learn." She backed out of the cage, making space between us. I could tell she wasn't comfortable tattling on the student, but then, I knew none of the employees liked Cheryl, and I suspected that in their own way they would be happy if she got in trouble, especially after what she had done to Greg's finches.

I thanked Maria for her candor and went to morning rounds. Cheryl was not at the table when I sat down, so I asked Stacey to go outside and get her.

"Do I have to?"

I said nothing, just gave her one of my looks. She grunted, spun around, and left the room.

Human drama aside, all of the patients were doing well. When we were finished with the medical discussions, Willy told us we had received a huge rebate check in the mail from workers' comp insurance, and Lisa announced that we had just hired a new receptionist to help out up front, a young Jamaican girl fluent in English, Spanish, and Jamaican patois.

"I needed to help her finish with the turtle." Stacey flicked her head toward Cheryl as the two reentered the room several minutes later.

"We're all finished here. But"—everybody started to stand but then froze—"Cheryl, can I talk to you for a moment? Please have a seat." She looked at me with an expression somewhere between annoyance and apprehension. Everybody else got up and immediately exited the room.

"So what did you think about the tortoise surgery yesterday?" I tried to look her in the eyes. She was looking down at the table.

"It was okay."

"Just okay? I thought you'd really like being part of that procedure." I kept up my one-way eye contact. "In fact, I was surprised that you didn't participate in the egg binding surgery."

"I needed to help Dave with the pond turtle." Finally, she looked up, met my eyes, then instantly looked back down at the pen she was twiddling between her fingers.

"Come on, Cheryl. You can work on pond turtles anywhere. According to your résumé, you do it all the time back home. How often do you get an opportunity to remove eggs from a tortoise?"

"I got to watch the first one." She spoke to the table.

"Those two surgeries are as different as night and day." I reached over toward her and gently tapped the table. "Please look at me."

"What?" She looked up with her eyes only, not lifting her head. I could see the long scar across her brow that went from her right temple to the top of her left ear. God, I could only hope that she had been unconscious when that happened.

"It's been a rough couple of weeks' start for you. I was really hoping that you would find your happy place with all the turtle work we do." She lifted her head a little. I smiled. "How many of these tortoise surgeries have you done?"

"None."

"Have you seen many of these performed?" I had seen her résumé. Nowhere did it show that she ever worked for anyone who did these specialty procedures.

"No."

I took a deep breath. "Okay, Cheryl. Then I have to ask you why you told Maria that I did not know what I was doing." It was direct, but it needed to be said if she was going to finish out her externship. I could not have a student being disrespectful.

"Because you were doing it wrong!" Her voice took on an aggressive edge, and she looked at me directly for the first time.

"So if you've never done one of these surgeries, never seen one of these surgeries, what makes you the expert? How can you judge my techniques? What makes you think I was doing it wrong?" I was exasperated. "Did you not see how well both tortoises were doing this morning?"

"No."

"Why didn't you check on the patients?"

"I was outside with the pond turtle."

"You didn't answer my question. What makes you such an expert that you can tell my staff I am doing everything wrong? I've done over three hundred of these procedures."

"Because that's not how I read it was done!" She actually slammed her fist down on the table, pen in hand.

I had to admit, I did not expect that answer.

"I was so excited about coming here that I read up on everything that's been published on tortoise surgery." She started to cry. "You did it all wrong. I just couldn't watch anymore."

"Cheryl, the article you're referring to was written over twenty years ago." I kept my tone calm, though I wanted to explode. "Dr. Frye, the one who wrote the article—"

"I *know* Dr. Frye wrote it!" she interrupted.

"Dr. Frye was my professor," I said calmly. "During my time in school and as a resident, I did several dozen of these surgeries with him. He's retired now, and the techniques and procedures have changed many times since that article was published.

"Part of the reason students do externships is so that they can experience how other experts and facilities do procedures. There are a lot of ways to skin a cat, so to speak."

The silence seemed to last an eternity.

"May I go, please?" She wiped away the tears from her eyes.

I wanted to talk to her as well about the way she had treated Dave, but I felt she'd had enough for one morning. "Okay, but I expect you to participate in the care of the hospitalized patients. I don't want you spending all of your time with the wildlife. We do the wildlife for free as a community service. The paying patients keep the lights on."

• • •

Greg left a note that he had not seen or heard Cheryl all weekend, but he knew that she was in her room because he saw the lights go on and off a few times.

She showed up for morning rounds and sat quietly while we all reviewed the hospitalized cases and the weekend's emergencies. As soon as we finished, she slipped out the back door without saying a word.

Lisa stopped me after rounds and said that Dave's wife had called and told her that he was still incapacitated with one of his migraines. I felt bad for him. His Vietnam injuries were tremendous and he hid them well, but nobody can run from a migraine.

My first client of the day was an unusual emergency walk-in, and I was looking forward to hearing what had actually happened. I looked around for Cheryl to see if she wanted to participate, but she was nowhere to be found.

The story: a woman was starting up her dishwasher after her kids left for school when she heard a funny sound coming from inside. At first she figured it was just a dish rattling around, but it dawned on her that it sounded less like glass touching glass and more like a frantic "knocking at the door." Stumped, she stopped the machine and opened the door. Steam flowed out from around the edges of the front panel as it cracked open and a ferret immediately jumped out the top and scrambled out of the room.

Her children's ferret had free roam of the house. Apparently it had hopped into the dishwasher while the door was open while she had turned away. The ferret likely was hiding in the back of the lower tray to "pre-clean" the dishes, and she did not see it when she closed the door. Fortunately, the ferret had been in the running machine for no more than a minute and was going to be just fine.

Ferrets as pets are illegal in the state of California. Private citizens are forbidden to own them. If you get caught with a ferret, you can be fined, and in almost all cases, the California Department of Fish and Game (the CDFG, which would later become the California Department of Fish and Wildlife) would confiscate the ferret and give the owner one of two options: you could have it euthanized, or you could pay a fee for a bonded courier to take the animal across state lines to a third party who would take responsibility for the animal, and sign a statement that you'd never bring it back to California or the animal would be euthanized and you'd face felony charges.

I had heard horror stories of officers going to people's homes, confiscating ferrets, and euthanizing them in front of the owners. I never verified these accounts, but there was not a ferret owner in California who had not heard them. As a result, ferret owners rarely brought their pets to veterinarians for fear that they would be turned in to the authorities. Fortunately, unlike human doctors, who are required to report things like child neglect or gunshot and stab wounds, veterinarians are not required to play police.

When veterinarians graduate from veterinary school we have to take an oath. Part of it reads, "*Being admitted to the profession of veterinary medicine, I solemnly swear to use my scientific knowledge and skills for the benefit of society through the protection of animal health and welfare, the prevention and relief of animal suffering . . .*" Because of this, veterinarians are allowed to administer care to a sick or injured ferret, even though ferrets are illegal in the state.

That's the key point: the ferret has to be sick or injured. Veterinarians are not allowed to perform preventive medicine such as vaccines or spays and neuters. It's splitting hairs, but we checked with our attorney, and in our yellow page advertisement we clearly state, "We Treat Ferrets." As a result, we had a significant number of ferret-owning clients.

After finishing with the superclean ferret, I asked around if anyone had seen Cheryl and was told that because Dave had called in sick, she was outside cleaning cages and treating the wildlife cases. She clearly preferred to work alone, so I let her be.

◆ ◆ ◆

I awoke feeling great. The fall weather had started to turn, and the air had a crispness to it that made you feel fresh when you walked outside. The morning fog had not been around for several weeks, and it seemed like the perfect day to ride my bicycle to work.

No sooner had I arrived when I was met by a very distraught Lisa. "Dave needs to talk to you. He's in the conference room."

Dave had been out sick for the past several days, and my first thought was that he was having serious medical problems with his head injuries. I passed both Stacey and Fred milling about in the treatment room, but they avoided eye contact when I walked by.

Dave was sitting alone, blankly staring at an envelope on the table, his hands in his lap when I entered.

"What's up, Dave? You feeling okay?"

"I need to turn in my resignation." He looked up, sliding the envelope across the table. "I'm really sorry I've let you down."

His statement stopped me cold in my tracks.

"What are you talking about?" I left the envelope on the table. "You've *never* let me down." I could tell he had been crying.

"It's all in there." He pointed to the white letter. "I need to go." He stood up.

I reached out and gently took his hand. "Please stay for a minute while I read this."

"I'd rather not. I feel I've taken too much of your time as it is." He pulled his arm away. "I need to leave before everybody else gets here."

"Dave, please do me a favor." I reached for his hand again. "As a friend,

I ask that you at least go upstairs to my office and wait for me to read this. As soon as rounds are over, we can talk about it."

"I don't think there's anything to talk about." He was in full tear mode now.

"Please, Dave. Give me a few minutes to process what is happening, and then we can talk." I let go of his hand. "Please, wait for me upstairs.

Dave nodded, turned, and headed out of the room.

As soon as he left, Stacey and Fred came in. I looked at them and they shrugged but said nothing. Morning rounds were hurried, and words were not wasted. Cheryl was there and once again asked if she could go take care of the wildlife as soon as we finished. The minute she left the room I got this terrible feeling.

I excused myself from the group and went immediately to the bathroom where I could get some privacy while I read Dave's letter. It was short and to the point.

Dear Dr. Mader and Staff,

I want to thank you all for allowing me to work with such a fine group of professionals. You have given me many wonderful opportunities to learn and have also opened your hearts and friendship to both my wife and me. I am so sorry that I have not lived up to your high expectations, but I do understand. Please accept my resignation.

May God bless you all.
Dave

Oh man. My head started spinning. We all knew that Dave lived with serious war injuries, and there had been times in the past when he had missed days due to medical problems. But he was a volunteer, and his work with us had never been expected, only appreciated. Any help he had given us had been a blessing. We all loved him.

I reread the letter several times. Each time, I started to get a clearer picture of what was happening, and I began to seethe. I took a minute to center myself, then went upstairs to my office. Dave was sitting at my desk, bent over, face buried in his hands.

I pulled Willy's desk chair next to Dave, and when he looked up, I handed him back the letter. "I can't accept this."

He was crying. He pushed the letter back toward me.

"I won't accept this," I said, tossing the envelope into the trash. "You are as much a part of the team as any paid employee. Your contributions are more valuable than I can put in words." I gently touched his hand, adding, "You know that I would pay you, but you won't let me."

"Yeah, Dr. Mader, but I've let you down." He was still crying, his eyes bloodshot from a combination of tears and migraine.

"Tell me why you think that." I was pretty sure I knew what he was going to say.

"Because I can't be depended on." He looked up at me. His moustache was wet with tears. "I'm not doing my job, and the wildlife is suffering."

"What did that student say to you?" I asked, taking a leap.

"She said that if I couldn't do my job and she had to keep covering for me, then there really was no need for me to come in anymore."

"When did she tell you this?"

"I called this morning and talked to Stacey to tell her I was not able to make it in. I was up vomiting all night and am so dizzy from the headache that I really shouldn't be driving." Dave pulled out a fancy red scarf from his back pocket and blew his nose. "The student got on the phone and told me not to bother anymore, that I was so irresponsible that she would take over."

Immediately my mind went into overdrive. I felt like my head was going to explode. Who the hell did she think she was, coming into my house and mistreating one of my employees? Especially when she had been no angel herself? My first thought was to storm downstairs, grab her by the scruff of the neck, shake her, and boot her ass out the door.

I've had to deal with a lot of really bad, mean people over the years. I learned years ago that losing your temper is not a productive way to handle situations. I realized that the most important action to take at that moment was to reassure Dave that he had done nothing wrong and that there was no way I was going to let him quit. I took a deep breath and sat back in the chair.

"Dave, you are one of my dearest friends in the world," I said. "I have no reason to mislead you. You are a huge asset to us, and you've given us much more than we've ever been able to give back. I ask you—no, I beg you—please reconsider your letter and stay on with us. The problem isn't yours, it's mine for not controlling the student." I continued. "She had no business talking to you the way she did. She has no say in how we operate our hospital. She was totally out of line." I leaned forward, adding, "And I will deal with her."

Dave looked up. "But she's right! I haven't been here for the past five days. The wildlife has not been getting taken care of!"

"Come on, Dave. Of course it has. We have paid staff that takes care of them when you're not here. They never suffer. Anything you give us is a blessing for us and the patients."

"I just don't know." He covered his face with his palms again. I sat back looking at this broken man. His life on a veteran's salary was nothing to boast about. He drove a twenty-year-old pickup truck, his wife worked as a day care provider, and he lived in chronic pain. His only passion was taking care of wildlife, and now he felt like a failure at that.

"Dave, I'll have Stacey give you a ride home so you can get some rest and take care of your headache. I'll come get you to pick up your truck when you're feeling better. Come back whenever you're ready." I kneeled down next to him. "I promise you that you won't have any more problems."

• • •

After Dave left, I took some time to digest what had transpired. I talked with Stacey and Fred. I also discussed what had happened with Willy. Fortunately, it was not that busy, so I asked Cliff to take my cases, which he willingly did. Finally, after getting all the facts, I brought Cheryl up to my office to get her side of the story.

Although she did admit to talking with Dave on the phone the day before, she said that all she told him was that she was really sorry he wasn't feeling well, that she knew what it was like to have chronic pain, and she was happy to help out with the wildlife, and for him to get better. She said that she had never told him he was unreliable or that he did not need to come back.

When I questioned Stacey again, she confirmed that she had been standing next to Cheryl while she was talking to Dave, and Cheryl had in fact told Dave that he was not dependable and that he should just quit if he could not be counted on.

More than fifty students had externed with me since I started Noah's Ark. I've had the occasional problems with students confusing medications, forgetting to write something in the record, or occasionally saying something that was misinterpreted by a client—all stuff you can expect from someone young in their career and still in the learning stages. Although sometimes frustrating and potentially awkward for the hospital, these offenses were all forgivable. To come into my workplace and abuse one of my staff members, however, was just inexcusable. After speaking with Cheryl, I called the dean of her veterinary school. He was in a meeting, and I left a message that it was urgent he call me back that day. Her school was on the East Coast, so it was three hours ahead of California time.

I stayed up late to discuss the situation with Matt Leonard, our attorney. Since Cheryl was not an employee, he said, I couldn't actually fire her, but I could certainly ask her to leave. I asked him whether we had any liability—could I be sued?

"Of course! This is California," he laughed.

I did not think it was funny.

"Seriously," he continued, "if she spent money to come spend time with you, if she had to hire a house sitter, pay for plane tickets, spend extra money for meals while here, and especially if it would affect her standing in school if she got asked to leave the externship early, she could sue you for costs and any related damages."

Great. Just what I wanted to hear.

Regardless, I had to make her leave. I could not let one person disrupt my house and staff, my family. To the best of my recollection, I transcribed all the details from the past few days into a narrative that I might have to use in court in the eventuality she decided to sue me somewhere down the road.

I finished my essay around 2:00 a.m. Wok was coiled up just behind me on the carpet, and Sidney was fast asleep on top of my neurology book next to my computer, enjoying the warm air blown out by the fan in the back.

When I got in to work the next morning, there was a message in my inbox from Greg to call the vet school dean right away. I excused myself from morning rounds and went up to the privacy of my office. Before I picked up the phone I looked out my window. The day was clear, and I could see the beautiful San Bernardino mountains off in the distance, a stark contrast to the graffiti-scarred walls on the windows and storefronts across the street. I knew what I had to do, despite the warning from Matt. I dialed the number, and to my surprise, the dean himself answered the phone. It must have been his private number.

After introducing myself, I described in detail what had transpired since Cheryl had joined us for the externship. I included the details about the finches, her reluctance to participate in daily treatments of hospitalized patients with the exception of the wildlife cases, her reluctance to go with me for my consultations at the research facility, and finally, the incident with Dave.

As soon as I finished my summary the dean's first words were "You need to excuse her."

"Excuse her?" I was confused by the possible ambiguity of his statement. "You mean forgive her?"

"*No!*" The dean's tone was adamant. "Excuse her, as in send her ass back here. Let us deal with this. This is a disciplinary situation." I could hear the frustration in his voice. "As the dean of this university, I don't want a student like Cheryl representing us to off-campus educators like yourself, and especially to the pet-owning public."

"Okay." I was relieved that he was supportive. "I have never had to excuse a student before. Is there anything special, meaning are there any legal issues, that I need to address before I tell her she has to leave?"

"No, Dr. Mader." The dean sounded like he was experienced with situations like this. "I will support your decision 100 percent. Just document everything that happened with specific details and timelines, including this phone conversation."

"I've already contacted our company attorney, and I have done that," I told him.

"Great. To make it easier on yourself, tell Cheryl that we spoke and I told you to terminate her externship." There was a slight pause. "Do it today."

I thanked him for taking my call and apologized that we had to meet on the phone over a situation like this. We exchanged pleasantries, and he finished by telling me to contact him anytime; if she did take legal action, they would get the university attorney involved.

I had Lisa call the airlines to check on flights back east and also contact the airport shuttle to come pick her up. Once everything was arranged, I met with Cheryl in my office, with Willy as witness, and told her she needed to leave. She immediately broke down into tears, sobbing uncontrollably, rambling on about her automobile accident, her mental state, and more. She promised to make things right if we let her stay. Please, could we give her a second chance?

Just yesterday I had watched Dave in the same chair, sobbing, ready to quit because of the way Cheryl had treated him. As much as I always want to give someone a chance, an opportunity to make amends, the writing on the wall was clear. The dean himself had spoken. And, more importantly, I had to honor my promise to Dave.

• • •

My first case of the morning was too cute to be legal. Dodo, a ten-week-old emu chick, came in with his owner, Mrs. Chissler, and her nine-year-old daughter, Jenny. Dodo, the young girl explained, got his name from the prehistoric flightless dinosaur.

Emus are the second largest bird in the world, only the ostrich being larger. Adult emus are mostly a dirty-brown color with a lighter neck skin, bluish-black face, bright red eyes, and long, powerful legs. In contrast, emu chicks look like little raindrops with tiny heads and disproportionately short legs. They have horizontal brown and white stripes that run from their neck to the tip of the tailless butt, and a brown-and-white speckled head with brown eyes.

If the diet is poor, as is often the case in captivity, the long legs on these giant birds don't grow correctly. Eventually, the legs splay out so badly that they cannot support their own body weight, the bird can no longer stand, and it will die. That was the case with Dodo: one of his legs was growing almost completely out to the side, and he could not stand or walk.

I explained the importance of diet to the owners and told them that the best way to handle this would be to put a comfortable hobble on the chick, essentially placing a strap around the legs from the "ankle" down to the foot, and confining it to a small, narrow crate while it was maturing through its rapid growth phase. The combination of the hobble with the narrow growth box would not only prevent the legs from splaying out any further but would force the lower legs to start growing back inward, underneath the bird, as it got older.

It seemed drastic to keep the bird locked in a box, but it really wasn't that bad, and it would not be forever. In fact, I told them that they could take Dodo out of the growth box for a few minutes a few times a day to play and stretch, but for the most part they needed to keep him confined.

I could tell that Mrs. Chissler and Jenny did not like this idea. When I was finished with my long explanation and detailed expectations, Mrs. Chissler asked me about a surgery that she had heard about, one where the leg bones could be cut, straightened, and then allowed to grow normally once healed.

I told the pair that I was very familiar with the procedure, called an osteotomy, and that I had done several, but that they were usually reserved for older birds that had passed their normal growth phase and had no other options. When the procedure was done in young growing birds that still had relatively soft bones, the complication rate was high, and there was a risk of death if things went badly. I assured them that although my plan using the growth box seemed cumbersome, it would in fact work. Redirecting the growth of the long leg bones was like putting a child in braces to straighten their teeth. It would work, but it would take time and patience.

"Okay," Mrs. Chissler said, not looking me in the eye. "I'll give it a try."

We made a recheck appointment for two weeks down the road. I promised the concerned mother and daughter that Dodo would be running around like a normal emu chick within a few months.

"Please trust me and be patient. He *is* going to get better," I assured them as they took the chick out to their car. Unfortunately, I had a feeling that nothing I said was going to be followed.

• • •

"Where's your student?" Dr. Kristin Sullivan asked as I greeted her in the parking lot just outside of the Los Angeles Herpetology Society meeting. Tonight was our big tag-team lecture to the reptile group on the dangers of salmonella, the topic that had come up after last month's meeting and the big bake sale.

I looked at her, puffed my face, rolled my eyes, let out a huff, and responded, "Don't ask."

"That bad?" She smiled.

"Now's not the time to get me started." I reached out and gave her a big hug. "Thanks for doing this."

"My pleasure!" Kristin had such a wonderful personality. I really enjoyed her company. We walked into the building and were immediately mobbed by society members. Kristin had never been to one of these meetings before, and I had neglected to warn her about the frenzy.

"Hey, Doc! Is this your student?" Bean was the first to greet us, motioning toward Kristin. Lizzie was hanging on his neck in her usual repose.

"Oh my!" Kristin said, putting her open palm over her heart when she noticed the big saurian.

"Don't worry, she's a sweetie!" said Bean as he turned his shoulders to position Lizzie's face directly in front of Kristin, its long, purple, snake-like tongue flicking the air.

"Your students are getting older!" Bean grinned.

"Bean! That's not polite!" I interjected as Kristin laughed. "And *no*, this isn't my student. This is Dr. Kristin Sullivan, our guest speaker." She held out her hand to shake Bean's, but instead he bowed, took her hand, and gave it a kiss. "An honor to meet you, Doctor," he said, standing straight. "Wow, a real doctor!"

Kristin looked at me and smiled. I just shook my head.

After all the normal pre-guest lecture business, Herb Paul—an icon of the herpetology world in Southern California, the owner of Herb's Herps and Pets (making him Bean's boss), and the current president of the LAHS—introduced us to the group. It was the largest crowd I had seen at a meeting since I joined three years prior.

I was the first to present and gave a brief history of the salmonella disease in reptiles. I talked about how it is spread, how it is managed, and how serious the nasty bacterium is.

Then the real star of the show, Kristin, took the stage and talked about how people catch the disease and what it can do to them. She kept her explanations simple and to the point. She was direct, not trying to scare anyone, but made a point to emphasize how important it was to prevent contamination—like mixing food and handling reptiles at the same time.

We talked for about thirty minutes, then opened the floor to questions.

"I have a question for the doctor." A frantic hand went up in the back.

"Which *doctor* would that be?" I asked, feigning hurt.

"Oh," the young girl said as she covered her mouth with her hand, "I meant the people doctor!" Everybody laughed.

The Q and A lasted for another several minutes. Most of the questions were for Kristin. I just stood back, watched, and listened. It was fun observing her be the center of attention—almost like a rock star surrounded by groupies.

◆ ◆ ◆

As a thank-you for her efforts, I took Kristin out for sushi after we finished. We enjoyed some great food, excellent company, and a couple of sakes until I was feeling guilty and knew I needed to get home and feed Wok, Sidney, and the fish.

As I was driving back home I had to pass through some not-so-nice parts of town. About two miles from my turn-off, traffic came to a standstill. I could see up ahead multiple emergency vehicles near the intersection.

Eventually the mass of autos slowly inched forward. At least a dozen emergency vehicles—police cars, two ambulances, a fire truck, and a van with large black-on-white block letters with "Coroner" emblazoned on the side—surrounded a McDonald's. A police helicopter was circling overhead, its spotlight flooding the parking lot, randomly drifting over nearby houses, illuminating yards and side streets. The myriad of flashing red, white, and blue lights made for a surreal scene.

As I got closer and finally passed by, I noticed what looked like two bodies covered by yellow plastic sheets lying on the ground next to a car in the drive-through lane.

I made it home just minutes after passing by the drama. As I always did when I walked in the front door, I gave each of my "kids" a big hug. I wondered if the bodies back at the McDonald's had pets still waiting for them at home.

•••

The next day, I entered through the back wildlife door and made my typical rounds, wishing everyone a good morning, calling each employee by name. When I got to the reception area, Lisa was there but wearing a long face and making some notes in a manila file. "I think we are going to have to let Bianca go."

Bianca was the new Jamaican receptionist that we had just hired two weeks before. She had turned out to be a fantastic worker: beautiful, pleasant, trilingual, always punctual, and self-motivated. She was also a great problem solver.

"What's the problem? I thought she was doing a great job."

"She *was,* when she actually showed up for work." Lisa was clearly frustrated. "I've had to cover for her for the last three days. She has not been in since last Thursday."

"Have you heard from her? Did she call in sick?"

"Not a word." She looked at me. I could tell she was really frustrated. "I've called and left several messages on her phone."

This wouldn't be the first time that an employee decided to quit and not tell us. It never seemed to bother them when they did, but many were surprised when potential future employers called and they didn't get a stellar reference.

Meanwhile, our November student, Morten Dennis, arrived two days early. He had called and said that he was in town visiting relatives and asked if he could come by before he started to tour the hospital and meet the staff. I let him know that the current student had to leave unexpectedly and that if he wanted to get a couple of extra days with us, the apartment was open. He jumped at the opportunity.

My initial impression was threefold. First, he was polite and proper. Second, he was a bodybuilder and had the physique of an Adonis, something not missed by the female staff. Finally, I suspected he came from money. Not only was he wearing a shiny Rolex, but he had driven out to California from the East Coast in his new BMW, a gift from his parents for getting into veterinary school.

• • •

I've always loved Halloween. Willy and I encourage the staff to dress up. At the end of the day, we get together and decide which employee had the best costume, giving the winner a $100 gift certificate to one of the nicer restaurants in the shore. As a result, we get some pretty creative characters, and each year the competition gets stiffer.

As usual, I had arrived early that morning. I wanted to see all the costumes when they came in the door. Student Mort joined right in with the team and was dressed up as a hillbilly, wearing overalls, no shirt, a red scarf, and a tattered, stained floppy hat. He was even sucking on a piece of straw. The shirtless outfit readily exposed his physique, highlighting each muscle as he moved his arms or flexed his broad chest.

Fred was dressed as a pimp; Maria, who had just found out she was in the maternal way, a very pregnant woman; Lisa, a witch; Stacey, a very sexy French maid; Robert, a vampire (what else?); Leanne, a hooker; and Peter was Elvis.

I was hanging out in the doorway to the treatment room surveying my costumed "family" when Lisa came up behind me, placed her hand on my shoulder, and whispered in my ear.

"Dr. Mader, can I talk to you for a moment?"

I turned, smiling at the scene and her costume, feeling great, then abruptly startled as I noticed her expression. "Of course, what's up?"

"It's Bianca," she said, motioning for me to follow her. We went into the conference room to talk in private. "She just called." Lisa wore an expression of total shock.

"I know now why she hasn't been at work. She couldn't tell me where she was. But she wanted to call to apologize."

"Go on."

"Last Thursday night she was out with friends. They were at a McDonald's, in the drive-through lane, when out of nowhere they were surrounded by a gang.

"She was in the back seat with her boyfriend. Her friend driving the car tried to back out, but there was a car behind them, essentially boxing them in. Suddenly two of the gang members pulled out guns and opened fire into her car, killing both front passengers, and wounding her boyfriend."

"Oh my God!" I immediately flashed back to the drive home last Thursday night after the herpetological meeting. It had to have been Bianca in that massacre at the McDonald's not far from my house. "Was she hurt?"

"She was cut by flying glass but not hit by any bullets." Lisa's eyes welled up. "Her boyfriend was in surgery all night, but they say he is going to make it."

"My God" was all I could mutter once again. I looked down at the floor while I was trying to come up with something more appropriate to say. "Is she going to come back to work?" I knew that was stupid as soon as it came out of my mouth.

"No. In fact, as I said, she couldn't even tell me where she was calling from. The police told her she needed to leave town for her own safety." Lisa's eyes were dilated from fear, and she trembled as she spoke.

My God. I reached out and gave Lisa a hug, holding tight, not letting go. She put her head on my shoulders.

"Mornin', everyone!" Cliff walked into the conference room, also dressed as a hillbilly. "Uh-oh—am I interrupting something?" He was laughing.

"No." I released my hug. Lisa wiped away a tear, turned, and walked out without saying anything.

Although I was distracted by Lisa's report, morning rounds brightened my mood. The best part was seeing the two hillbillies Mort and Cliff sitting side by side. Apparently they had planned it. The contrast between Mort's Arnold Schwarzenegger physique and Cliff's Pillsbury Doughboy body was like night and day.

The occasional client came in dressed for Halloween, and more than one pet arrived incognito. My favorite was Checkers the squirrel dressed up in a camouflaged uniform as Rambo, complete with a plastic rifle strapped to his back.

I was upstairs in my office eating lunch when Lisa paged up that I needed to get downstairs right away. I dropped my sandwich and headed down to find Stacey holding a large, whimpering dog, her French maid outfit covered with blood.

"I was coming back to work and I saw this dog run across the road and get hit by a car!" She was holding a bloody towel over the side of the struggling dog's face. It had a long cut down the left flank, road rash from the shoulder to the hip, and its left rear leg was dangling at an odd, ninety-degree angle from the shinbone.

"Was there an owner?" I reached down to examine the dog, and it violently snapped at my hand, screaming in pain as it did.

"Careful!" Stacey pulled the dog back, struggling to hold it down.

"Get me some morphine!" I commanded to no one in particular. The pimp handed me a muzzle, and I cautiously slipped it on the dog, trying to avoid the laceration over its left eye. I noticed that the entire sclera, the white part, was completely filled with blood.

Hillbilly Mort handed me a syringe and, assuming that it was the morphine I had asked for, I quickly administered it into the dog's shoulder muscle while the French maid held her grip on the frightened animal. The dog was so amped with adrenaline that it took longer than usual for the drug to take effect, but finally the terrified animal started to relax. The hillbilly and French maid lifted the large black Labrador onto the treatment table, and I carefully removed the muzzle. Once it relaxed, maid Stacey was able to remove the towel covering the side of the face. Hidden under all the clotted blood was a collar with a well-worn tag.

I was not able to read the name etched on the tag because of all the blood, so I removed the collar and handed it to the pregnant Maria. She immediately took it to the sink to wash it off, eventually uncovering both a pet and owner name as well as a phone number. Lisa the witch took the info and tried to call an E. Azarov, but the number was out of service.

"What should we do?" Stacey the maid asked. The dog was resting comfortably after the morphine shot. Fred the pimp and Mort the hillbilly had packed all the open wounds with sterile gauze to stop the bleeding. Most of these wounds would need to be sutured closed, but I could not legally take the dog to surgery without the owner's permission. For now, I planned on just continuing with pain control so he would not suffer, supportive care, hemorrhage control, and efforts to find the owner. Hillbilly Mort pulled up a stool next to the treatment table from which to monitor the dog.

I was impressed at how Mort had jumped right in with the team. Clearly he had some previous clinical experience. The other characters went back to their normal duties, and things seemed to be under control, at least for the moment. Suddenly the front lobby erupted in screams from both Mai Tai, a sulfur-breasted toucan that was our clinic mascot, and what sounded like a wounded person. We all looked at each other with alarm, and then I ran toward the front. Before I could round the corner, a large woman filled the doorway, screaming and yelling, as Lisa the witch tried to restrain her by holding on to her arm.

"I tried to stop her, Dr. Mader!"

"Let the fuck go of me, you stupid bitch. I want my dog!" the hulking woman snarled, yanking her arm free.

"It's okay, Lisa." I stood in the middle of the hall blocking the woman's passage, hands in front of me. The woman was built like a professional linebacker and was wearing soiled, tawny slacks, wet around the crotch, and a sleeveless, braless black vest, buttoned halfway up the front. She was shoeless and reeked of alcohol. As she moved, her large breasts peaked out from the sides and front of her filthy garment, especially when she bent over.

"I'm Dr. Mader. Your dog is going to be fine." I wanted to start with something positive. "We have him sedated and—"

"I don't give a fuck who you are," she interrupted. She then grabbed my arms and threw me full force against the hallway wall. My elbow smashed against a framed picture, shattering the glass front. "I just want my goddamn dog!"

She charged toward Mort, who was sitting with the injured, sedated Labrador. When she got to the bloodied dog she burst out in tears, bending over the table, hugging it, and crying uncontrollably. At least for the moment, there was no imminent danger of her hurting anyone.

I turned to Stacey, whose sexy French maid costume was covered with dog's blood, but before I could say anything she mouthed, "I called 911."

I glanced around the room at all the Halloween characters looking on from behind tables and peeking around corners. The pirate and the Pillsbury hillbilly had disappeared. Hillbilly Mort was still sitting near the table with the dog, having pushed his stool back a couple of feet to get out of reach of the owner.

"Go!" I whispered, motioning the staff to give us space. Hillbilly Mort looked at me inquiringly, tacitly asking if I wanted him to stay. Odd—here was this brand-new student, thrust into this somewhat violent, dramatic scene, and he was the only one willing to have my back. I looked at him and nodded.

I walked over to the woman slowly, approaching her directly so she didn't think I was sneaking up on her, and said quietly, "Viktor"—the dog's name on its tag—"is injured, but we have him stabilized right now. He's on morphine to keep him calm and help with his pain."

"I don't give a fuck," she snarled, her alcoholic breath toxic at such close range. "I just want to take my Viktor and go home." She looked up. Blood was smeared on her face, in her greasy hair, on her vest, and down her arms.

"Ms. Azarov," I said, taking a guess that was her name, since it was on the dog tag, "Viktor needs more vet care. He's in no shape to go home right now." I reached out to pat her shoulder, but just before touching I thought better of it.

"I just want to take him home." She buried her face back into her critically injured pet, crying.

"Viktor really needs some serious medical care. I can tend to his injuries for you if you give me permission." I took a chance and bent over, closer to her so she could hear me through the sobs.

Still no response. Mort the hillbilly stood up and pushed his stool over to Ms. Azarov. "Here you go, ma'am." She looked up, so bloody now that she looked like she'd been beaten. She nodded and took the stool, still hugging her dog.

Just as she sat down, I looked up to see a policewoman enter the treatment room. She looked at me and motioned me over. The officer had no partner but was just as large as Ms. Azarov—at least six feet tall and a couple of hundred pounds. She had on a bulletproof vest, and her hair was pulled back in a tight bun, giving her something like the mean face of a sumo wrestler. I was glad she was on our side.

"Your office manager said she assaulted you?" The policewoman phrased the statement like a question.

"It was no big deal. She was upset," I replied, though my elbow was killing me where it had hit the wall. "My biggest concern is that she wants to take the dog home. She appears to be intoxicated. I really don't think she should be driving, but more importantly, the dog is in critical condition and should not leave the hospital."

"Do you want to press charges?" She was all business.

"No. I just want what's best for the dog," I replied, looking over my shoulder at the owner. Our buff hillbilly was still sitting quietly next to the Russian woman, who was sobbing and rocking back and forth.

The policewoman nodded. "I can give the woman a ride home if you're willing to keep the dog here, or I can call animal control and have them come pick it up, and I'll take her to jail."

"I'm concerned about getting the dog proper care. We can care for it here." I turned and slowly, quietly, approached Ms. Azarov.

"Ms. Azarov," I said, and she looked up. Her hair was matted on the bloodied side of her face, her eyes red from tears and alcohol. "The officer here has offered to give you a ride home. I'll take care of Viktor." I paused to let the idea sink in. "He really needs to have his wounds stitched."

"Please, ma'am," the policewoman finally said, speaking directly to the distraught woman. "Let me take you home so that the doctor can help your dog." She walked over and put her hand on the owner's shoulder.

I was just about to say, "I wouldn't do that!" when all of a sudden the Russian jumped to her feet and took a swing at the cop.

Deftly the policewoman parried the roundhouse, grabbing the woman's arm, twisting it behind her back, and tossing her to the floor in a slick judo move. The cop landed on the Russian's back, holding her to the floor.

"Now, why did you do that?" The cop yelled at the woman.

"Get the fuck off me!" Ms. Azarov screamed at the top of her lungs. And then again, "Get the fuck off me!"

"Not until you calm down!" The policewoman had an arm lock on the struggling woman. I think between the two there had to be at least four hundred pounds of muscle. We all stood back, stunned.

"Please listen to me, Ms. Azarov," the policewoman said with amazing calm. "The doctors are going to take care of Viktor, and I am going to take you home to get cleaned up." She continued. "Do you hear me?"

"Of course I fuckin' hear you! I'm not deaf. Get off my fuckin' back,

bitch!" After what seemed like forever, Ms. Azarov finally stopped struggling and cursing.

"I'm going to let you up if you promise to behave." The cop admonished. Blood was now spattered all over the tile, and there was a yellow
puddle under the Russian's midsection.

"I promise," Ms. Azarov reluctantly acquiesced. The cop waited a few
moments, then cautiously released her grip on the woman's arm and lifted
herself from Ms. Azarov's back.

The treatment room was once again lined with a buff hillbilly, a pregnant woman, a vampire, a pimp, a prostitute, a bloodstained French maid,
and a witch. Still no Pillsbury hillbilly or pirate to be seen.

The Russian slowly rolled over and righted herself, scooting her backside up against the wall for support.

"We'll take good care of Viktor." I bent down to be at her level. The cop
put her hand on my shoulder, a tacit warning for me not to get too close. I
feigned a smile. "I'll make sure of it."

She looked at me, eyes filled with tears. Her left eye was partially
swollen shut from hitting her head on the floor when the cop wrestled her
down. Was the blood on her face all from the dog, or had she cut her brow
when she hit the tile?

"Come on, Ms. Azarov," the policewoman offered her hand. "Let me
help you up." The Russian looked up and took the cop's hand and, with her
help, stood. She was wobbly on her feet, and before I knew it, hillbilly Mort
had stepped over and grabbed her other elbow, steadying her as she rose.

"Why don't you come with me over to the sink so you can wash the
blood off your hands?" The officer gently led her across the room.

As soon as Ms. Azarov put her two hands under the water, the cop
slapped a pair of handcuffs on her wrists. Immediately the handcuffed
woman went ballistic again. She let out a ferocious scream and took an
arching swing at the officer's head with her arms. The blow hit the policewoman on the temple, knocking her off her feet and sending her flying

back against the treatment table. The stool rolled across the room, crashing against the wall.

Hillbilly Mort and I immediately jumped on the large woman, knocking her back to the ground. The cop scrambled to her knees and joined in the fracas, expletives flying.

The policewoman pulled a stout cable tie from her belt and secured the woman's feet and legs while Hillbilly Mort and I held her down. Just when I was wondering how we were going to get her out of the hospital, I looked up and saw two uniformed male officers standing in the doorway.

They immediately rushed in and took control of the Russian woman, who was really putting up a struggle. They kept yelling at her to calm down, but that just infuriated her more.

Ms. Azarov refused to stand, instead struggling and fighting, kicking, and spitting at the officers. Everybody else in the room stood far back while they fought. Finally, the three officers wore her out and literally carried her lengthwise out of the building.

After they left I stood in the middle of my treatment room, silently taking in the carnage—stools knocked over, tables pushed aside, blood on the walls and counters, dog and human urine and blood on the floor. A witch, a pregnant woman, a pimp, a prostitute, the buff hillbilly, a vampire, and a bloody, sexy French maid. What a day—certainly a Halloween I would not soon forget.

My elbow was screaming with pain. I looked at my arm, and it was covered with blood down to the wrist. I went over to the sink to rinse it off and noticed that the blood was my own and that it was coming from a four-inch slice through my forearm.

As I was mindlessly rinsing off my battle wound, I heard a voice coming at me from behind. I turned to see a pirate and the Pillsbury hillbilly walking in the door.

"What happened here?" they asked in unison.

NOVEMBER

Mort the Conqueror

Around midday, Fred returned from lunch bragging that a woman had just hit on him while he was walking back from McDonald's. Gene pointed out, to Fred's chagrin, that the woman in question was actually a hooker, not an admirer. With the exception of Fred, we all got a good laugh out of the incident.

After the brief amusement, Lisa came to me with a concern that in the past few weeks a prostitute had been aggressively approaching our male clients when they left the hospital after dark. In the past few days the complaints seemed to have escalated, and the description of the woman was always the same. We had no off-street parking, so owners and pets had to walk up and down the block to get to their cars. Having my clients harassed by a lady of the night was not the experience we wanted them to have, so I decided to confront her before I left work.

The sun had started to set, leaving the evening somewhere between daylight and streetlight. I had only to walk a few steps out our front door to find the lady in question, leaning against the corner street sign. A cinnamon complexion complemented her silver-and-black hair pulled back in a tight bun, she had on skin-tight gold Lycra pants and a gossamer, dirty-gray braless top cut mid-belly, and she was adorned with excessive jewelry that looked like it came from a ninety-nine-cent store. She drew a long, pensive drag on her cigarette as I approached, then dropped and crushed it into the sidewalk with a sideways twist of her scuffed black pumps.

"Looking for a date, Doctor?"

"What's your name?"

"Whatever you want, honey." She smiled—a Cheshire grin that lacked the four upper middle incisors.

"We need to talk."

"Whatever you want. It's your money."

"I respect your right to run your business," I paused briefly, for effect. "I ask that you respect mine."

"What are you talking about?" Her eyes got large, the color blanched from around her pursed lips, head slightly cocked to the side, and she leaned forward into my personal space.

"Some of my clients object to your confronting them. I'm concerned that they may choose another veterinarian where they don't feel uncomfortable walking to their cars after dark. That takes money out of my pocket." I maintained a flat, businesslike tone. "Leave my clients alone, and I won't call the police."

She stared at me for a moment, then took a baby step backward. "I can respect that." She smiled and lit another cigarette. I watched her ignite it, and then I turned and headed back toward my office. Two steps away I heard a soft voice: "It's Harriett."

I stopped and turned to face her.

"You can call me Harriett." She looked me in the eyes, took a long drag, then focused her gaze far down the street. Garbled music poured out the door of the China Girl, the strip club a block away. I could see a bouncer hanging out by the entrance, leaning backward with a foot up against the jam, also smoking a cigarette. His tattoos were obvious even in the dim light.

At some point during the silence she looked down at her feet, and I noticed that a small clump of hair was missing from the top of her head, almost as if it had been yanked out.

"Well, Harriett, I suppose it's nice to meet you." I extended my hand. "You can call me Doug." For a brief a moment I felt like I was talking to a friend.

"*Dr.* Doug," she said with emphasis on the "Dr." She took my hand and held it gently. "The *pleasure* is all mine." She smiled again and gave a little squeeze. "From this night on, I promise to respect your right to business." She let go and started to walk off. "We *both* have business to do," she proclaimed as she sashayed down the street.

Was she being genuine or working me? I watched her for a brief moment and couldn't help but wonder who would be attracted to a character like Harriett. To each his own. I shook my head and went back into the brightly lit office.

◆ ◆ ◆

I was excited when I looked at the appointment books that morning because Dodo, the emu chick, was due to come back for its two-week recheck (albeit a little late). I hoped the cute little bird was doing better. These large ratites grow several ounces a day, which is one of the reasons they suffer problems with their long bones the way they do. I had filled Mort in on the case, and we entered the room together.

To my disbelief, the little bird, which was twice the size as when I saw it just eighteen days earlier, was balancing on the floor with the hobble tightly wrapped around just one leg, the other leg trailing behind. The bird's right leg, the one without the hobble attached, was pointed nearly forty-five degrees out to the side.

"When did the hobble come off?" I asked, trying my best not to show my frustration.

"It's been on the whole time," Mrs. Chissler responded. Her daughter, Jenny, stared at the floor.

Mort picked up the now much larger chick and placed it on the exam table. The hobble was tangled around the good leg so tightly that the skin was crimped at the site. A day or two longer and it would have cut off circulation to the foot. The portion of the hobble dragging on the ground was so worn and soiled that I could tell it had probably been off the whole time since they had last seen me.

"Can't you just cut the leg and straighten it?" the owner asked.

"Yes, it can be done," I said, looking at the legs, "but as I told you, that surgery has a very high rate of failure, meaning death." I paused a moment. "Mrs. Chissler, the left leg looks great. I still think we can get the right leg to turn back to the front using the hobble. This is the preferred technique. Since they grow so fast, it *will* correct in just a few weeks." I looked directly at her, then down at Jenny. As soon as I looked at the young girl, she turned away. She was wearing a lime-green shirt with a pink ostrich on the front.

"Please, let's try one more time to straighten out the leg with a hobble." I reached down and gently turned the right foot to face forward. "If it doesn't help, I will do the surgery."

The owner looked disappointed. "He hates the hobble, and he seems so miserable in the box." I was sure she hadn't been keeping the chick in the box as instructed.

"Yes, but it's temporary and safe. Much less risk than the surgery." I petted the chick's head. It was so cute, pecking at my watch and the round silver end of my stethoscope. They like shiny objects. "A couple of weeks of tough love and your bird will be running around the backyard and playing with your daughter! Wouldn't you like that?" I looked at Jenny. She finally looked up at me, smiling.

"Well, okay," Mrs. Chissler answered quietly but, like her daughter, not looking at me when she spoke. "I just want him to get better."

"Please fix Dodo." The freckled little girl finally spoke.

"I'll do my best, sweetie." I smiled back.

Mort and I took Dodo to the treatment room, where I fabricated an elaborate hobble out of wide rubber bands. By the time I was done, the bird was standing perfectly straight and was able to hold itself upright.

"Come back in two weeks so I can assess the leg and, hopefully, remove the hobbles at that time!" I knew that if she followed my instructions, Dodo would respond well and go back to being a normal emu.

◆ ◆ ◆

A couple from Palos Verdes Estates, one of the wealthier neighborhoods in the Los Angeles metropolitan area, brought in a black-capped capuchin monkey. They had a large home and sizable property on the western side of the peninsula overlooking Catalina Island, where they kept multiple animals, including horses, a donkey, several dogs, and two monkeys. About eight weeks earlier this particular monkey had stopped being able to use its legs. It could look around with its head, move its arms and hands, but was a paraplegic from the waist down. The little primate was only three years old, not old for a capuchin, a primate that can easily live into its late twenties.

Mort helped Stacey take X-rays, from which I was able to immediately make a diagnosis. Mikey had a broken back. The fracture was brought about from the monkey having weak, brittle bones. This is a common result of not getting proper calcium and vitamin D in its diet, or enough natural sunlight—a condition called rickets in humans. Mikey had probably been jumping around his large indoor cage the way a normal monkey would do but, because of the nature of the diseased bones, had fractured his fragile spine.

Unfortunately, because Mikey was two months into the condition, he stood little chance of ever regaining use of his legs. I gave his owners, the Keplins, the bad news. Nevertheless, the family had no financial concerns and wanted to do everything possible to try to fix Mikey's back and restore the use of his legs. I told them that I did not do spinal surgery, but I would make some calls.

Since Mikey had become incontinent and had been wearing a diaper since the injury, he had developed diaper rash and urine scald. I gave them some salves and liquids to help with the skin and some pain medication for his back, and I told them I would call them as soon as I came up with a treatment plan.

After my morning appointments were finished, I called my surgeon friend Dr. Elliott Roberts, the specialist who had treated Wok's hips. I figured if anybody could fix Mikey, it would be Elliott. When I described the unusual case, however, he pointed out that he had never worked on a monkey. "You may want to consult a human pediatric surgeon, someone who has done this type of thing on children before," he said.

As soon as he said that, I had an epiphany. I would call Ellen's boss, an orthopedic surgeon, first thing Monday morning and see if he'd be interested in helping me with Mikey's surgery. If he couldn't or wasn't interested, he certainly might know a human surgeon who might be willing to try.

I was so amped up about trying to help Mikey that I couldn't sleep all night. When Ellen got home from work in the morning, I told her about the adorable little monkey and asked her if she thought her boss might be interested in helping. She offered her boss's home phone number, and although I felt bad about bothering him on a Sunday, I gave him a ring.

Dr. Abraham Goldstein had been an orthopedic surgeon at Long Beach Memorial Medical Center for over three decades. He told me that he had actually done spine surgery on several monkeys back when he was in his training during his residency, but that was over thirty years ago. In recent times, he had limited his surgical practice to hip and knee replacements. But he did give me the name and number of one of his young associates who specialized in spine and neck surgery.

As soon as morning rounds were finished, I put in a call to Dr. Goldstein's associate, who, it turned out, was his son, Adam Goldstein. His father had already called him and brought him up to speed on Mikey's case, and the young Dr. Goldstein was more than willing to help. He would come to my office on Thursday morning for the surgery and would bring the specialty spine instruments that he needed with him.

The Keplins were ecstatic something might be done to help little Mikey. The plan was for them to bring Mikey in on Wednesday for the necessary pre-op preparations like blood tests and chest X-rays. Since the condition affecting Mikey was most likely due to improper diet, I explained to the Keplins that there was a good chance their other monkey had similar issues and should also be examined. Further, Dr. Goldstein had recommended that we have some spare monkey blood available, just in case we needed to do a transfusion on Mikey during the complicated surgery. We could use his cage mate as a possible donor.

◆ ◆ ◆

One of my favorite clients, Mr. Knight, came in for a Tuesday-morning allergy shot appointment with his little white poodle, Cindy. He was all smiles when he arrived, pushing his walker with his right hand, while coddling Cindy in the other. Cindy was almost ten years old, about the same age in doggy years as her owner. She had a history of severe allergic skin disease that was getting worse as time went along.

Mr. Knight paid immaculate attention to Cindy's medical needs. Both she and Mr. Knight's mother lived with him. He subsisted on Social Security and a small pension that he had accrued from working as a cobbler for forty years until his arthritis would no longer allow him to hold the tools of his trade. Standing over a workbench his entire life had left him hunched over, with the kind of dowager's hump so often associated with older women.

Cindy was extremely sensitive to house dust, pollens, fabrics, and cigarette smoke. Mr. Knight had been a smoker his entire life, but as soon as he found out Cindy was allergic to cigarette smoke, he had quit cold turkey. For the rest of her allergies, Cindy needed a weekly allergy shot, especially in spring and summer. Mr. Knight was not able to administer the injections, so he budgeted the cost of the weekly veterinary visits into his limited income and, like clockwork, showed up every Tuesday for Cindy's treatments. Mr. Knight cared about only two things: Cindy and his mother. I never asked, but I suspected that was also the order of his priorities.

Although any of my technicians could administer Cindy's allergy injection, I preferred to do it myself. I really admired Mr. Knight. Especially on a busy or rough day, I got personal pleasure from taking a few minutes to chat with the kind man. During one of those Tuesday chats, I learned that Mr. Knight's mother had fallen in the shower and broken her hip but was being denied hip surgery on account of her age. The county hospital where Mr. Knight had taken his mother said that she should instead be sent to a rehab facility to see if she would heal on her own.

Age was not a disease, I told Mr. Knight, surprised that his mother's doctors wouldn't help her. Unless she had some coexisting medical condition that precluded anesthesia, I didn't see why they couldn't perform surgery to fix the hip. I suspected that the hospital was worried about getting paid. I told him that my wife, who as a nurse worked for some of the top orthopedic surgeons here in the city, could consult with one of the specialists about his mother's situation.

Luckily, the outcome of my intervention was successful. Mr. Knight's mother got her hip surgery, and he was overjoyed when he came in to see me that Tuesday morning.

"Morning, Cindy. Morning, Mr. Knight," I greeted the older man and his poodle. It was my tradition to always address his dog first. I patted her on the head and she squirmed with excitement, tail wagging against Mr. Knight's chest.

"I've got to tell you, Dr. Mader, my mother is doing *great*! I am so thankful to you and your wife for helping her." His big smile wrinkled the skin around his entire face. He held tight to Cindy, petting her as he spoke. "She's home again now after rehab, and walking better than me!"

• • •

"Big day!" I said as I opened Mrs. Keplin's door when she, her husband, and the two monkeys pulled up out front in their Mercedes.

"Yeah, a bit nervous." She looked at me as she stood, surprised to see me at the curb. Mort walked around and shook Mr. Keplin's hand as he exited the vehicle. Mikey was wrapped in a blanket in Mrs. Keplin's arms, and their other capuchin, Bali, was bouncing around in a stout metal transport cage in the back seat.

Mr. Keplin opened the rear door, but before he could say anything, Mort reached in and grabbed the cage, putting his fingers through the top bars to get a firm hold. As soon as he did, Bali pounced on the opportunity and sank his teeth into Mort's knuckles.

It all happened so fast: Mort initially reaching for the cage, Mr. Keplin yelling "Don't!", me screaming "No!", the feisty monkey howling "Aaaack!", then Mort reacting with a piercing "Yooow!" Even Mikey, who was swathed in his security blanket, screeched out a monkey yowl.

Mort tried to release his grip on the cage, but the ferocious, hairy little monster would not relinquish Mort's finger. Mr. Keplin started banging on the top of the cage with his fist and yelling at Bali to stop, but that just seemed to antagonize the monkey more. I reached between the front seats, grabbed a coffee mug, and tossed the contents into the face of the attacking beast. The splash caught the caged cannibal by surprise, and it immediately released its bite, allowing Mort to pull his fingers out from between the bars, blood splattering everywhere.

Stacey had been inside and saw what was happening, and so she dashed outside and wrapped Mort's hand in a towel. Mr. and Mrs. Keplin were stressed out and apologizing, Bali jumped up and down triumphantly in his cage, and Mikey looked around and mumbled monkey words, clearly shaken.

"Let's get inside," I instructed, then ushered Mort, who was grimacing while he held the towel around his injured hand, directly back to the treatment sink. Meanwhile, Stacey ran ahead and got the water running in the sink and some first aid supplies at the ready.

I unwrapped Mort's hand and washed the blood from his fingers. Luckily the wounds were fairly minor, but they had bled a lot, making quite a mess of the light-gray leather seat of the Keplins' Mercedes. Most of Mort's pain was from the teeth crushing his fingers, not from lacerations in the skin.

Stacey helped him scrub the wounds with antiseptic soap, and I recommended that he go to an emergency room to have it looked at, but he refused: he was current on his tetanus, and the wound didn't look like it needed sutures. Besides, he said, he wanted to stick around to help with the monkeys.

Once things settled down and the Keplins left, we sedated the attack monkey, took X-rays, and performed blood tests. Although Bali's bones were thin, they were nowhere near as bad as Mikey's, and correcting the diet should easily take care of the problem.

"Hey, Mort!" Lisa announced to the treatment room crew over the intercom. "There's something for you up front."

We all looked at him and headed en masse to the reception area. On the counter was a huge vase of flowers and a large box of chocolates with a bright-yellow card shaped like a banana:

Dear Mort,
I'm sorry I bit you—I really didn't mean it!
Signed, Bali

I had stopped at a Jack in the Box and got a chicken teriyaki rice bowl on the way home from work. After feeding Wok, Sidney, Dewe and Traci, my tortoises, and the fish, I snarfed down the takeout, grabbed one of my surgery books, and hunkered down on the ugly olive-green recliner in my home office to review the chapter on spinal surgery. I had never met the young Dr. Goldstein, and I really didn't want to look stupid. "Real" doctors generally don't have a lot of respect for veterinarians.

Also, the reading was a perfect way to start studying for my upcoming specialty boards.

Mikey was awake in his cage, still wrapped in his blanket, when I arrived in the treatment room in the morning. Greg said that the patient had slept well most of the night. Bali, on the other hand, would rattle his cage and toss feces out through the bars whenever he walked by. It seems it's always the nice pets that get sick!

Everybody arrived to work pumped up for the big surgery day. We had our usual morning rounds. The plan was to have Fred as anesthetist, Stacey as surgical room technician, Dr. Goldstein as spinal surgeon, and me as his assistant. Mort, with his bandaged hand, would be in the room just to observe.

I was surprised when Dr. Goldstein arrived at nine, as scheduled. For some illogical reason I was expecting a stately older gentleman like his father, but he looked to be about my age, shorter than me at about five foot six, with dark hair and black rimmed bifocals. He was wearing green surgical scrubs that read "Long Beach Memorial Medical Center" across the back.

"Hi, I'm Adam." He extended his hand. His grip was neither firm nor weak, his hands were soft, and his nails were perfect. I later learned from Ellen that he went to a manicurist every week and insured his hands for several million dollars.

"I'm Doug. Welcome to my humble hospital."

"I've heard a lot about it from my dad." His dad had never been here, but I suspect that Ellen had talked about it.

"I would imagine you won't find it nearly as sophisticated as what you're used to," I noted.

"Oh no. I can tell already that this place is great!" He looked around as we walked back toward treatment to meet his patient, introducing himself as Adam to all the employees as we passed.

"Is that him?" Adam looked incredulously at the bouncing Bali.

"No," I laughed, as did all in the treatment area. "In fact, don't get too close." I could see Bali feeling around the bottom of his cage for some feces to toss. Fortunately, Peter and Maria had just cleaned it moments before we entered the room. "He's our blood donor."

"I was gonna say, he's looking pretty strong for having a broken back."

"This is our patient." I pointed to the pathetic-looking capuchin wrapped in a Casper the Friendly Ghost blanket. "His name is Mikey." I opened the door and carefully lifted the paralyzed little monkey and blanket up out of his cage.

Adam reached out and gently took Mikey's tiny palm between his own thumb and index finger. The monkey grabbed the tip of the doctor's finger as if shaking his hand and let out a soft "Eew, eew."

"Wow. I've never touched a monkey before." Adam smiled. All the techs stood around in a semicircle watching. "He's so much smaller than my usual patients."

"It's hard not to feel for the little guy." I slowly reached over and stroked the curly hair on the monkey's head. "I hope we can help him."

"We'll do our best." He let Mikey's hand slip from his finger. "I've got a bunch of equipment in my car. Can someone help me bring it in?"

"I'll help." Mort was the first to respond, even with his hand wrapped in a white gauze bandage, covered with a large blue latex glove.

While Mikey was getting his pre-op preparations, Mort helped Adam set up his equipment in the surgery room. I was amazed how many boxes he had brought, and I suspected that his instruments cost more than my car.

As soon as Mikey was anesthetized, Adam injected a radio-contrast dye into Mikey's spine, a procedure called a myelogram. The iodine highlighted the injured area of the little monkey's spinal cord, allowing Adam to know exactly where to make his incision.

"That's not good." The black-and-white image of the X-ray reflected off the front of the surgeon's glasses. "The damage is right here." He pointed to an area on the X-ray with the tip of his pen that showed where the injury was most severe.

"Do you think we can help him?" I could clearly see the impairment.

"Put it this way," he said, looking at me, "if we do nothing, he'll always be paralyzed and will most likely die in less than a year from kidney failure. That's the most common cause of death in human paraplegics. If we take him to surgery and we can't fix the back, he'll be no worse off than he is now, but at least he'll live with less spinal pain." Adam turned back to the myelogram and tapped the nasty damage with his pen. "Let's do this," he said.

"This is just like my hospital," Adam stated as we entered the surgery suite, "except my patients aren't quite so hairy." Mikey was all set on the operating table, while a constant background *beep, beep, beep* of the EKG machine reassured me that the patient was stable.

"I'll bet your patients don't bite and throw crap at you."

"Wanna bet?" he laughed.

For the next two hours it was all business, no more joking.

"Whoa," Adam muttered to no one in particular as he concentrated on his task. I could sense dismay in his voice. "These bones are *really* soft."

"That's the rickets," I stated, realizing as soon as I did that of course he already knew that.

"In today's society we rarely ever see this disease." He was busy working on the spine. I noticed that some bright red blood had started to well up in the incision. "I belong to Doctors Without Borders, and I still occasionally see it when I go to third-world countries." He spoke while clearly concentrating on finding the source of the bleeding.

"Normally, if this were a traumatic back fracture in a child, I would attach one or two metal plates onto the spine to help stabilize the bones while they healed." He took a break and looked across the table at me. "But Mikey's bones are so soft they won't hold a screw, much less a plate."

"What can we do?" I said "we," but he was doing all the work.

"I've done it," he said. Using the tip of one of the instruments, he pointed to the area of the spine he had been working on for the past ninety minutes. "I've done what's called a laminectomy."

I could see where he had removed essentially the entire top of the vertebral column over the soft, snake-like spinal cord. "Normally the actual spinal cord is off-white, covered by a thick outer layer called the dura mater." Adam continued to point at the surgical area. The cord wasn't white, but dark purple.

"It's discolored because of bruising, caused by the damage from the broken vertebra. Essentially the shattered bones have crushed what's left of the cord." He gently blotted away a small dollop of blood that was oozing up from behind the cord once again.

"Any thoughts on prognosis?" I asked, handing him another gauze sponge.

"Not good." He turned to Stacey. Before he could say anything else, she reached up and carefully blotted sweat away from his brow. I could see he was impressed with her attentiveness. "I seriously doubt that our little friend will ever walk again." Just as he said that, the area where Adam had just dabbed the small amount of blood suddenly started to rapidly well up a pool of red.

"Damn!" Adam grabbed more gauze and packed it around the cord. "It's one of the spinal arteries from the fractured bones." Nothing more was said as he concentrated on stopping the bleeding, and we all just watched. He took more dry gauze and packed the surgical area and applied pressure over the spine. For a moment he just stood there, staring at the surgical site, blood soaking into the gauze. Rather than remove the gauze and replace it with fresh, clean gauze, he just packed more gauze on top. As the gauze turned bright red he continued to place even more on top of the layers.

"Want me to start the transfusion?" Fred asked. Bali's blood was gently rocking back and forth in the collection bag inside the incubator in the corner of the surgery room.

I looked at Adam.

"Yes, please," he said.

Stacey grabbed the clear bag containing the dark-red blood, and within seconds the fresh fluid was flowing into Mikey's IV line, bringing with it new red blood cells, platelets, and clotting factors.

When the transfusion bag was about half finished, Adam carefully removed the blood-soaked gauze from the spinal cord incision, saying as he did, "Cross your fingers."

Everybody held their breath. Time stood still as we all watched and waited to see if the bleeding would start again.

Fortunately, the transfusion did its job. The hemorrhage had stopped.

After what seemed like hours, we all took a collective deep breath.

"Okay, time to finish this up," said Adam. With precision he sutured closed the several layers of tissue that he had to incise to expose the broken back and repair the damaged spine.

Once the procedure was complete, we stood back from the table and let Fred, Stacey, and Mort place a sterile dressing over the incision and take Mikey back to his recovery cage.

I looked at the clock. It was after two. Including the myelogram, we'd been in surgery for four hours.

"I'll bet you're hungry." I patted Adam on the back for a job well done. "How about I treat you to lunch and we can go over what I need to do post-op for our patient."

"That would be fantastic. I'm famished!"

We changed into our street clothes, and I took him to Lili's Country Kitchen, a Korean diner a short walk up the street from the hospital, just on the cusp of the bad part of town. Nothing fancy, but Lili had some of the best burgers I've ever eaten. I know, burgers aren't Korean, but who cares? It was perfect post-monkey-surgery comfort food.

The Keplins came by to visit in the late afternoon, but Mikey was still sound asleep from the pain drugs. The couple stood outside his cage for about a half hour, stroking the fur on top of his head and talking softly to him. I showed them the preoperative myelogram that demonstrated the severe damage to the spinal cord, and the postoperative X-rays that clearly showed what Dr. Goldstein had done to try to alleviate the injury. I explained that it was highly unlikely Mikey would ever walk again, but I assured them that Dr. Goldstein felt that if nothing else, the surgery would alleviate any pain Mikey was surely experiencing.

They were extremely thankful for all we had done. Mrs. Keplin gave Greg and me a big hug and cheek kiss then headed out for the night. We promised to call them if there were any changes in Mikey's condition. The best part was, they took the little monster Bali with them when they left.

Around 9:00 p.m., Mikey awoke from his stupor and started cooing. Greg and I immediately went over, and he reached out for my hand. While I was holding his little fingers, Greg warmed up some baby food and mixed vegetables. Mikey readily grabbed the spoon and started sucking the orange-green paste.

"Yum!" Greg smiled and reloaded the spoon. Mikey reached out for more. "He's got a good appetite."

Riding the high from the day's back surgery with Adam and my normal insomnia, I slept in fits, if at all. I was so worried about Mikey that I got up, fed all of my sleepy critters, and headed into work about an hour earlier than usual.

Greg was still on shift, but to my surprise Adam was in the treatment room checking on his patient when I arrived.

"Good morning! I didn't expect to see you here." I reached out and shook Adam's hand. He was wearing a set of green hospital scrubs like the ones from yesterday.

"I've got a full day of procedures scheduled today, but I wanted to stop by to check on my patient before I went into the hospital. I hope that's okay?"

"Of course! Beyond the call of duty." I patted him on the shoulder. "What do you think?"

"Well, considering that we cut away about 25 percent of his spine, I think he's looking pretty good." He glanced through the bottom of his thick bifocals at a graph of Mikey's vital signs from throughout the night. The line connecting all the dots representing his breathing, heart rate, and temperature was nice and level.

Adam lifted Mikey's blanket. Greg had changed out the Casper blanket to one with a Donald Duck motif. Adam looked at the incision and then felt the pulses in Mikey's feet.

"I think everything looks good." He carefully replaced the blanket. Mikey was awake, cooing, and looking up at Adam. "He sure is cute."

Adam and I discussed a few more details about the monkey's aftercare and potential discharge instructions, and then I asked him if he could step aside with me, away from Greg, for a moment.

"Adam, I really appreciate all you have done, as I've said, above and beyond."

"Oh, it's really my pleasure."

"Seriously, though, I never asked you what I owe you for your time. I can only imagine what this would cost in your hospital. The Keplins are so thankful and will pay whatever you decide," I told him.

"You owe me nothing." He smiled. "Doug, really, it is my pleasure. I am glad to help, and now I've made a new friend outside of my work." I was honored. "All I ask is that you keep me posted on his status."

The Keplins came by later in the day for another visit. This time they brought a huge goody basket for the staff that included chocolates, candy, popcorn, fruit, and more.

Mikey was much more alert and responded with a loud "Hoot, hoot" when he heard their voices. When they entered the room, he lifted his upper body using only his hands and arms, propping himself up on his elbows while he chattered away.

Everybody was just thrilled. Maybe there was hope.

◆ ◆ ◆

The little monkey's parents came by the next day to take him home. He didn't have any sensation in his feet or legs, but his attitude was bright, alert, and very responsive. The plan was for them to bring Mikey back the following Saturday for a recheck and suture removal. Adam had asked for us to schedule it for a Saturday because he wanted to be here when Mikey came back in.

After they left I sat at my desk reviewing charts and came across the medical record for Dodo, the emu chick. It was supposed to come in Monday for its two-week follow-up. Rather than wait until then, I decided to give a call and check with the Chisslers to see if they had any questions or concerns.

"Hello?" a quiet voice answered.

"Hi. This is Dr. Mader, from the vet hospital." There was a long pause on the other end. I was waiting for a response. "Is this Mrs. Chissler?"

"Yes." The word trailed off almost to the point where I couldn't hear it.

"I'm just calling to check on Dodo. How is he doing?"

Silence.

"Mrs. Chissler?" I had a really bad feeling. "Is everything all right?"

"No."

"What's the matter?" Immediately I thought that somehow the little chick had become tangled in the hobble, caught in the box, or something else horrible, and that it was all my doing.

"I'd rather not talk about it." She was louder now, almost curt.

"Are you upset with something I did?" Now I was really concerned. "How is Dodo? Is he all right?"

"*No*. He's *dead*!" she pretty much screamed into the phone.

My heart stopped. What could have happened? I have done hobbles dozens of times, and they had always worked.

"I am so sorry." Now I was fretful. I am sure she could hear it in my voice, if she was at all perceptive. "Please tell me, what happened?"

"I took him to a specialist to have the surgery to straighten the leg."

"And?" I asked, but I knew what she was going to say.

"After the surgery the leg was perfect." Her voice started to break up. "But that night when I got him home, the leg bone broke right above the surgery site where the pins were. The doctor said it couldn't be fixed, so he had to put Dodo to sleep."

Before I could say anything she slammed the phone down.

My job can be an emotional rollercoaster. There was the high of sending Mikey home with happy, compliant owners, followed by the gut punch of the phone call with Dodo's owner, who was too impatient to listen to my advice, and now her cute little bird was dead.

She didn't mention the name of the exotic specialist who had done the surgery, but I had a good idea who it was. His ego was so large that I could see him jumping at the opportunity to show off. "Dr. Mader did what? Put your bird in a box? How stupid! Hey, I can do a little surgery and straighten those legs." I could picture him holding his hands up over his head, palms open, as if celebrating a victory when he finished explaining the procedure. "Simple!"

I took Wok for his evening stroll that night and couldn't help but dwell on the day. My own emotions were a torture of happiness, sadness, and abject anger.

My best friend and personal confidant made his normal rounds, peeing on his favorite bushes, trees, and the like, then as usual ended up back on the bench while I told him about my day. He knew I was upset. Suddenly, he leaned over and gave me a sloppy dog lick on the side of my face, his lips curled in a subtle "I love you, master" dog smile.

"I love you, Wok." I reached over and embraced my furry black bear with a hug. His curly tail went into overdrive.

◆ ◆ ◆

Mort accompanied me on a visit to one of my commercial clients. I was the veterinarian of record for a large research facility that specialized in eye care products like contact lenses.

Our first task was to evaluate an ongoing project that involved six crab-eating macaques. The animals had been trained to sit in primate restraint chairs for a drug trial. These custom metal chairs have historically received a lot of bad publicity from animal rights groups. The primates' feet, legs, arms, and hands are free to move about, but the head and neck are loosely restrained in a yoke that is fastened to the back of the chair. This allows the monkey ample movement while in the chair. It can eat, drink, urinate, and defecate, but because the head is restrained, it cannot get up and run away.

No matter how you spin it, it looks harsh. I've always hated seeing these intelligent animals in these chairs. But I can tell you, they are never hurt or injured when they are in the chairs, and in fact, they are trained to voluntarily go, without any coercion, from their cages to the chairs, and then back to their cages, when the procedures are finished. They are only permitted to be in the chairs for a few hours a day and are constantly being rewarded with treats.

In this project the primates were getting eye drops every two hours, drops that were being evaluated for use in humans to treat glaucoma. If the medication was proven to be safe and effective, it would help treat millions of people.

It didn't matter what I felt about the chairs, it was my job to ensure that animal welfare guidelines were being followed and to make sure that the monkeys were all being handled properly and not stressed or in any discomfort. I checked the heart rates, respiratory rates, and blood pressures of all the animals. After each exam the handler gave the monkey a treat. Basically, they were all in great shape and actually seemed excited to see me and get their physicals.

Mort seemed to enjoy the morning, but most importantly, not a single monkey tried to bite us or throw feces at us.

It was a beautiful fall day. We finished up at the lab building, and rather than head directly to NAVH via the 405 freeway, I decided to take the Pacific Coast Highway. We stopped at the deli where I had taken the two Karens last summer and sat out on the seawall to watch the waves while we ate lunch. I enjoyed Mort's company. He was definitely one of the better students I had supervised in a long time. We talked about his small veterinary school, where he lived, and his family. It turned out that his father was a real estate developer back in Virginia and had done quite well for himself. To my surprise, Mort had a part-time job working in the pharmacy at the university. Although his parents paid for his school expenses, he had to cover any other costs. No wonder he seemed so self-possessed.

• • •

When it came time for Mikey's sutures to come out, I arranged for the Keplins to bring Mikey in at noon, and I told Dr. Goldstein to arrive around 12:30, figuring that most likely I would be running a few minutes late as I almost always do on busy Saturday mornings.

Sure enough, the Keplins arrived right on time, with Mikey wrapped in a Popeye the Sailor blanket and happily screeching as they walked in the front door. As soon as Mai Tai saw Mikey, Mai Tai let out his jungle scream—some secret rain forest welcome, I supposed.

Dr. Adam Goldstein arrived moments later. He felt that Mikey's incision had healed beautifully. Mikey still could not use his legs, but he could twist around at the waist and would grab at the scissors every time Adam tried to remove one of the stiches. Fred was able to hold Mikey's arms so that the surgeon would not get his million-dollar hands bitten.

"I'll bet your patients don't do that!" I greeted Adam as I entered the room. He had just finished removing the last suture.

"Hi, Doug." He set the instruments on the counter and shook my hand. "Our patient is looking good." While the Keplins watched, Stacey held Mikey up and Dr. Goldstein tested Mikey's reflexes in his legs and feet. Unfortunately, still nothing.

The big thing that we all noticed was that Mikey had developed pressure sores—the type seen in elderly patients in nursing homes.

"Are you turning Mikey over frequently?" Dr. Goldstein asked the Keplins. They looked at each other as if deciding who was going to accept responsibility for the wounds.

Mrs. Keplin answered, "Probably not as much as we should." She looked guilty. In my experience, that meant "no."

"We need to get these bedsores under control." Adam looked up at me. "That's Dr. Mader's area of expertise." He smiled. "As far as Mikey's spine is concerned, I think it's healing well." He slid his hand down the scar on the little monkey's back, ultimately holding on to the flaccid feet. "I was hoping for some signs that the nerves to his legs would be returning, but I think we just need to give it a little more time."

Mikey let out a "Hoot, hoot" and chattered his teeth. We all laughed. It was almost as if he understood what Adam had said.

After Adam left, I attended to Mikey's bedsores and instructed the Keplins how to clean and dress the wounds. They had a hot tub at home, so I also advised them to start carefully soaking him every day once his wounds healed.

♦ ♦ ♦

Tina Scheelings's large Rottweiler, Max, was my first appointment of the day. It seemed like everybody called their Rottie Max, just like everybody calls their cocker spaniel Buffy, or their poodle Fifi. Max weighed in at 122 pounds, easily fifteen pounds heavier than his petite owner. Amazingly, the dog was so well trained that Tina had experienced no issues handling such a large beast.

The first words out of Tina's mouth today: "Dr. Mader, I'm pregnant!" Her expression, however, did not mirror the ebullience you would expect from a woman in the family way.

"That's fantastic!" I smiled, but I had a feeling that there was more to come.

"Yeah." Tina forced a smile.

"I sense something's rotten in Denmark. What aren't you telling me?"

"My doctor said I have to get rid of Max." I noticed her eyes were red. She had been crying.

"Why? Because you're pregnant?"

"Well," she said, pulling a tissue out of her purse. Max sat attentively at her side, alternately looking between his owner and me. He was a solid Rottie, broad forehead, proud face, and clearly protective of his mom.

"I don't have a spleen." She wiped her nose and tucked the tissue back into her purse. "I was kicked by a horse when I was a little girl, and it had to be removed."

"Oh . . ." I've never considered myself particularly smart, but I have a strange propensity to remember really unusual diseases and other weird things. "Your obstetrician is worried about *Capnocytophaga canimorsus,* the bacteria that lives in dogs' mouths."

"Yeah, I think that was it." She looked surprised that I knew about it.

"No worries." It was coming back to me. "All dogs normally carry this in their mouth. Your spleen acts kinda like a fuel filter in a car; it filters out certain bacteria that can cause disease. If your spleen isn't working, or if you don't have one, you are more susceptible to infections by those bacteria."

"Yeah. She's worried that if I get sick from the dog, it may affect the baby." She placed her hand on her as of yet swollen belly.

"I constantly hear from my clients with AIDS that their doctors tell them they have to get rid of their pets." I shook my head. "Bless their hearts, human docs just don't understand. It is easier for them just to tell people to get rid of their pets than make an effort to preserve that all-important human-animal bond."

"That's sad." Tina looked down and rubbed Max's head. He licked the air and gave his tail a wag.

"Let me ask you this: how long have you owned Max?"

"I've had him for six years now."

"Did you have any other pets before him, since after you lost your spleen?"

"Yes." She looked slightly confused about my line of questioning.

"Have you ever gotten sick from any of your pets?"

"No." I could see that she was starting to get the picture.

"Personally, I don't think you need to get rid of Max." I changed my serious look into a confident smile. "Obviously, I'm not an obstetrician, and I don't do human babies. But I do know animals and infectious disease." I walked around the table and bent down to examine Max. "Let me check out this big fella and make sure that he's healthy, and I will write a letter for you to take to your doctor."

"Can we test for the bacteria?" Tina queried.

"Yes, but it's best to assume that all dogs have it. If you accept that premise, and take precautions, I really don't think you need to worry."

I gave Max my best physical ever. I took blood and evaluated his feces for parasites, looking for anything that might be problematic for a pregnant woman.

Since we regularly saw so many clients with AIDS, we had prepared a handout for them on how to avoid contracting disease from their pet. It was composed of simple reminders like washing your hands after playing with your pet, cleaning any wound, and going to a doctor for antibiotics if you get scratched accidentally.

Max checked out perfectly healthy. I knew that he would be a great guardian for Tina and her little baby someday not too far down the road. I encouraged her to make an appointment with an infectious disease specialist and not just take my word for it.

• • •

Mark and Brian, KLOS's morning goofball DJs, weren't their normal good-humored selves while I listened to them on my way into work. As I rounded the traffic circle on Pacific Coast Highway, they were talking about the fact that a superior court judge had ordered the trial of the four officers charged in the Rodney King beating the previous March to be moved to Simi Valley.

Rodney King was the black motorist who had been severely beaten by four white Los Angeles police officers after a traffic stop earlier in the year. Seventeen other cops had stood around the melee in a large circle and watched. The beating was captured on film by a private citizen who recorded the entire horrendous incident from his balcony. The following day he gave the tape to the Los Angeles television station KTLA.

Over the next several days the video went viral—quite a feat back then—and was shown on every television station, seemingly twenty-four hours a day. People of all colors were outraged. About two weeks later the four police officers seen beating King, who had been down on the ground and not fighting back, were all indicted by the grand jury. However, the same grand jury refused to indict the seventeen officers who had stood around watching the beating and did nothing to stop it.

The announcement of the change of venue came as a shock and a blatant slap in the face of justice. Moving the trial out of Los Angeles to the predominantly white, upper-middle-class Simi Valley clearly prejudiced the case in favor of the four police officers.

◆ ◆ ◆

NAVH was not open for regular appointments on Thanksgiving; however, I took ER calls so that Drs. Nordic and Furtano could have time off to be with their friends and family. Willy was out of town for the long weekend with his buddies. Ellen had opted to work, as she was getting paid double time. That meant that it was just Wok, Sidney, the tortoises, the fish, and me sharing a turkey TV dinner for the holiday. Well, maybe not so much the fish; they more or less just watched.

Even though the examination for my specialty boards was still seven months away, I took every chance I had to get in some studying. After my aluminum-tasting dinner, I grabbed a cardiology textbook and got comfortable in my ugly recliner for some exciting reading.

Somewhere around midnight, midway through a chapter on supraventricular arrhythmias, my pager went off. I had it set to buzzer and beep, so the combination not only startled me but also caused Sidney, who was sleeping on my lap, to jump straight up in the air.

"911." I spoke out loud, as if to explain it to Sidney, and now Wok, who had heard the commotion and came running into my office. A second page came in as soon as I looked at the small digital screen, this time with a phone number that I didn't recognize.

"Dr. Mader!" Greg answered my call, clearly upset. "It's Stacey—she's been stabbed!"

"What?" I was still in the cardiac fog of monitoring irregular EKGs. Greg's alarming news flash was totally out of context.

"Stacey! She's been stabbed. Outside the hospital!" He yelled into the phone.

"Okay, Greg. Calm down and tell me what happened. Is she okay? Where are you?"

"I'm at the emergency room. She's in surgery. I'm sorry I didn't call you sooner, but I had to get her to the ER as soon as possible."

"You did the right thing. I'll come right over."

I grabbed my keys and headed to my car, peeling rubber down my street. My head was pounding, thoughts racing. As I sped off, I suddenly realized that I did not know where Greg was calling from. Which ER hospital did he take Stacey to? I didn't want to waste time and go back home and call the number on the pager, so I kept driving.

My initial thought was that he would take Stacey to Long Beach hospital and that most likely Ellen would be one of the nurses taking care of her. But as I started heading in that direction, I realized there was a much smaller hospital only two blocks from NAVH, and if it were me in that situation, I would have taken her directly there. I took a chance, turned back toward work, and headed to the community hospital ER.

My instinct paid off. I saw Greg's car parked diagonally across two spaces, just feet from the entrance to the ER, clearly left there in a rush. I locked my car and ran to the entrance but was immediately stopped by two large, armed security officers.

"I'm Dr. Mader. One of my nurses was stabbed and brought here a few minutes ago!" I wasn't about to let them stop me.

"Okay, sir." The guards stepped aside. "Down that hall!" The larger of the two pointed toward the surgery wing.

As I arrived Greg was pacing back and forth. He was covered with blood, his eyes wide with fright.

"Are you okay?"

"I'm fine." Greg gestured to his shirt. "This is all Stacey's."

"How is she? What happened? Where did this occur?" I had so many questions.

"I haven't heard anything yet." He was very upset.

"Just tell me what you know." I grabbed Greg by the shoulders and forced him to look at me.

"She offered to cover for me tonight so I could have dinner with my family. I got back to work about 11:30 and noticed blood all over the sidewalk, and a trail leading into the front door. I figured it must have been from a hurt dog or something. But when I got inside, I found Stacey slumped down against the wall, under the phone. There was blood on the wall, like she tried to call someone." He was fidgeting as he relayed the story. "I was going to call an ambulance, but she wouldn't let me!" Greg almost seemed apologetic. "So I helped her into my car and I drove her here as fast as I could."

"You did well, Greg. How bad is it?"

"I don't know. She was conscious, but it looked like she lost a lot of blood. She was stabbed right here in her stomach." He pointed to his mid-section. "They literally rushed her right to surgery."

While we waited anxiously, he told me the rest of the story as Stacey had related it to him on their way to the ER. Apparently at about ten o'clock she got hungry and decided to drive down the street to the local twenty-four-hour McDonald's for a late-night snack. When she returned to NAVH, as she was getting out of her car she reached back in to grab her radio, the kind that slid in and out of a slot on the dashboard. When she turned around, a man, who seemed to have come from out of nowhere, stabbed her in the stomach, grabbed at the radio, and tried to flee. Stacey, not wanting to let go of her radio, fought with him, screaming and punching him in the face with her free hand. That was enough to make him run off.

She collapsed to the ground and crawled the twenty yards to the hospital, opened the front door, and then pulled herself over to the phone. She hadn't turned on the alarm when she left, so to get help she had to call someone, but she didn't have the strength to stand and reach the wall phone.

She must have passed out. Fortunately, Greg got back from his dinner shortly thereafter and found her. She was holding her stomach with one hand and her radio in her lap with the other.

At three in the morning Stacey's trauma surgeon came out to say that Stacey was going to be just fine. She had lost a lot of blood, but by some miracle there was no damage to any internal organs.

◆ ◆ ◆

It was eerily quiet in the hospital all the following day. Even though we were open as usual, it was still a long holiday weekend, and a lot of people and their pets were away traveling.

The police were there at first light taking pictures of Stacey's car and the blood trail leading into the hospital. The blood-covered radio was still in the receptionist office, so they took that to try to get fingerprints.

Once the cops left, Maria mopped and scrubbed the blood from the tile, walls, and phone, while Robert hosed down the sidewalk and washed the dark red smears off Stacey's car.

Brenna and the Skunk

Brenna Halvorson, our new student, arrived on the second of December. Mort was such an excellent extern, she was going to have big shoes to fill. Brenna was of Scandinavian descent. Her blond hair was pulled back, French braids along each side over each ear then joined in back of her head and continuing in a single, larger French braid down to the middle of her back. She looked physically fit and was tall, easily six feet.

Stacey had been released from the hospital. She was doing great, but quite sore. We were all worried that she would be afraid to go out alone or at night, fearing that she might encounter the man who'd stabbed her. She said she wasn't afraid—rather, she was *pissed*, and she remembered exactly what he looked like and said if she saw him she was going to kick his ass. I didn't doubt it—if anyone on our staff had to get stabbed, she was the one who could best handle it.

After rounds I had Lisa call the Keplins. Mikey was doing well, and they said that they were keeping up with the physical therapy and that his bedsores were already better.

Dave was in working with the wildlife. He was on a high because he had been accepted as a member into the Hollywood Magic Castle, a private club for magicians that required an audition after which you had to get voted in. It was a very exclusive club.

Shortly after lunch, Lisa paged me and said that Dean Farnsworth, from Mort's veterinary school, was on the phone.

"I'm sorry to bother you, Dr. Mader." The dean was very formal. "But I'm just checking on Mort. He did not show up at the university this morning. I was just calling to see if he was still there?"

"No, sir. Mort left here last Wednesday evening." Mort had departed after the last appointment was finished and planned on driving the twenty-seven hundred miles over the next four days in order to be back at school for classes on Monday.

"I'm sure it's nothing. Maybe he had some car trouble." The dean paused. "His parents have not heard from him either, which is why I called. Sorry to bother you."

"No bother. Please let me know if you hear anything." I was about to hang up. "By the way, Mort was an excellent student. I told him that if he wanted to move to California, I'd offer him a job when he graduated."

• • •

I can usually tell the day of the week without a calendar. For instance, Mr. Knight was waiting for me in the room with Cindy for her weekly allergy shot, so it had to be Tuesday.

"Good morning, Cindy! How are we today?" It was my usual greeting, always to the little dog first.

"Good morning, Dr. Mader!" Mr. Knight was full of smiles. Cindy's nearly hairless tail was wagging full throttle.

I was about to administer the injection when all of a sudden I heard a panicked, baritone voice screaming, "I need help!" from the front reception area. Mai Tai let out an almost simultaneous squawk.

"Excuse me!" I set the syringe down on the exam table and bolted for the reception area.

Mr. Rockwell's backlit silhouette filled the frame of the open front door, and he was hugging one of his little Pomeranians close to his chest. The dog's head was lolling off to one side, its swollen and blue tongue hanging out of its mouth.

Stacey grabbed the limp, furry, little pointy-nosed dog and dashed back toward treatment.

"Follow me," I said, motioning to Mr. Rockwell. "What happened?" I called back over my shoulder as I chased behind Stacey and the dog. Fred and Peter had already set up the oxygen mask, and as soon as Stacey set the dog on the table, they put the cone over its face.

"I think she ate this!" Mr. Rockwell held out a nine-volt battery. It was covered with saliva and had chew marks all over the case. "Is Lucy going to die?"

In what seemed like only a matter of minutes of aggressive emergency care, we got the little dog stabilized and breathing on its own. In actuality, two hours had passed.

Just as I was feeling pretty good about what we had done, Lisa came up from behind and tapped me on the shoulder.

"Dr. Mader," Lisa said, shaking her finger at me, "did you forget Mr. Knight and Cindy are still in Room 2?"

◆ ◆ ◆

That Thursday, Brenna was sitting next to the cage watching a tortoise recover from anesthesia while I finished my operatory notes. A call came in from a Mr. Dennis. I didn't recognize the name at first, until it dawned on me that Mr. Dennis was Mort's father.

It turned out that Mort had fallen asleep at the wheel on his marathon cross-country drive over the holiday weekend and crashed into a ravine. It occurred at night, and no one had seen it happen.

It wasn't until days later, after the highway patrol put out an alert for the missing car and driver, that someone noticed the skid marks leading off the road and found him. He was conscious but had broken both of his legs and was not able to crawl out for help. He was taken to a local hospital where he was treated. Once he was stabilized, his family drove out to bring him home.

Life can be so unpredictable. You just can't count on tomorrow.

◆ ◆ ◆

Even more than usual, I didn't sleep much that whole week. For one thing, I was thinking about Mikey, who was scheduled to come in for his recheck on Saturday. I had kept almost daily contact with the Keplins. I could tell by the tone in their voice over the past few days that they were beginning to lose hope. Mikey still was not using his legs, and his bedsores were not healing. Dr. Goldstein and I had told them it was unlikely that Mikey would ever be normal again, but I don't think they realized how hard it was going to be to care for such an invalid pet.

As soon as the Keplins arrived, I could see in their expressions that they were ready to give up. Mikey looked like a skeleton wrapped in his Superman blanket. He had lost so much weight that you could count his bones. His face was gaunt, eyes sunken, and the Superman images on the blanket showed stains from the open sores. Before I could even say anything, Mr. Keplin, the quiet half, spoke, almost in a broken whisper. "Do you think it's time for us to say goodbye?"

My first thought was *Oh my God, yes.* We needed to end this suffering. Lying in your own feces and urine and wasting away, covered with bedsores, is no way to die with dignity.

Before I spoke, however, Mikey looked at me with his tired, sad eyes and uttered a barely perceptible "Hoot, hoot." In that moment of nearly tacit communication, the little monkey sent me a clear message. In spite of his sunken eyes and sallow expression, he didn't want to die.

My sleepless night came back to me. I had one of those microprocessor moments where a zillion thoughts crossed my mind. I knew I needed one more try. Mikey wasn't ready to give up, and I was not going to quit on him; I just needed the Keplins to believe in me.

I managed to convince them to leave Mikey with us over the weekend. I felt it was the best for Mikey and would also give them a much-needed break from his constant care. We then gave Mikey multiple warm emollient baths, gently cleaning and debriding his decubitus ulcers. After drying him, we packed the open bedsores with a poultice of medications to assist healing and started him on systemic antibiotics and some strong pain medication.

By the next morning I could see a huge improvement in his appearance and attitude. As soon as he saw me, he lifted his torso with his arms, something he had not done in over a week according to his owners, and let out a solid "Hoot, hoot!"

"Look at you, little man!" I reached in the cage and scratched the top of his head. He looked up at me and started to coo, balancing on one arm and grabbing for my hand with the other, as if trying to shake it hello.

I had spent the weekend working on a project that I hoped would make life better for the little trooper, and at morning rounds I told everybody about it. The apparatus resembled a baby's high chair. I had replaced the seat with a padded sling designed to wrap around Mikey's upper thighs, suspending him like a person wearing a climber's harness. Doing so not only kept the weight off his knees, hips, and buttocks, relieving pressure on the bedsores, but also kept his bottom free so that the urine and feces would fall into an easily changeable tray filled with kitty litter to allay any odor between cleanings.

I had built in adjustable, padded curved sides. The pads acted like the vest of a man's suit, but open in front and back to keep him from falling forward while sitting in the chair. The pads were soft but waterproof so they could be readily cleaned and disinfected.

In front of the seat was a small tray like a high chair would have, with padded elbow supports. The central portion was made of a high-impact Lexan polycarbonate plastic that would handle scratches, bites, and constant pounding from a monkey.

My contraption was met with praise from the staff. But now it had to pass the real test. Robert carefully got Mikey from his cage. The little monkey knew something was up because of all the people gathered around staring at him. As soon as Robert picked him up, he started a series of happy screeches, waving his arms back and forth and flashing his teeth in a typical "monkey smile."

I helped guide his emaciated body into the chair, carefully placing each leg into the harness. Once I had him aligned so that the sling did not interfere with the sores on his hips and knees, I gently tightened the straps to make sure he was sitting evenly. Next I adjusted the side panels so he could move his torso comfortably, but I made sure they were not so loose that he would lose his balance and fall forward onto the tray. I slid the tray back so it was just about an inch from his chest. His arms were free to move anywhere, and he was able to turn his head in all directions.

At first he just sat there, staring at the tray, the arm rests, at us, then back at the chair. "Hoot." He looked up at me with questioning eyes. "Hoot." He rubbed his palms slowly over the smooth, clear surface of the tray. He kept looking up at me as if seeking my approval. I smiled each time. Then, suddenly, his hands started moving much faster, quickly in progressively larger circles, as if he were cleaning or sanding something. "Aaaack!" He pounded the tray with both palms, looking up, and monkey smiling. "Aaaack, aaack, hoot, aaack!"

Everybody started clapping. The more we did, the more Mikey hollered and slapped the table.

Was that monkey talk for "I like this!"? This was the first time in three months the little fellow had sat up on his own. His skinny, nearly hairless legs dangled lifelessly beneath the bottom of the chair, but from the waist up he looked like a normal monkey.

Peter handed Mikey a piece of banana, which he grabbed with both hands. Immediately he stuffed it into his mouth and reached for another.

Maria gave him a small baby bottle filled with orange-flavored Tang.

Mikey took it, gave a quick suckle on the nipple, then tossed it on the floor, monkey laughing as he did.

I think we hit a home run.

• • •

I held off calling the Keplins about Mikey's chair and told the staff not to tell them anything over the phone. I wanted the new chair to be a surprise, but I also wanted to make sure that Mikey was in fact adjusting to it.

Sometimes my good judgment pays off. Even though the day was busy with surgeries and appointments, I made sure that there was a staff member watching Mikey in his new chair at all times. As the day progressed I felt more and more confident about the new device. Each time I checked in on Mikey, he seemed to be resting comfortably, eating or playing with the rubber dinosaurs and baby rattle that Maria had given him. Then, about four in the afternoon, Fred came to get me between cases. "Dr. Mader, I think you need to come take a look at Mikey. Something's not right."

I headed immediately back to the treatment area and stopped in my tracks as soon as I turned the corner. Mikey was slumped forward in his chair, not moving, arms dangling to the side, drool leaking out his lips in a short, bubbly string to the top of the clear Lexan.

"What happened?" I rushed over and lifted Mikey's head. "When did he collapse?" I looked at his eyes. His pupils were almost completely dilated. As I lifted his head, his jaw dropped open, mouth agape, mucous membranes pale.

"He was fine, Dr. Mader!" Fred sounded almost defensive. "He just suddenly slumped over—for no reason, I swear!"

"Help me get him out of the chair." I slid the tray forward and lifted him out. "Get me some oxygen!"

Wonderful. Here I thought I had invented something that would save our patient, and now it looked like he was going to die. I listened to his heart, and it was slow and weak. He was barely breathing, and his body was totally limp.

No time to panic. Just think. It looked like he had fainted. He was pale, no blood to his head. Just as with humans, I raised his feet so blood would return. In the meantime, Stacey prepped his left arm and placed an IV catheter in the vein running over the top of his wrist while I rubbed his body to try to stimulate circulation.

Within minutes Mikey started to blink and move his head. A few seconds later he was grabbing at the oxygen mask trying to dislodge it.

"Aaack!" he screamed, weakly at first, but then more and more loudly. His breathing picked up and his heartbeat got stronger. I could actually see the jugular veins in his skinny neck start to pulsate.

"You scared the crap out of me, little buddy!" I rubbed his head. He insisted we remove the oxygen mask, which we did, but I had Stacey continue the IV drip.

Once I felt he was stable, I had Fred put him back in his regular cage. Enough chair time for one day. I told Fred to stay with Mikey and come get me immediately if there were any changes. Then I headed upstairs to my office to think this through. I did not understand what had gone wrong, though clearly we somehow overdid it.

I paged Adam Goldstein, hoping to get his thoughts, and he called back immediately. He surmised that Mikey had experienced a condition called "orthostatic, or postural, hypotension." This happens, for instance, when a person with low blood pressure stands up too quickly. They get lightheaded and sometimes even see "stars." The blood leaves the circulation to the brain, momentarily cutting off oxygen and causing dizziness. If it happens too fast, the person can faint.

He went on to explain that patients who have been in the prone position for extended periods are often not able to adjust to being upright for any length of time. Since Mikey had been essentially on his back or side for the past three months, a few hours of sitting up had overwhelmed his circulatory system, and he had developed hypotension—more simply, low blood pressure.

Adam was excited about the chair and encouraged me to continue to adapt Mikey to it, but to do it gradually, adding a few minutes to the daily schedule. Mikey should still sleep in his bed at night, because the body needs to lie flat and rest naturally every day. Eventually, however, Mikey should have no problem staying in the chair for ten to twelve hours a day, just like a person in a wheelchair.

It was interesting, Adam pointed out, that a common torture of prisoners during wars was to strap them upright to a pole and not allow them to lie down. The constant upright position would eventually wear the prisoners to the point where they would tell their captors what they wanted to know, pass out, or die.

Here I thought I was doing something good. Instead I had been subjecting my patient to torture!

♦ ♦ ♦

Mrs. Keplin broke down in tears. Mr. Keplin, no surprise, was speechless.

Mikey, on the other hand, was not. He screeched and hooted the moment he saw his mom and dad enter the room. He had a toy soldier in one hand, a piece of banana in the other, and was *holding* a red dinosaur in his left foot! The techs had been doing physical therapy on his legs and feet several times a day, and one of the exercises was to place objects in his feet. He was still a long way from ever walking again, but we were moving in the right direction. Mrs. Keplin couldn't stop crying happy tears as she walked over to the high chair and gave Mikey a big hug. He returned the gesture by slobbering banana spit down the side of her face. Before they left I got a photograph of Mikey, sitting in his chair, with his parents standing next to him on either side, so I could send it to Dr. Goldstein.

What a great day.

♦ ♦ ♦

I received a surprise Christmas package from my friend Dr. Elliott Roberts, Wok's surgeon. Inside the bright, shiny red-and-green holiday color wrapping was a *Self-Assessment: Internal Medicine* textbook.

The book was formatted like a test, containing three hundred questions. Most had images like X-rays, pictures of disease conditions, EKGs, and the like. Each image had a question associated with it, and there were five possible answer choices. The best feature of the book was the section at the end of each question with a thorough explanation of both the correct and the incorrect answers. So regardless of whether or not you got the question right, you were able to get a detailed review of the subject matter.

Tucked inside the front cover was a note:

Doug –
Go through this book now and get an idea where your strengths and
weaknesses are. Then, when you start studying (which you should have
already), concentrate on your weak areas. It is easy to study the stuff
you already know!
Happy Holidays,
Elliott

With Christmas just around the corner, I decided to take a short break at lunch and do some shopping for Ellen. We were both scheduled to work on Christmas Day, so our plans were to try to have our own little private family Christmas with Wok, Sidney, the turtles, and the fish this coming Sunday, when we were both scheduled off.

I hated that Ellen worked in such a dangerous part of town. Granted, she loved the adrenaline rush of her ER job, and she really couldn't do it at the intensity she did if she worked anywhere else (Long Beach Memorial Medical Center was a Level I, or top tier, trauma center). The area around the trauma center was not one where you wanted to be walking alone after dark, and she had to drive through the roughest part of the city to get to and from the hospital every morning and night.

Cellular phones had been all over the news. Pagers were great if someone needed to get ahold of you, but you had no way of getting back to whoever was trying to reach you unless you could get to a pay phone. Mr. Rockwell, the ex-football player with all the Pomeranians, kept a portable phone in his Jaguar. When Dr. Goldstein came to work on Mikey, he carried with him a very cool portable phone, a "cell phone," as he called it. No matter where he was, he could call or be called if the phone was turned on. It was compact—just slightly larger than a brick!—and he kept it in his briefcase. When he needed to use it he took it out, attached the antenna, and made the call.

I thought this would be a perfect gift for Ellen. That way, if she ever broke down she wouldn't have to leave the safety of her car; she could just call for help.

The only place that sold these new phones was RadioShack. I made the short drive to the nearest store, which was down by the shore, only to be disappointed when I arrived. All the cellular phones had sold out—apparently a rush on them for Christmas. I begged the salesclerk to put me on the wait list, but he said that the phones were in such high demand that there was no way I'd be able to get one before the holiday.

Crap.

I had been so excited about this new kind of phone and felt it was really important for Ellen to have one. Dejected, I wandered aimlessly around the store. After a few minutes of fruitless meandering, I decided I had best get back to work and headed out to where I had left my car. I'd had to park a couple of blocks away because of all of the holiday shopping and traffic. As I approached the car I ran into Package talking to a couple of unsavory types in front of one of the closed bars. As always, his fluffy white guinea pig, Powder, was snuggled in the bend of his elbow.

"Doc!" Package turned from his associates and reached out with his free arm for a handshake.

"Guys," he said, looking back at his acquaintances, "this is Dr. Mader, the *best* veterinarian in the world!"

"Hey." The first one shook my hand.

"Hey." The second just looked at me and nodded.

"Nice to meet you." I smiled, reaching over and stroking Powder.

"What brings you down in my neighborhood, Doc?" He turned his attention from his street buddies.

"Oh, just trying to do a little Christmas shopping for the missus."

"Empty hands, not too successful?" Package was astute. His contacts nodded in silence and turned away down the street. One of them tucked what looked like a roll of money into his hip pocket.

"Hey," I motioned toward the pair. "I didn't mean to interrupt."

"Oh, no worries." He waved them off like annoying flies. "Just a little business meeting. Nothing that can't wait."

"I was hoping to get one of those new cellular phones for my wife. She works in a crappy part of town. Nights. I thought it would be a good safety thing for her to carry in her car."

"Oh man." Package reached into a leather satchel hung around his neck and pulled out a portable phone. It had a furred, white-and-brown cowhide cover. "These things are the best! I couldn't do business without one." He handed it to me. The antenna was screwed on, making it almost sixteen inches tall. The faceplate was lit up with digital numbers as if he was expecting a call. I could imagine how handy having a portable phone would be in his line of work.

"Unfortunately, because of the holidays, RadioShack said they're on back order until next year." I handed it back. "No phone for Ellen this holiday."

"Doc!" Package smiled. A beam of sunlight glinted off the diamond in his tooth. "You want a cellular phone, I can get you a cellular phone!"

"Really?" I was ecstatic. Then realized I was talking to a drug dealer. "Is it legal?" As soon as I said this, I realized it probably was not the best thing to ask.

"Doc! Doc! Doc! Of course it's legal." He leaned closer, way too far into my personal space. "You hurt my feelings when you say things like that." All I could do was focus on the tooth. "I know people who know people who may owe me favors."

"Yeah, but how can you get me one if they're on back order?" I really didn't want to buy a stolen phone for my wife.

"Let's put it this way . . ." He put his free arm around my shoulder, gently turning me back in the direction that I was heading. Powder was clearly comfortable riding in his elbow and I'm sure had been witness to this type of interaction many times. "Tomorrow, I want you to walk back into RadioShack and ask for Tommy." He pointed down the street to the same store from which I'd just been turned away.

"Tommy. You ask for Tommy." He smiled, stepping back out of my zone, now petting Powder. "Tommy will have a brand-new cellular, portable phone, in its brand-new, unopened box, with your name on it."

I must have looked totally confused.

"Tommy owes me one. I'll make sure that your name gets moved to the top of the list."

"Are you sure?" Of course he was sure. That's what he did.

"Mrs. Mader will have her cellular phone for Christmas. All you have to do is go to RadioShack and pay for it, just like normal." He gave a thumbs-up. "Ask for Tommy."

Just as Package promised, Tommy had a brand-new, portable cellular phone waiting for me, still in its unopened box, when I went into RadioShack over lunch the next day.

The phone was on sale at a special Christmas price of only $827, which included the AC and car adapters. If the phone wasn't turned on, the battery lasted almost ten hours, and if left on, nearly three. For a monthly service fee of $65 you got fifteen minutes of total talk time. Extra minutes were available at $5 a minute. Any leftover minutes at the end of the month could not be carried over, so Tommy recommended I make sure I use up all fifteen minutes each month.

I was beside myself with excitement! I had bought Ellen the perfect Christmas present that I hoped she would never have to use.

◆ ◆ ◆

The week before Christmas, and not a creature was stirring. . . . It was really dead at NAVH. With just a couple of days left before Christmas, people were getting ready for the big day, not spending on pets and vets. Willy had left prior to the weekend to be with his family. I had sent Dr. Furtano home because she had family in town. Cliff was finishing up on a routine puppy spay with Fred. I had grabbed a stack of X-rays and was going through them with Brenna, reviewing each case and using them as a learning tool.

Suddenly Lisa paged back to the conference room and almost screamed into the intercom: "Dr. Mader, we need you up front, *stat*!" Brenna looked at me with alarm. We dropped the X-rays on the table and headed to the reception area.

A man was holding a limp boa constrictor in his arms. The snake looked to be about eight feet long. The man was crying and trying to talk to Gene at the same time. I approached and reached for the lifeless snake. The first thing I noticed was that he reeked of smoke—burned wood smoke.

"What happened?" I lifted the snake. It was actually hot, not warm, and dangled like a limp rope.

"My apartment burned down." He choked out between tears. "Is he dead?"

"Brenna, take him to the back and grab the Doppler." I handed her the snake. Stacey and Maria were standing next to her by this time.

"I'll check." I put a hand on his shoulder. My initial assessment was not good.

We took the snake to the treatment room and attached the ultrasonic Doppler to the scales directly over its heart and listened for a heartbeat.

Nothing.

Everybody watched in silence as I carefully slid the sensor from side to side and from front to back over the area of the heart. It seemed like I had been searching forever when all of a sudden we heard a very faint but clearly distinguishable *whoosh* sound.

"That was a beat!" I stated, hoping for a miracle. "Stacey, get me—"

She handed me a syringe before I could get the words out. "One milligram epinephrine." Stacey was always one step ahead of everybody else. As with Mickey the mouse, I injected the epinephrine directly into the snake's heart and started CPR.

In the meantime, Stacey had grabbed a small breathing tube and placed it into the snake's windpipe, hooked it to an oxygen bag, and started pumping oxygen into the snake's lungs. About two minutes into the CPR the speaker on the Doppler monitor emitted another *whoosh*. Sure enough, a few seconds later, another *whoosh*. This was followed just seconds apart with another *whoosh*, then another, and another. Within a minute, the *whoosh*es were becoming more frequent and stronger, a sign that the heart, lungs, and brain were getting the much-needed blood flow and oxygen that had been choked off in the fire.

Cheers and claps emerged around the room. Right about then I noticed that the snake was beginning to make voluntary movements with its tail. Within a couple of minutes it began to breathe on its own.

The owner of the snake was waiting for me in the conference room. Like the snake, he reeked of smoke. The acrid smell made my nose cringe. "How is he, Doc?"

"I have good news, Mr. . . . " I realized that I had never got the man's name.

"Williams. LeRoy Williams." He held out his hand to shake mine.

I started to return the gesture, but noticed blisters all over his hand—some filled with fluid, some burst open and bloody, some blackened.

"You're burned!" Rather than shake his hand, I gently held it and looked at the blistered skin. "You need to see a doctor."

"Never mind me." He pulled his hand back, covering the injuries with his other hand. "How's my snake?" He looked behind himself, found a chair, and sat down.

"The good news is that he's alive. He has a strong heartbeat and is breathing well on his own now." I gave my best reassuring look.

"That's good." He looked down at the floor, rubbing the back of his burned hand with the other. Stacey entered the room with a damp wash-cloth wrapped around some ice and handed it to the man.

"How much is this all gonna cost?" He didn't look up.

"The important thing is that he's still alive, though I suspect his lungs have sustained some damage from the heat and smoke. He's not out of the woods yet." I looked at the man's despondent expression. "He's still going to need more care."

"That's what I'm worried about." He used his good hand and wiped his nose, tears in his eyes. "I ain't got no money. I just lost everything I own." He started to sob.

"Tell me what happened, Mr. Williams." I patted him on the shoulder.

When he got home from his nightshift that morning his apartment had been cold so he had turned on his space heater while he made breakfast, not realizing it was too close to his small Christmas tree. Before he knew it, the tree was burning and so were the curtains, the couch, and the rug. The snake's cage was on the other side of the tree, which fell over and landed on it. Mr. Williams pulled the tree off the cage with his bare hand and grabbed the snake out of the cage.

Several other apartments had also burned in the blaze by the time the fire department arrived, and now his neighbors were all blaming him. Fortunately, no one other than Mr. Williams was injured in the fire, but several families lost everything.

"Mr. Williams," I squatted down to be at his level. "Let's worry about you and your snake." How could I possibly add to this man's burdens? "You go get your hand looked at. I'll take care of your snake. It's on me."

• • •

On Christmas Eve, I did not expect it to be busy. The plan was to be open for only a half day so the staff could go home and be with their families. Since it was Tuesday, Mr. Knight and Cindy came in for their weekly allergy shot. Cindy was dressed up in a bright Christmas scarf, and her toenails were painted an alternating red and green. Mr. Williams's snake had made it through the night and was looking good. I had Brenna give it a bath to remove some of the smoke stench. Its skin was starting to blister, but I wasn't worried, as the snake could just naturally shed the damaged skin.

Lisa told me that there was a woman from Texas on the phone wanting to talk with me. She had gone to two different veterinarians with her large python, and they had tried treating it with various antibiotics, to no avail. She was afraid that it was going to die and needed my help.

Her seven-year-old daughter wanted only one thing for Christmas—for Santa to make her snake better! The woman described the snake's symptoms: unable to crawl, rolling over on its back, lolling of its head from side to side. To top it off, it had not eaten in four months.

The lack of appetite did not bother me. Big snakes can go as long as a year between meals in some situations. However, the other symptoms were extremely serious. I explained this to the owner and apologized that there really wasn't anything that I could do for her or her snake over the phone.

The snake had belonged to her husband, she told me. He was a cross-country trucker and would keep the snake in his cab, much the same way many truckers keep dogs in their trucks for company during the long hauls. Apparently on Christmas Eve the year before, the husband had fallen asleep at the wheel on his way home for the holidays. The truck went off the road, crashing and killing him instantly. The highway patrol officers had found the snake alive in the cab. That snake was the family's last link to their loved one.

The woman asked if I would look at the snake if she could get it to me.

Of course I could take a look, I told her, but even if I did see the snake, judging by the symptoms that she was describing, the prognosis sounded grave. I told her I was very sorry, and I wished her the best before I hung up the phone. I felt bad for them.

The next thing I knew it was after one and we were officially closed for the holiday. All our employees had left for the day. Brenna had gone to spend Christmas with Stacey. The only patient we had in the hospital was the burned snake, and it did not need any overnight care, so I told Greg to take the night off and I would just field any emergency calls myself.

After everybody left I walked around the empty hospital, turning off the holiday lights, randomly organizing things as I meandered about, not really in any hurry. The normal buzz of the busy hospital seemed so distant when nobody was around. Suddenly I remembered that Wok was nearly out of food and I needed to bring some home. I grabbed a bag of dog food for him and headed out the front door.

Christmas Eve. Cold and damp. The chill penetrated my coat, gloves, and scarf. A steam ghost danced from a street vent as I approached my car, passing by a large dumpster behind the China Girl strip club. I tossed the bag of food onto the passenger's seat and started the engine. The windows were all fogged up, so I sat in the car while I waited for it to warm up inside, allowing the defroster to clear the windows. While I waited, I lamented my long, difficult day, the fact that so few of my clients had any money to pay their bills, and the knowledge that it was going to be another lonely night, despite the special holiday.

Out of the corner of my eye I noted a figure step out from behind the dumpster. A man, hunched over at the shoulders, was standing on his tiptoes peering inside the rusty metal container. He fished around for a few moments, then jumped back from the garbage, holding what looked like some old trash. Through my foggy windows I was able to see that the man appeared to be talking, but I couldn't see anyone with him. I wiped the window with my sleeve. Then I saw it.

Attached to the end of an old rope was a scraggly little dog, some type of terrier mix. The man unwrapped a wad of aluminum foil that he had just pulled from the dumpster and held it out for his companion. The scruffy mutt dove into the rubbish, chomping away. The man sat on the cold sidewalk curb and reveled in his dog's delight.

I reached down to the floorboard of my SUV and gathered up several empty Diet Coke cans, about a half dozen in total. As I rolled down the window, the cold air shocked my warmed face.

"Excuse me, sir." I spoke through the night.

"What?" The man looked up, spooked. His dog stopped eating and quickly hid behind him. "I ain't doing nothin'." His eyes were wide, voice trembling. He had obviously been in this situation before and, I am confident, was used to life on the mean streets.

"No, of course not," I reassured him. "I was wondering if you had any use for these?" I held up the cans.

"Oh, yes!" He smiled, showing his yellow peg teeth. With fingerless gloves he grasped all six cans at once. "I can get twenty-five cents a pound for these babies!"

I watched as he stuffed the cans into a soiled, tattered sack and snugly tightened the drawstring.

I thought about my day and my troubles. I couldn't help but contrast them with the tough life that this man and his dog had to deal with on a daily basis. I watched as he fed his little dog some more scraps from the garbage. I thought about going home to my warm house and spending Christmas Eve with Wok, my best friend in the whole world.

"Sir," I beckoned one more time, "my dog, Wok, and I would like to share some Christmas cheer with your little buddy." I held out the bag of dog food through the window.

"Thank you, Mister!" He hugged the bag at first, then held it down to show his dog. The little terrier's tail went crazy. "You have a very merry Christmas!"

• • •

On Christmas Day, as much as I wanted to sleep in, I got up early so I would be awake when Ellen got home from her overnight shift. I was excited to give her my Christmas present, thanks to a little help from a drug dealer.

I put the wrapped gift under our small tree, turned on the lights, lit some pine logs in the fireplace, and got out some cider to warm up on the stove. Christmas stockings with the names Ellen, Wok, Sidney, Dewe, Traci, and Fish were hanging on the mantle.

I looked around the living room. Sidney was sitting in front of the fire, and Wok was lying on the floor next to him. The tortoises were still asleep in their night boxes (at this time of year, it was too cold for them to be up this early). The fish were swimming about, oblivious to anything and everything other than food.

I looked at my watch. Just as I was thinking that Ellen should be coming home any minute, my pager went off. It was the hospital. The screen read "911." I picked up the phone.

"Dr. Mader, you need to come right away." Peter was the technician who had drawn the short straw and had to work Christmas morning.

Christmas? What was that? Was Christmas supposed to be something special? Excited to spend the morning hours with my wife? Not today.

"I'll come right in."

Waiting for me at NAVH were a woman, her daughter, and their snake. "We drove all night. We left El Paso as soon as I got off the phone with you." The woman's skin was pale, and dark circles were under her eyes. Her daughter, sporting red pigtails and a puffy, pink down jacket, was asleep on the bench in the reception area when I arrived. "We only stopped for gas and something to eat."

The little girl's head was resting on the edge of a large burlap sack. Inside was a motionless hump. Coiled up inside was a cold, very thin, nearly lifeless reticulated python, just short of eighteen feet long.

I examined the snake from the slowly flicking tongue to the tip of the tail, all six yards of it. Once I finished, Peter helped me take a blood sample and get some X-rays.

After reviewing all the information with the owner, I gave her the bad news. "It looks like your pet has viral encephalitis—an infection in the brain. This is a very serious condition, one that usually ends up with the snake being humanely euthanized," I told the woman and her daughter.

"You have to do something, Doctor. I drove out all the way from Texas. It was my Christmas present for my daughter." As tears moistened her eyes, she added, "It's her only memory of her father." I don't think the little girl understood the gravity of what I had just said, but she reacted to her mother's show of emotion with tears of her own.

I looked at them both, and my heart just fell out.

I took the snake to the treatment area. Peter and I placed an intravenous catheter in the snake's jugular vein, started it on warm IV fluids, initiated antibiotics and antiviral drugs, and placed it in a large cage with several heat lamps in order to warm its lifeless body.

A couple of hours later, I went back to the reception area to find both mom and daughter sound asleep. I woke them with an update, then offered to take the pair to lunch. Since it was Christmas, there wasn't much to choose from, so we celebrated the holiday at a Jack in the Box.

I finally made it home around three in the afternoon and noticed that a truck that had been parked out in front on my curb all week was still there. I didn't recognize it. I also noticed that it had two parking tickets tucked under one of the wipers.

Once inside the house, I found Ellen fast asleep on the couch. Her present was opened, the phone and the Christmas card tucked next to her chest. Wok was lying next to her on the floor, his tail wagging a million miles an hour, and Sidney was curled up between her legs on top of a throw blanket.

"Merry Christmas." I sat next to her on the couch and gave her a kiss on the cheek.

"I love it!" She woke up, bleary eyed. "Sorry, I fell asleep."

"No worries." I gave her a big hug. Wok got up and stuck his short nose into our faces and gave us each a big lick with his black tongue. "I'm sorry I got called out."

Ellen was scheduled to work again, so we had a quick early dinner and spent about an hour talking. I decided to tell her about all the snakes that had come in the past few days and the story behind the phone from Package.

While she was getting ready for her night shift, I decided to take Wok for a stroll. As soon as I got out the front door he started pulling me toward the truck parked at the curb. That was odd, as he was usually very well mannered and never tugged when he was on leash.

I let him lead me over to the truck. About ten feet away he stopped, stood rigid in a protective stance, and barked.

"What, Wok?" He inched forward with cautious little steps.

The camper's windows were closed from the inside, so I couldn't see in. When we arrived at the rear of the truck, Wok started to lick something off the bumper.

"Stop that." I pulled him back. I kept a tight leash and moved in for a closer look.

A foul smelling, reddish-brown liquid was dripping from the bottom right corner of the tailgate. I bent over and touched it with my finger. As soon as I did, I knew what it was: blood.

The second I got inside I washed my hands with the hottest water I could tolerate and then took a hot washcloth and wiped Wok's mouth and face.

When my hands were dry I called 911, then went to tell Ellen what I'd seen. Within twenty minutes my street was swarming with several cop cars, an ambulance, and a fire truck. By this time all the neighbors had come out to see what the big ruckus was about. A fireman took a large crowbar and broke open the back door of the camper. Two policemen were standing at the ready, guns drawn. As soon as the door popped open, one of the officers turned away, covering his mouth with one hand and holstering his gun with the other.

The second officer cautiously stepped up to the open door and looked inside with a flashlight. I watched him replace his weapon, turn back to the rest of the group, and make a slashing motion across his throat.

I walked over to the truck, and an officer immediately stepped in front of me.

"It's my house. I'm the one who called." I looked at the officer. He looked at me as well, but not like a stranger.

"Dr. Mader!" The cop relaxed and smiled. "I'm Roy, from the snake club." He grabbed my hand and gave it a shake even before I could register what was happening.

"Of course," I said, smiling as I tried to remember him. "You have all the colorful king snakes?" I was guessing.

"Yeah, that's me." He seemed pleased that I remembered him. "I didn't know it was you that called this in."

"What happened? There's blood dripping from the back."

"It's bad, man." Roy shook his head. "Some poor fuck blew his head off with a shotgun." He pointed his finger into his open mouth and pulled the trigger of an imaginary gun. "Brains all over the place."

Great. Wok had been licking some bloody brain juice, and I had stuck my finger in it. It had been unseasonably cold all week. That's why we hadn't smelled anything.

Wok and I sat on the porch, watching the drama. What a sad day. What a sad situation. How could things be so bad that one would want to take their own life, much less in such a violent fashion? What message was he sending to the people whom he left behind?

The commotion lasted for several hours, long after dark. After the emergency vehicles, the detectives, and coroner departed, Wok, Sidney, the fish, and I sat by the fire until the last ember died out. Pondering the sad situation that unfolded in my front yard on this afternoon, I knew that even though my wife was not here, I was still fortunate to be surrounded by family, albeit covered with scales and fur.

♦ ♦ ♦

We got a nice Christmas card from Mort. He was still in a wheelchair, but he was starting physical therapy and beginning to use a walker to start building up his legs. He said he'd been hitting the gym for upper-body workouts almost daily.

I took Brenna to lunch for her last day. Unfortunately, it was cold and rainy, so we couldn't go to the beach, but I took her to the diner at the end of the Seal Beach Pier so she could watch the big waves crashing against the shore. She was from Michigan and was headed back to snow and ice, so I figured an ocean day was a good send-off.

When we got back to the office, we both did a double take. Since NAVH was in the middle of town, right between the slums and the affluent neighborhood, we attracted all types of clientele, from families living in poverty to the very rich. However, I don't think I could recall ever before seeing a Bentley parked at the green curb in front of the hospital. What looked to be a chauffeur was leaning against the back bumper, puffing a smoke.

Lisa grabbed me at the door and said that there was an emergency waiting. I asked her why the other doctors hadn't taken the case. Lisa shrugged and replied, "They didn't want it."

When I entered the room, I saw an extremely beautiful platinum blond woman, elegantly dressed, perhaps in her midfifties, with a hairdo that was clearly the work of a high-end salon. Expensive but tasteful jewelry accented her outfit, and some type of fur coat was draped over the back of the nearby stool. But the most striking aspect of this vision was the very fat black-and-white skunk sitting in her lap.

"Hi, I'm Dr. Mader," I said, motioning to my side, "and this is my senior student, Brenna." I reached out to shake the stylish woman's hand.

"Hello, I'm Carol Shaughnessy," she said as she looked down in her lap, "and this poor girl is Bouquet."

"Is she friendly?" I liked to ask before touching any exotic.

"Oh, yeah." She hoisted the hefty beast onto the exam table. "Especially today, I don't think she'd have the energy to bite even if she desired."

I did my examination with Brenna. Aside from the skunk's morbid obesity, I noticed an irregular heartbeat. It was obvious, and Brenna noticed it immediately as well.

"Mrs. Shaughnessy, I think Bouquet may have heart disease." I paused to let her digest what I'd just said. "I am going to need to get an EKG and some X-rays of her chest." I was petting Bouquet as I spoke. The depressed skunk just lay prone on the table. In fact, Bouquet had made no effort to move during the entire exam. "May I have permission to do that?"

"Please, and it's Carol. Of course you can do whatever you need. Finances are of no concern."

Whenever a client says "Money is no object," it's usually because they don't have any. However, I didn't recall anyone ever saying it with such eloquence. "Finances are of no concern." Given the Bentley parked at the curb and her sophisticated manners, I believed her implicitly.

Just as Brenna hoisted Bouquet to take her back to the treatment area, I remembered to ask an important question.

"She *has* been de-scented, right?"

"Oh my!" Carol covered her mouth as if stifling a laugh. "Absolutely!"

I had Brenna help Stacey get the EKG and chest X-rays. The tests gave me the answer.

Brenna and I left the obtunded skunk in the treatment room with Stacey to prepare an overnight cage.

"Carol," I said, flipping off the overhead light switch and slipping the X-rays onto the lighted view box, "I'm afraid I don't have very good news." The worried woman stood to get a closer look.

"How bad is it, Doctor?" She reached into her Louis Vuitton purse and retrieved a laced, monogramed handkerchief. "Is Bouquet going to be okay?"

"Bouquet has a form of heart disease called dilated cardiomyopathy, more commonly called DCM. The heart muscle is stretched out and becomes dilated like a large, flabby balloon, and can no longer beat effectively."

"My God." She looked down, dabbing her eyes, being careful not to smear her makeup. "Is it something I did?"

"Of course not." Actually, it *was* most likely something she did. DCM in dogs and cats commonly stems from an improper diet. Even if Bouquet was overweight, it did not mean that she was getting the right type of calories. However, I was not about to tell her that right now. First we needed to get Bouquet through this crisis. Later I would have a thorough discussion with her about proper nutrition.

"DCM has a congenital basis," I continued. I wasn't lying. Certain breeds of dogs and cats were more prone to this type of heart disease than others. It had also been reported several times in skunks. "But right now the most important thing is for us to try to get her heart stabilized."

"Of course, Doctor. How do we do that?" She folded her hands over her heart.

"Right now her heart is beating irregularly. She's experiencing what's known as 'atrial fibrillation.'" I could see that the big words went right over her head, not surprising, as few people knew what that meant. "For example, rather than beating like a healthy heart, with the normal *lub-dub*, Bouquet's heart is more or less vibrating like a bowl of Jell-O. That's very inefficient, and the heart cannot pump blood to the lungs and brain effectively. That's why she's so weak."

"That sounds most serious. Can you help her?" Her voice was clearly strained. I think she was doing her best to hold back tears.

"I can sure try my best." I reached over and patted the back of her hand. "In order to do so, I'd like to ask that you leave her with me so I can start her on some medications that will help her heart beat more regularly, and stronger."

"Oh my." She sat down. I could see the color leave her face. "Do I *have* to leave her?"

"It would be best. That way we can start her on the heart medication and monitor her response overnight.

"Can't I just start her on the medication at home?"

I could tell she was scared. An owner's biggest fear when faced with an ill pet and the necessity to hospitalize it is that their loved one will pass during the night when they are not with them.

"Yes, Mrs. Shaughnessy, you certainly can. However, you have no way to monitor her, and, if she had a problem, you would not be able to administer any emergency treatment like oxygen, epinephrine, or the like." I paused to let her process what I was saying. "We have someone here all night, checking on her."

"I live upstairs, Mrs. Shaughnessy." Brenna suddenly spoke up. "I'll keep an eye on her all night, and I promise to call if anything happens."

"Oh, you sweet thing!" Mrs. Shaughnessy stood up and hugged Brenna. "Okay, then," she said, letting out a sigh, "you do what you have to do. Thank you!"

She reached into her Louis Vuitton purse. "I have a portable phone that I keep with me at all times." Her case was white leather, studded in diamonds. "I'll keep this on and you can call me anytime, day or night."

"I won't let her out of my sight," Brenna responded. "Why don't I take you back to the treatment area where Bouquet will be staying so you can give her a kiss before you go?" Brenna was all smiles. She also towered a good foot over Mrs. Shaughnessy.

Wow. That was the most interaction with a client I had seen from Brenna all month.

After Mrs. Shaughnessy bade adieu to Bouquet, I pulled Brenna aside.

"Thanks for stepping up in the room." I looked directly at her. "But you said that you would not let her out of your sight." I was stumped. "Aren't you leaving tomorrow?"

"I heard that you don't have another student until January fifth."

"Yep, but what does that have to do with you?"

"Well, I was going to ask if I could stay an extra week until the new student gets here." She pursed her lips, waiting for my response.

I was surprised, as she had been so neutral all month, and this request seemed to come out of nowhere. "That's fine."

"Awesome!" She hopped up and down and gave me a big hug. "Thank you." She stepped back and smiled. "I better go get started on Bouquet. I have a promise to keep."

We worked on Bouquet until late at night, starting the obese skunk on Digoxin, a cardiac medication designed to support a weak heart. An EKG monitor allowed us to follow the effect of the treatment.

Even though Greg was there to take over the night care, I stayed long enough to ensure that the skunk was stabilized. Brenna, true to her promise, wanted to stay by the patient's side and make progress reports to the owner. Around midnight I felt that the skunk's heart rate was as controlled as it was going to be, so I said my good nights and headed home.

I arrived my usual early self in the morning and went straight to the treatment room. Brenna was sitting on a stool in front of Bouquet's cage, drinking coffee. To my surprise, Bouquet was standing and munching on some kibble. The corpulent skunk paused only long enough to take a quick glance in my direction, then buried its short, pointy nose back in the food bowl.

"She's doing so great!" Brenna immediately hopped off the stool when I entered the room and gave me another big good morning hug.

"I'm impressed." I stepped up to the cage. It looked like a different skunk. "Were you up all night?"

"Uh, not really." She smiled and lifted a large cup of coffee. "I went to bed around half past two." She didn't look like a person going on just a few hours of sleep.

"Mrs. Shaughnessy called a little after midnight to check on Bouquet, and I got the feeling that she needed to talk. I think she was really nervous, because we ended up talking until after one!"

"What did you talk about?"

"Oh, it was pretty interesting." She smiled, animated. "I found out all about her, and why 'finances are of no concern.'"

"She does look like she comes from money. Tell me."

Brenna went on to explain that Mrs. Shaughnessy was an heir to the Charlie perfume legacy. Charlie, a fragrance marketed by Revlon back in the early '70s, was the world's top-selling perfume.

I found it ironic that a woman whose entire world revolved around beautiful scents kept a skunk as a pet.

◆ ◆ ◆

Another year was almost finished. I had a few appointments the morning of New Year's Eve. Of course, because it was Tuesday, Mr. Knight and Cindy were first up. Both were doing great.

The biggest news was that Brenna and I had released Bouquet to Mrs. Shaughnessy the previous morning. It was the kind of success story that made me thankful to be a veterinarian. For Brenna, it was the most significant case of the month. Not only that, but Mrs. Shaughnessy was so impressed with Brenna that she offered to pay for all of her books during her last year in veterinary school. Brenna of course declined, but Mrs. Shaughnessy insisted.

Mr. Williams's Christmas-tree burn snake healed well and also went home. The Texan snake was much more active and crawling around its cage.

About noon I bade everybody a happy New Year and took off for the rest of the day. I was not scheduled to come in New Year's Day, and I was not on call that night or the next, so I had no intention to come back unless it was a dire emergency.

Unfortunately, Ellen was scheduled to work the night shift. I feared it would be a bad night, since it was New Year's Eve. Lots of parties and lots of drinking meant lots of auto accidents and other bad stuff. I worried about her working in the ER, but it was her choice and she loved it. At least now she had a super-cool mobile phone she could use if she needed anything.

Wok, Sidney, the fish, and I watched some stupid television after she left for work, until about eleven at night. Then I decided to take Wok out again for his last stroll of 1991.

There was a ton of traffic on the thoroughfare that ran past the park. New Year's revelers heading for their midnight celebrations, I presumed. I wondered how many of them were already legally drunk.

I sat on my favorite bench while Wok did his rounds in the park, marking his usual bushes. It didn't take much for my mind to wander. The drunks on the road made me think about my own auto accident years ago. I found myself unconsciously rubbing my badly injured elbow, running my fingers over the nearly two feet of scars. From there my mind went to the surgical scars on Mikey the monkey's back, the unnecessary death of Dodo the emu, to Dr. Woakes at the conference, and on and on. Mindless thoughts jumped from one topic to another, connected by tendrils of both similarity and irony.

As usual, Wok finished his rounds and came to join me on the bench. He hopped up the short jump with his bad hips and sat next to me, leaning against my side as he did. He looked at me, panting, his hot breath making whitish puffs in the cold night air. It didn't matter that I was a person and he wasn't; our tacit communication crossed species. Sometimes the best conversations between friends were the words never spoken.

We sat on the bench as the year ticked down. We watched as the traffic just about vanished in the minutes before midnight. Throughout the city you could hear the crescendo of fireworks as the midnight hour neared, the bottle rockets, the whistlers, spinners, and poppers. You could easily tell the difference between the firecrackers and the M-80s, the latter sounding like pipe bombs.

Wok always hated loud noises, including thunder, and would bark incessantly at the cracks and bangs. But sitting next to me, he didn't make a sound. He looked around in all directions trying to locate the sources of the different night noises, as did I. Finally, the clock struck midnight, the sounds intensified, and a new sound intruded on the celebratory cacophony—the sound of bullets being shot into the night. It was not uncommon for morons to shoot their rifles and pistols into the air.

I suspect that most of the individuals indulging in this stupid behavior had also been indulging in various substances affecting their judgment. They seemed to forget that what goes up must come down. Every year, at least one person would end up in the ER with a bullet through the top of his head. I suspected that Ellen would have some horror stories to share tomorrow. Fortunately, none of the gunshots seemed to be anywhere near where we were sitting, although I suspected that plenty of bullets were falling all around NAVH.

About fifteen minutes into the New Year the machine gun-like pops and bangs had almost died out, and Wok and I decided to head home.

It seemed like the past year had been extra tough. The hospital was growing, but so too were the problems associated with running a business. I knew already that 1992 was going to bring new challenges, both in life and work. I had my goal of passing the specialty boards, and no matter what life decided to throw at me, I was going to make that dream a reality.

JANUARY

Big Mac

Living in the greater Los Angeles area, we have our share of famous clients. It's always fun to have a movie, television, or sports star's pet as a patient. Most of the time it's the star's personal assistant who brings the animal, but on occasion, a big-name celebrity would personally come in with a pet. While animal patients are not covered under HIPAA, their medical information is still protected by law in many states, including California. It was hospital policy to respect their privacy, and it was forbidden, under any circumstance, to ask for an autograph or photo.

My first appointment of the morning—an emergency walk-in—was probably one of the biggest celebrities in town, having been featured on television commercials all over the world. In the past few days it was impossible to turn on the television and not see this celebrity, perhaps multiple times on multiple stations. And New Year's Day called for several guest appearances, most notably at the 77th annual Rose Bowl Parade and the championship football game in Pasadena. I'm talking about the bull terrier Spuds MacKenzie, the mascot for Bud Light. In actuality, Spuds, who played a "he" on television, was a she.

The white-and-black terrier came in extremely lethargic with a fever of 104.5 degrees; by contrast, a normal temperature for a dog is rarely ever over 102.5 degrees. The owner brought in Spuds because she had refused to eat breakfast, something she never did.

As I conducted my initial exam I noticed makeup leftover from her appearances the day before: Spuds's TV look was slightly exaggerated by the face paint. All the while, poor Spuds just lay on the exam table, too weak to stand. There was not so much as a tail wag from the world-famous party animal.

We took blood and determined that she was dehydrated. Too much activity and not enough to drink—water, not beer. After reviewing my findings with the owner, he agreed to let me keep the celebrity overnight for IV fluid therapy and some much-needed R & R away from the lights, cameras, and action.

Spuds's dad wanted to know what security we had to ensure her safety. I told him that we had a whole-building security system, that we were silent-wired to the 911 operators and, more importantly, we had two people on premises all night. I also told him that if he did not let anyone know that Spuds was here, there should be no one coming around asking for him. I let him know that he could come visit or call any time. He thanked me profusely and kissed the very despondent Spuds on the top of her head before leaving.

After the owner left, Stacey and I got Spuds started on treatments. As soon as we got the exhausted superstar in her cage, she fell fast asleep.

I stood in front of the cage watching my patient. Robert came up and broke my reverie. "How do you know that's the real Spuds MacKenzie?"

I started to answer, then stopped myself. He was right. How did we know this was the real Spuds MacKenzie? Couldn't anyone with a white female bull terrier paint up their dog to look like the celebrity and take it to a party? They would for sure be the hit of the event. Not only that, but I had a suspicion that Spuds, like most other animal TV stars, was not unique—that Budweiser used a number of Spuds look-alikes for marketing at parties all around the country at the same time.

What a buzzkill. I could be staring at a fake Spuds.

Then again, what did it matter if this was the real Spuds or not? The poor dog was really sick, and helping her was my number one priority.

"You're right, Robert." I looked at my tattooed kennel helper. "I have no idea."

The only hospitalized patients were the big snake and Spuds MacKenzie, so morning rounds did not take long. We rechecked Spuds's blood test, and although she was looking and acting more alive this morning, her kidney values were still high as a result of dehydration. I called the owner to give him an update, and although I knew that he really wanted to take Spuds home today, I recommended he let us keep the celebrity dog on IV fluids for at least one more night.

The handler agreed, knowing that it was in the best interest of his megastar. He did say, however, that he was really hoping that Spuds would be back up to speed, because she had a series of appearances coming up to start promoting the Super Bowl at the end of the month in Minnesota.

The owner certainly talked like his dog was the real Spuds MacKenzie.

♦ ♦ ♦

That Saturday was Brenna's real last day. I had her call the big snake's owner with an update, and also Mrs. Shaughnessy to check on Bouquet. The obese skunk with the bad heart was doing spectacularly, and the wealthy owner was thrilled. She told Brenna that she was planning on getting a new skunk and would send pictures. Before hanging up, Mrs. Shaughnessy reminded Brenna to forward all of her book receipts so she could pay for them as promised.

I was sitting in my office upstairs finishing my records when Lisa paged. "Dr. Mader, you gotta come down here!" I could hear the smile in her voice.

I made it down the center stairway to find a huge crowd of staffers and others in the receptionist area. Spuds's owner was up front with two drop-dead-gorgeous Budweiser cheerleaders, or Spudettes, as they were called, in full costume. They each had several goody bags in their arms. In addition, there was a man taking photographs of the hospital, girls, and staff.

Spuds was sitting on one of the benches, and my employees were taking turns being photographed with him. On either side was a Spudette. Once each employee finished getting their picture taken, one of the beautiful models would give them a goody bag filled with Spuds merchandise (stuffed Spuds MacKenzie dolls, sunglasses, T-shirts, etc.). I made sure that Brenna got in there for a photo and Spuds memorabilia as well.

After the impromptu festivities, Spuds and his entourage headed out. His owner said that they would be sending us the photographs in the next few days, and we could use them however we chose. He did ask, however, that we not mention that Spuds had to spend any sick time in the hospital.

Fair enough.

"So," I said to Robert, stopping him as the party was breaking up, "do you still think that was *not* the real Spuds MacKenzie?"

◆ ◆ ◆

Saturday was a carnival, but Sunday was a circus.

William "Big Mac" MacDonald, our newest student, arrived late in the afternoon, about the time that the technician shifts were changing. I suspect that the day shift was in a hurry to get home and did not spend much time briefing Mac when he arrived. Instead, they just gave him a key to the building and took off. Greg was working the night shift, but since Mac had arrived before the day techs left, he had assumed that they had instructed the new student on what to do and what not to do.

In his midforties, Mac was older than most other veterinary students. He had served twenty years in the army before entering veterinary school, using his G.I. Bill to pay for tuition. He was called "Big Mac" because he towered well over six feet tall and weighed at least 250 pounds.

A perfect storm of errors led to my pager going off around 10:30 p.m.

I got the page from Steve, the owner of the alarm company, not someone from the night shift. Action Alarm had received notification of a perimeter violation at the hospital around 10:15. Following proper protocols, the alarm company had called the office to see if the alarm was real or false. If the latter, the person answering the call would give the alarm company the safe word and the alarm would be turned off. If no one answered, or if the person answering did not know the safe word, the alarm company both responded in person and also called 911 to solicit police assistance.

I arrived at the hospital in a flash to find the building surrounded by police cars and flashing lights. Immediately my heart was in the back of my throat. Where was Greg? Why didn't he call me? Where was the student?

To my shock, as I approached the building I saw a large, older man wearing only his underwear, sitting on the stairs leading up to the office and apartments, being questioned by two policemen.

Steve from the alarm company stopped me just before I entered. "I think it's a false alarm. Just a big misunderstanding." I didn't recognize Steve when I first arrived, as I rarely saw him at night when he wasn't wearing his hat, face mask, and gloves. He was an interesting character—an albino with a condition called cutaneous porphyria—also known as "vampire disease." People with porphyria suffer when exposed to daylight, so during the day Steve always covered his head, hands, and any exposed skin.

I thanked Steve for paging me, and he introduced me to the supervising officer on the scene. "Do you know this individual?" the officer asked, referring to the nearly naked man sitting on my stairs.

"The honest answer is 'no,' but I can make an educated guess." I smiled. "Are you William MacDonald?"

"Yes!" William tried to stand, but an officer pushed him back down on the steps. It was cold, and he was only wearing his skivvies. The front door was open, and I am sure he was freezing.

"It's okay. He's my new student."

"Are you sure, Doctor?" The senior cop reached out and touched my shoulder, as if in a tacit warning not to approach the stranger. "He didn't seem to know much about what he was doing here."

I was tempted to drag out the scenario, but I figured the poor guy should have a chance to get some clothes on. "Can you please let him get dressed?" I asked.

"If you're sure, then, yes."

Just about then Greg walked up. He asked what was going on and then provided his side of the story. After finishing his evening treatments, Greg had told Mac that he had to run over to the university library to check out a book he needed for a class. His leaving was not against protocol: I had mandated that there always be at least one person in the hospital at all times, so it wasn't uncommon for the night technician to leave for a moment to run out and get food or fulfill an errand. It was fine as long as the student was in the building.

Greg, however, had turned on the alarm when he left the hospital. The alarm was sensitive to both motion and the door opening or closing. If you left the building the alarm would not trigger. However, if you entered the building without typing the code on the keypad within forty-five seconds, the alarm would go off. It was a silent alarm, so a person triggering it would not know they'd done so until the police arrived or they got a call from the alarm company.

Greg had assumed that the day technicians had properly informed Mac about how to disable the alarm. They hadn't. Mac, not knowing that he was not supposed to leave when no one else was in the building, decided to walk down the street to get some fast food. When he returned shortly after 10:00 p.m., he entered the building through the front door with his key. Not realizing that he was supposed to enter the security code on the keypad, he set off the silent alarm. The "break-in" seemed legitimate when he failed to answer the phone call from the alarm company. Even if he had answered, he wouldn't have known the safe word.

Unaware of all this, Mac had shed his clothes as soon as he got back to the apartment in anticipation of taking a shower before going to bed. The next thing he knew, a police dog came running upstairs, cornering him in the back of the student's living room. With his military training, he knew enough not to move. Within moments two police officers, guns drawn, ran into the room, called off the dog, and forced him to lie on the floor until the police backup arrived.

Welcome to NAVH!

♦ ♦ ♦

My first patient visit of the day called for me to give a second opinion on an iguana with "mental distress." That was a new one to me. Physical stress was certainly a huge problem with captive exotic patients. But mental distress? Did the iguana need a psychiatrist?

Before I entered the room I took a look at the chart. On the "new client" form the owner had filled in "movie producer" as his occupation. In addition, there were some patient medical records from a veterinarian in Hollywood whom I knew practiced good, solid medicine.

"I'm Dr. Mader, and this is my senior student, Mac," I said after walking in and extending my hand to the couple in front of me, my new clients. The man whom I assumed to be the husband was bedecked in multiple gold chains around his neck and wrists, and he wore an ostentatious gold Rolex watch. He had a five-o'clock shadow that looked to be deliberate and was wearing a diamond earring in his left lobe.

The woman was wearing skintight white jeans hung low on her hips, with matching Salvatore Ferragamo shoes, belt, and sunglasses. A midriff-cut, sheer-white, deep-V-neck blouse exposed ample, braless cleavage, and a small gold ring pierced her belly button. Her breasts were accented by imprints of small, circular nipple rings readily apparent through the thin fabric.

At the center of attention was a pale, rust-colored, three-foot-long iguana, coiled up like an apostrophe on the exam table. The iguana, like the male owner, was also wearing a gold chain around its neck.

"I'm René." The man spoke first.

"And I'm Lana, and this is Iggy," the woman added with a smile.

"A pleasure to meet you both. I understand that Iggy is having some mental distress?" I could clearly see that its posture wasn't normal. An iguana should not be curled up like a snake. In addition, green iguanas get their name because they are green. This animal was clearly the color of rust, like an old nail that had been left out in the rain. Not a good sign.

"It's a long story, Doc." The man opened the conversation. "We took him to a doctor up in Hollywood because he wasn't feeling well. We noticed he wasn't eating, and his color changed."

"Okay," I said as I reached down and gently lifted the iguana from the table. As soon as I did, I noticed that its toes started to twitch, as if it were playing an air piano. "So where does the mental distress come in?"

"Look at her!" Lana blurted out, almost yelling. She reached into her purse and grabbed a tissue. "She's all twisted up in a knot." The woman turned her face toward the corner of the room. "I can't even look at her like this."

"Honey, the doctor's going to help." The man reached his arm around her, hugging her tightly.

I gently straightened the lizard while it was resting on the exam table. As soon as I relaxed my grip, it would coil back up in a circle, as if spring-loaded. It was clear to me what was going on before I finished my exam, but I still did not understand the talk of mental distress.

"Lana and René, if I may, I'd like to get some X-rays and a blood test on Iggy to help confirm my diagnosis. May I have your permission to do that?"

"Only if I can come with you!" the woman nearly screamed as she turned to face me. Mac was standing quietly in the back of the room like a soldier poised at attention.

"I'm afraid that's not possible for the X-rays, ma'am." I was still holding the iguana. "State law does not allow an owner to be in the X-ray room while

X-rays are being taken." I made sure that she saw how gently I was holding Iggy. "But you can come back with me. I'll show you the room, demonstrate how we take X-rays, then ask you to step out momentarily while I expose the film. The moment after, you can come back in to be with Iggy."

"That will be fine, Doctor," René assured me. "Won't it, honey?"

"What about the blood test?" She was clearly crying now. "That is so dangerous!"

"No, ma'am. I assure you, it's very safe."

"That's the problem, Doc." René stepped closer to me, as if attempting a private, man-to-man conversation. "That's why Iggy's so stressed. The last veterinarian, who claimed to be an expert, was too rough when he got the blood sample, and now look at him." He pointed to the coiled lizard.

"How about we go get the X-ray first; there's no stress involved whatsoever. Then, after we all look at the X-rays, if you'll let me, I'll take the blood sample myself. I've done it literally thousands of times, and you're welcome to watch how gentle I am." I bent over and spoke to Iggy: "I promise, it won't hurt at all."

"Okay." Lana grabbed another tissue from her purse. "Just go do it." She flicked her wrist like she was waving away a fly. "I trust you. Get the damn X-rays!"

"Okay, we'll be right back." I nodded to René and turned to leave.

"Just don't hurt him!" she admonished.

I had Mac help Stacey get the X-rays. As I anticipated, Iggy was female, not a male as the owners thought, and she was full of eggs.

"I have good news for you," I announced as Mac and I reentered the room with Iggy. Lana grabbed the lizard out of my arms and started hugging and kissing it on the lips.

"Please, tell us the good news, Doctor." René reached over and touched my shoulder.

"Well, to start with"—I put on my happy face smile—"Iggy is *not* a he. Iggy is a she!"

"*What?*" they exclaimed in unison.

"How can that be?" Lana challenged.

I showed them Iggy's X-ray and pointed out the eggs in her belly with the tip of my pen. They were obvious, but for emphasis I started counting. I stopped the pen at thirty and looked directly at Lana. "These are all eggs." I gave her a how-dare-you-question-me look.

"Iggy is definitely a female."

"That's just not possible!" She stepped close to the bright fluorescent viewing box, as if I might have switched X-rays on her.

"He, ah, she has *never* been with a boy! How could *she* be pregnant?" Lana looked at me, incredulous. I could tell that even René was stumped.

"Iguanas are like chickens," I explained. Mac was paying close attention as well. "Once they reach maturity, they start laying eggs. They don't need to be with a male." I pointed to Iggy's swollen belly. "They only need the male for the eggs to become fertile."

"Oh my God!" Lana hugged Iggy up to her face and once again turned away from us toward the corner.

"I still need to confirm why she's having problems being coiled up."

"It's because the other asshole vet stressed her getting the blood test!" Lana turned back to face me.

I did not like to hear any badmouthing of veterinarians, especially since I knew the other vet well, and he was a good doctor. "I'm confident that the other vet didn't cause this." Tentatively, I reached out to take Iggy from the owner. "Please allow me to get some blood." Reluctantly, she handed me the twisted iguana.

"He never did get the blood, Doc." This time when René spoke I could hear a bit of an edge to his voice. "He tried a number of times, and I think that is why she's so stressed." He looked at me. "He must've poked her with the big needle at least a dozen times. Is this really necessary?"

"No and yes." I looked directly at René. "I'm pretty certain what's wrong, but I really prefer to have proper documentation of Iggy's calcium status before starting her on supplementation." I took a syringe out of my pocket. "I'd like your permission to do what I need to do so that I can give her the best possible treatment."

"You're the doc." He flicked his hand at me like Lana had before. "Do what you gotta do."

"Do you want me to do it here with you watching, or do you want me to take her to my treatment area? Your call."

"Here," the man commanded. "I want to watch."

"I can't watch!" Lana turned back into the corner of the room, staring at the floor and covering her ears. Iguanas don't vocalize like cats or dogs, so I'm not sure why she did that.

I placed a soft towel on the table and had Mac hold Iggy on the edge with her tail hanging over the side. I knelt down, used a very small needle to collect my sample from a vein on the underside of the tail, and then stood up.

"All done!" I was thankful it had gone so smoothly.

"That's it?" René was surprised.

"She's . . . she's done? I didn't even hear anything." Lana picked up the lizard and continued hugging and kissing it where she had left off moments before.

"Yup." I smiled. I showed her the syringe full of purple-red blood. Just as I was about to hand the syringe to Mac, Stacey opened the door and grabbed it. I looked at her. How did she always do that?

"You didn't even turn Iggy on her back to get the blood." René remained surprised at how simple the procedure was.

"I never do. They're more comfortable in their natural position."

I explained to them that Iggy's twitching and coiling were likely hypocalcemia, or dangerously low blood calcium levels. In captivity, this was often secondary to improper housing and poor nutrition and was complicated by being full of eggs—the body needs extra calcium to produce the shells.

René and Lana seemed insulted by my explanation. Defensively, they protested that the lizard lived in a huge room in their Hollywood mansion and got only the best diet. I tried to explain that iguanas in the wild lived in ninety-plus-degree weather in the direct sunshine, not behind a big picture window, and ate fresh flowers and leaves all day long. The direct sunshine enhanced the lizard's natural vitamin D production, and the natural diet provided all the necessary vitamins and minerals, like calcium, that the iguana needed to not only grow but to reproduce and lay eggs.

I'm sure that in their minds they were doing what was best for their lizard, and I was not about to argue with them. Instead, I gave them some handouts I'd made for the herpetology society on iguana care, along with a prescription for a calcium supplement. It was the same prescription I had given Mikey the monkey.

Finally, I told Lana and René I'd call them in a couple of days when the test results came back from the lab, and that unless they planned on actually breeding Iggy—which I thought was a bad idea—they should consider having her spayed like a puppy or kitten.

As I'd anticipated, the mere idea of surgery was met with immediate negativity. At least I had planted the thought. The best hope for this iguana was to get it fixed—have her ovaries and uterus removed. That way, this problem would never happen again.

I escorted them to the reception area, stayed with them until they paid, and then walked them out to their red Ferrari.

I called Iggy's owners the next day and informed them that, as suspected, her calcium levels were dangerously low. René told me that after ingesting the calcium supplements, Iggy already looked a lot better and was nowhere near as crooked as yesterday.

I reiterated that they really should consider having her spayed so that this problem would never happen again. René said he would talk it over with Lana and let me know. I alerted him that I was leaving in a couple of days to lecture at a conference in Florida, but we could schedule the surgery for when I got back.

Before I left for the day I stopped by the operatory to check in on Cliff. He was just finishing a declaw procedure on a young kitten and was putting bandages on the front feet. I noticed the removed claws on the surgery table, scooped them up, and tossed them in the trash.

"What are you doing?" Cliff looked up at me over his surgical mask. He liked to draw pictures on the front of his facemask. Today he was a rat.

"Just cleaning up." I looked at him. I don't like leaving anything that isn't sterile on the surgical table. He seemed a little put out that I had touched his cat claws.

"Don't toss those. Robert collects them."

"What?"

"Robert saves the claws."

"Why?" This was the first I'd heard of it.

"He gives them to a witch who grinds them up and makes powders and potions with them." Cliff stated this as if it were a normal thing to do.

I should not have been surprised. I knew that Robert was a devil worshiper. One look at his tattoos had told me that. But I didn't know he actually dabbled in the dark arts.

That said, I was not too happy to think that some necromancer was taking discarded body parts from our hospital and using them to make potions. How would that look if it ever got out to the newspapers? I could see the headline: "Noah's Ark Vets Sell Patients' Body Parts to Local Sorcerer."

"I didn't know about this." I had expected to just check up on Cliff's surgery, but now I was glad that I had come in to talk to him.

"Fred, did—"

"I didn't know anything about it, Dr. Mader," Fred said, cutting me off, and then immediately left the room.

Liar.

"I can't allow this to continue." I put on my boss tone of voice. "No more giving Robert body parts." I waited for Cliff to look up, but he deliberately avoided eye contact. "In fact, all body tissues must be disposed of in biohazard bags, understood?" I turned my head toward the surgery prep area. "That goes for you too, Fred."

◆ ◆ ◆

My God, the conference was huge. I had first attended the North American Veterinary Conference in 1988 when it was nowhere near this large. It had grown logarithmically over the past few years, with more than 4,000 people at the meeting. My lectures were filled to capacity, with nearly 250 attendees in the rooms.

I love going to conferences. I love teaching and learning. I love the face time with all the attendees and my friends.

But I also hate coming back to a mountain of work and a whole bunch of little brush fires that need extinguishing. Such is life.

I arrived at work extra early on my first day back, intending to riffle through the stack of messages that always awaited my return. To my surprise, when I walked into the reception area René, Lana, and Iggy were waiting.

"Morning, Doctor." René stood and extended his arm. Lana then stood, Iggy clinging to her shoulder and, without saying a word, came over and gave me a big hug.

"Morning." I felt her perfume already clinging to my surgical scrubs.

"I didn't expect to see you here today." I reached out and scratched the back of Iggy's neck.

"We decided just to get this done," René stated in his subdued tone. "Do you think this surgery is really necessary, Doctor?" Lana still did not say a word.

"Yes, I do. Iggy's body is in crisis. It's a common consequence of living in captivity in Southern California. This may be the place for beautiful beach bodies, but not tropical lizards." As soon as I said this, I realized that it might have come across as an insult.

"The lack of equatorial sun and natural diet is a killer. Our only equalizer is to remove her reproductive tract, the source of the body's largest demand for calcium."

"And you are sure that she will be okay. She will live?" René looked me directly in the eyes. Lana looked up momentarily, then went back to petting Iggy.

"I never make guarantees in medicine." I held out my left arm and exposed all the surgical scars running the length of my arm. "I'm fit, not a big drinker, don't do drugs. When I went in for my surgery, I still had to sign a statement that I might not wake up from anesthesia." I held up my arm even higher. Lana reached out with her fingers and gently traced her manicured nails down the ugly scars on my arm.

"My point is, I had surgery for a traumatic wound, but my body was healthy. Iggy, unfortunately, is very ill. So she's at much greater anesthetic risk than, say, a young iguana coming in for a routine spay."

Lana turned away.

"I don't know, Doctor," René spoke in a whisper. "Maybe we shouldn't do this." He reached over and put his arm around Lana, pulling her and Iggy closer. "Are you *sure* that there is nothing else we can do?"

"You've had her on calcium supplements the whole time I was gone and she's still not eating, right?" I paused, then added, "And she isn't going to lay those retained eggs. So regardless of whether or not you have her spayed, she is going to need at least a C-section."

They whispered to each other for a moment. Finally, Lana spoke. "And you've done these before?"

"Many." I spoke with confidence. "If I don't know how to do something, I'm the first to admit it. I have no problem referring a procedure out to someone with more experience."

"Okay. We trust you." Lana handed me Iggy. Her eyes welled up with tears, causing her makeup to start running at the corners. Stacey appeared out of nowhere and handed them a clipboard with several forms they needed to fill out.

Just as I was about to take Iggy to the surgical suite, Lana cried out, "Stop!" It was so loud that it startled Mai Tai, who let out a deafening scream. At first I thought she was going to change her mind again. Instead, she stepped over and gave Iggy a big kiss on the top of her green head, leaving a bright red lipstick mark where her lips contacted the scales. Then she looked up, leaned over, and gave me a kiss on the cheek. It happened so fast I didn't have time to react.

"Please take good care of her, Doctor."

"Of course, Lana." I stepped back.

"I have a mobile phone," René said as he pulled his black leather phone from his man purse. "I'll give you the number. We're not leaving town. We'll just go get some breakfast and stay close by."

I told them about Lili's Country Kitchen. They thanked me many times and stepped out.

I had several surgeries on my list that were awaiting my return, but I promised René and Lana that I would do Iggy's surgery first. Big Mac helped Fred prep the iguana. I had done literally hundreds of these procedures, but I never took them for granted, no matter how common. No two surgeries are ever the same.

Using the radio scalpel, I cut through the gray-green scales covering Iggy's belly. Once I opened the body cavity, I was shocked to see not only dozens of eggs as expected but several eggs that had ruptured. This had not shown up on the original X-rays, so it must have happened during the week I was gone. The simple twenty-minute procedure instantly morphed into a nightmare. Instead of performing a quick spay as I had hoped, I had to deal with a yellow, gelatinous goo gluing all the internal parts together.

Fortunately, it went well and I was able to remove all the bad eggs and even clean away all the gross, thick yellow soup. Iggy looked pathetically skinny lying on the recovery table now that all that badness had been taken out. I had removed a total of fifty-two eggs from her swollen belly.

As soon as she was awake enough to swallow, I had Big Mac and Stacey give her some warm vegetable soup spiked with extra calcium. It had been a long time since she had eaten anything substantial, and she badly needed the calories.

The entire procedure took a little over an hour. Rather than call the owners right away, I decided to wait to make sure she was stable, as I knew that they would want to come see her.

Fred and I completed the remaining procedures on my schedule. As I was finishing up my last surgery Lisa came to me and said, "Those wacky Hollywood people have called multiple times!" She handed me a piece of paper with their mobile phone number scribble on it. "Can you please give them a call so I can get some work done?"

"Of course." I went over to the exotics cage and checked on Iggy. She looked good considering what she had just endured.

"By the way," Lisa laughed, pointing at my face, "you've got lipstick on your cheek."

◆ ◆ ◆

It was a red-letter day. Ellen and I actually had a night off at the same time. It wasn't by accident—she had to swap shifts with another nurse—but it was worth it. Dave had a performance at the Magic Castle in Hollywood. He was appearing in the Close-Up Room and got us two VIP guest passes to come see his act. Not only was the Magic Castle exclusive, it was also black-tie. A date night, a visit to a private club with Hollywood's beautiful people, and a chance to get dressed up: life didn't get much better.

Just before we were about to leave, I decided to get our picture together wearing our fancy attire. I grabbed my camera, attached it to the tripod, and set the self-timer. Quickly I ran around in front of the camera to stand next to Ellen as the blinking light counted down. A nanosecond before the camera flashed, there was a frantic pounding at our front door.

We both turned to look, and Wok let out a ferocious bark just as the flash fired. We looked at each other, tacitly asking whether we were expecting anyone. A quick shrug of the shoulders, and I headed up the hall to the continuous pounding at the door.

I peered through the security port, Wok growling by my side. It was still light out, but I could not see anything, as if someone was deliberately blocking the viewer.

"Who is it?" I called through the door.

"It's Norbert. I need to know what this is." A high-pitched, cranky voice echoed from outside the front door. Norbert was our obnoxious neighbor from three doors down. He had an ancient, severely arthritic Dalmatian that was covered with fatty tumors. I had spoken with him on several occasions about bringing his dog by my office so I could evaluate the tumors and, if needed, remove them. At least, if nothing else, I could also prescribe medication for the arthritis.

His response was always the same. "He's just a dog. I ain't spendin' no money on him." Then he would wave his arm as if brushing off the very notion of veterinary care.

I opened the door in my tuxedo, my beautiful wife standing behind me in a gorgeous dress, and there, in my face, was Norbert holding a clear baggie filled with bloody feces.

"What's this?" Norbert barked. Not a hello, how are you, you look marvelous, anything. Just a bag full of poop in my face.

"Looks like shit." I wasn't too pleased by this intrusion. Usually I would help any of my neighbors at any time. But Norbert was not a close friend, and it certainly was not an appropriate time. "What do you expect me to do with it?"

"You're a vetranarian," he said, mispronouncing the noun.

"Norbert, I'm about to head out." I turned and gestured to my wife.

"I'm not equipped at the moment to evaluate your dog's feces, nor am I planning on heading into work any time soon."

"Can't you give me somethin' for him?" He lifted the bag closer to my face. Norbert was probably in his late seventies, in dog years about the same age as his charge. He had been a smoker his entire life, and his face was badly wrinkled, his sclera and teeth both yellow, and there were a number of ominous skin tags on his balding pate.

I was really irritated. He never so much as nodded hello when we saw him outside, yet here he was on a Saturday evening, just as we were about to go out, holding a bag full of bloody dog excrement in my personal space.

"Norbert," I said, pushing the bag away, "I am leaving my house right now. Put the baggie in your refrigerator, and on Monday morning drop it off at my office. I'll have it evaluated and, if necessary, will bring some medicine home for your dog." The dog was sitting patiently by the owner's side. When I said "dog," he gave a little wag of his old graying tail.

"So you ain't gonna do anything?"

"Give him some Kaopectate, one tablespoon every six hours." I started to close the door in his face. "And bring the sample *to my office* Monday morning." I shut the door.

"Oh my God!" Ellen and I both laughed.

I looked out the peephole to make sure he was gone. Once satisfied that the way was clear, we headed out for our night of magic.

◆ ◆ ◆

Dave greeted Ellen and me at the door of the Magic Castle and escorted us inside. We were treated like VIPs by all the employees. The three of us sat at a large, round table with a half dozen others, all magicians and their guests, and by the end of the repast, we felt as if we'd been friends forever.

Afterward we got a tour of the castle and, finally, attended Dave's magic show, sitting in the front of the small, intimate room. It was incredible to watch the transformation on stage of this man, whom I had only ever seen while working with wildlife, as he put on a spectacular performance. I acquired a whole new respect for Dave.

On Monday morning when I left for work I just about tripped going out my door. There, on the top step, was a baggie full of bloody feces. Norbert!

◆ ◆ ◆

Mr. Knight and Cindy were not on the schedule for her weekly allergy shot, which was odd since he never missed their appointments. I asked Lisa to call the older gentleman to see if he was okay.

I finally got a chance to sit down with Robert and talk about the cat claws. He was truly apologetic. He had reckoned that since we were throwing the claws away, it would be okay to take them.

Mac took the Christmas snake out of its cage that morning, and it actually put up a fight, not wanting to be restrained. This was the most activity that we had seen from it since it had arrived almost a month ago. The python was still receiving daily fluids and antibiotics via IV, and we had been assist-feeding it with a six-foot-long stomach tube used for treating horses. The snake was gaining strength, starting to crawl in a straight line, and had put on several pounds.

"Do you de-scent skunks?" Lisa asked me after I finished struggling with the large python.

"Why?" I felt like I had done my workout for the day. Wrestling 110 pounds of muscle made me realize that I had not been to the gym since Mort's stay with us. "Why?" I repeated.

"Mrs. Shaughnessy got a new . . . kit, I think she called it."

"A kit is a baby skunk." I had a sudden flash of dread. "Did Bouquet die?"

"No!" She smiled. "In fact, she said that Bouquet was doing marvelous and she loves you for it. She just wanted to get a new baby, realizing that Bouquet will not be here forever."

It is illegal to keep skunks as pets in California. As with ferrets, however, it is not illegal for a veterinarian to treat them. I really have no problem treating any animal if it is ill or injured, but there is that fine line between treating a sick animal that's illegal to own and performing elective procedures, like spays and neuters, for it. I think most people would consider de-scenting a skunk to be over the line.

"Tell her I'll do it." I shook my head, knowing that I shouldn't, but Mrs. Shaughnessy had treated Brenna so well, how could I say no? "She needs to bring the skunk in *after hours*, to the back door. She can call us from her mobile phone when she arrives, and we will meet her outside in the wildlife yard."

◆ ◆ ◆

"Where were you last week, Cindy?" I rubbed the little dog's head. Her tail was wagging at hyper speed. As always, I addressed my first comments to the poodle. "You had us all worried when you didn't show up and we couldn't get ahold of you!"

"Oh, Doc Mader, I'm so embarrassed," Mr. Knight spoke. "I just, plain and simple, forgot to make my appointment."

"No worries, Mr. Knight." I shook his arthritic hand, the one he used to push the walker. He always held Cindy in his good arm.

"You are always so busy!" I was trying to make light of his overlooking his regular time slot. "My gosh, we all forget things."

"Yeah, that's nice of you to say." He looked down at his companion. "But I've been forgetting a lot lately." He looked back up at me. I could definitely see that he had aged since we first met. "I'm just getting old."

"Nonsense! You are more spry than most of my young employees. I don't know how you do it!" Stacey came in the room and handed me Cindy's allergy injection.

"I'll tell you what. I know how busy you are taking care of your mother and Cindy. Why don't I have one of my girls give you a call every Monday to remind you of your appointment the next morning?"

"Oh, that would be lovely, Dr. Mader." He looked his little poodle in the face. "Isn't that a good idea, Cindy?"

"Woof!"

• • •

"I think I'm going to need some help."

CDFG officer Kelly Pinkett did not look the part. The young, attractive, green-eyed blond resembled more a character from an action TV show than a real-life, gun-toting crime fighter. She had a natural beauty, wore no makeup, and her skin showed none of the typical signs of someone who worked outside in the Southern California sun. But the cargo pants, long-sleeved shirt replete with official patches on the shoulders, gun belt, and Kevlar vest painted a different picture.

She was struggling to hold on to a large dog carrier. The front bars were covered with a bloody towel.

"I've got a badly hurt fox," she announced. "I'm not sure if it can be saved."

I was working in the treatment room when they entered with the large cage.

"Hi, Doc!" Kelly was always cheerful. Even the day she saw the bald eagle feather tacked to the corkboard in my office, she smiled as she advised me I could go to jail for having part of a federally protected species in my possession.

"This little bugger didn't hear the 'Fore!' at the country club and got smacked right in the middle of its front leg. I think it's shattered." She slowly lifted the towel covering the carrier. "I'm not sure if you can fix it."

Cowering in the back of the carrier was an adult red fox. Its face was smeared with both fresh and clotted blood, giving it the look of one of those rabid, dog-like creatures from a horror movie that attack innocent children in the middle of the night.

The left front leg was grotesquely twisted near the shoulder, and approximately two inches of bloodstained, ivory-colored bone protruded through the skin.

"What's the chance of it having rabies?" I did not want to put any of my staff, or myself, at risk.

"Virtually zero." Kelly said, straight-faced. "I wouldn't have brought it here if there was."

"I figured. Just had to ask." Stacey handed me a flashlight. She always knew what I needed.

I shone the light on the fox's injured leg. The lower limb still looked viable, but the fracture itself was another story. The wound was obviously traumatic, and it appeared that some pieces of shattered bone were missing.

"I'll need to get some X-rays, but I'm pretty sure I can fix it." I handed the flashlight to Big Mac so he could get a better look. "But the real question is, why?"

"That's a toughie, Doc." I could sense it was a contentious point. "Normally we would not treat an injured fox. We would just have it humanely euthanized."

"This animal was injured at the country club. The injury was witnessed by some very wealthy, very politically connected individuals." Kelly spoke in a squeamish tone. "The guy who hit it feels super guilty and is offering to pay whatever it costs to fix it."

"Yeah, but this is not going to be an easy fix." I pointed to the leg. "You are looking at weeks to months for proper healing. Do you think it will be releasable?" I shook my head in the negative. "I don't."

"I agree." She grimaced. "But the upper-ups, the movers and shakers at CDFG, the ones who tee off with the country clubbers, are getting pressure and want it fixed. It's a PR thing now."

"Okay. Leave it with me. I'll see what I can do."

"You have to save it, Doc." Kelly flashed one of her killer smiles. "You're the best."

After Kelly left we sedated the fox to evaluate the injury. X-rays revealed a shattered humerus, the largest bone on the upper part of the front leg.

The damage was worse than I had initially assessed. The bone was fragmented into a dozen or more pieces right in the middle of the shaft. I estimated that a good inch or two of bone was missing where the sharp edges of the break poked grotesquely through the muscle and skin.

This did not look like a blunt projectile injury to me, as an errant golf ball would inflict. I suspected that the fox, probably looking for a handout, had gotten too close to one of the golfers at the course and was struck by a mighty swing of a club.

Regardless, I was looking at an orthopedic mess. If this were a dog, I was sure that I could repair the break. However, healing time would be prolonged. The golden rule of wildlife medicine is get them in and out as quickly as possible. This was not going to be "quickly."

I got to work before sunrise the next day and went upstairs to my office where I could have some quiet time to ponder what needed to be done. I just didn't feel right about repairing the fracture. The sad reality was it was a red fox, the most common fox on the planet. There were too many red foxes in captivity, and even if I repaired the leg, no zoo would take it.

It was a remarkably clear morning. From my window I could look out over the city and watch the sunrise above the snow-covered San Gabriel Mountains to the east. I sat there, staring at the mountains, trying to make a decision on the best course of action. I had briefly chatted with the other docs during daily rounds, and they unanimously agreed that the most humane thing to do would be to euthanize it.

Part of me agreed, but a bigger part of me hates to euthanize anything that has a chance, and besides, I was under advisement from Kelly—representing the CDFG—that they wanted me to "fix it."

I talked with Dave as well, and of course he also wanted me to try to save it. He said he was willing to do the post-fracture-repair rehab work and keep the human contact to a minimum. If anyone could do it, it was Dave.

I was mulling over the situation, gazing out the window through the morning haze at the snow seventy-five miles in the distance, when I remembered a fox I once saw while working in Alaska. I recalled that it was missing a hind foot, and I assumed that it had been caught in a steel leg trap. However, that fox was running around like it didn't have a care in the world.

By the time I got downstairs most of the morning staff had arrived. "We're amputating the leg!" I instructed anyone in the treatment room who would listen.

"What? You can't do that? How is it going to live in the wild?" Cliff was skeptical.

"We see amputee dogs and cats all the time. Tripods do great." I had made up my mind. Kelly asked me to save it. She didn't say I had to save the leg. My promise was "I'll see what I can do," to which her response had been, "You're the best."

That was the only green light I needed.

After rounds, during which I announced my decision and was lambasted by all the other docs, I had Big Mac and Fred prep the fox for surgery. Meanwhile, I called Officer Pinkett to tell her my plan.

"Wow." She seemed a bit shocked by my decision. "I never anticipated that."

"You asked me to save the fox, Kelly," I stated, businesslike, being as objective as possible. "If I repair the fracture, which is a severely, badly damaged bone that has been out in the muck and covered with dirt, and more than likely infected, and if there are no complications with the implant or bone graft, after rehab, we may be lucky to release the animal in at best eight to ten weeks or, realistically, three to four *months*, and then hope that it isn't so imprinted on humans that it goes right back to the country club looking for food because it has forgotten how to hunt." I paused to catch my breath after the super-long sentence.

"If I amputate this leg, the fox will heal and can be released in seven to ten *days*."

There was silence on the other end of the line.

"Well?"

"I'm not so sure that he'll make it in the wild with three legs." Kelly paused. "But you're the doc. That's why we come to you."

As soon as I hung up I went directly to surgery. Dave was in the prep room when I arrived.

"I think this is a great idea, Dr. Mader." Dave gave me both thumbs-up.

"Thanks, Dave." My mind was running ahead of my body, ready for the surgery. "I think you are the only one who's on my side."

As far as surgeries go, the amputation was routine. For all intents and purposes, the small fox was like any of the hundreds of dogs and cats whose limbs I had amputated. The only difference was that where I usually use skin sutures for my final closure of the surgical site, this time I buried absorbable stitches under the skin so that I wouldn't have to catch the fox to take them out when the incision was healed. The less we handled the animal, the better its chances were for survival once released.

Tanya and the Snake

The big buzz of the morning was that the infamous Rodney King police beating trial was supposed to start today in Simi Valley. It was all the news stations could talk about, and even Mark and Brian, the sunrise radio goofballs on KLOS, normally wild and crazy, were all serious about the onset of the trial over this racially charged incident.

Four white Los Angeles police officers were accused of beating a black motorist, Rodney King, after a traffic stop. Further consternation had arisen when the courts transferred the location of the trial to the affluent and predominantly white city of Simi Valley, north of Los Angeles. Few people thought it would be a fair trial, but hope remained that the court proceedings would be just and there would not be any repercussions in the streets.

Tanya, our new student, came to us from Tuskegee University's College of Veterinary Medicine, the nation's first and only African American veterinary college. It opened in 1945 and has since graduated over 70 percent of all African American veterinarians in the United States. Tanya's parents lived in South Central Los Angeles, so she passed on using our student apartment and opted to stay with her family, even though it meant a daily fifteen-mile drive south on the horrific 405 freeway.

"Don't you know that black people don't like snakes!" were Tanya's first words when she met the large python.

I wasn't sure how to respond.

"But," she paused, "that's why I'm here. I gotta learn." She bent down close to the cage. "I just figured my first snake would be, oh, like a foot long or something."

She clearly had a good sense of humor.

The big constrictor was getting stronger every day. It was still on IV fluids, antibiotics, and vitamins, and with us assist-feeding it with the horse tube every three days, it was gaining about a pound a week. It still had a long way to go, but it already looked like a different snake from the one that arrived on Christmas morning.

Dave had set the fox up in our largest wildlife enclosure in the backyard. He covered the front of the cage with cardboard so that it could not see people and arranged schedules so that he was the only one to care for it.

I filled Tanya in on the fox's situation, both medically and politically. We went out to the wildlife yard and peeked through a small portal that Dave had vented into the cardboard. The fox was standing in the corner, chomping on a mouse that had been tossed into the cage moments before.

We were able to medicate the patient by hiding the drugs in its food. A small doggy door connected the fox's run with the adjacent cage. There was no need to handle the fox, and it had virtually no human interaction.

I called Officer Pinkett with an update. Her response was anything but expected. "My supervisor is not too happy with me right now." Kelly sounded somber. "They're telling me now to euthanize it."

"Why?" I asked, but I already knew.

"Because they expected that you would fix the leg and we could return it to the country club golf course." Her voice was the edgiest I had ever heard it.

"We can still return it to the golf course!" I was a bit miffed. I had spent many hours worrying about this case and, on my own, had made a difficult decision that would keep the animal alive. I was hoping it might be appreciated.

"I agree with you, Doc." I could hear her swallow. "But the money people, the ones paying for it, were expecting you to fix the fox, not cut off its leg."

"I did fix the fox!" I hoped Kelly realized that I was upset with her supervisor, not with her. "And I won't charge them. Money isn't important—the fox is what matters."

"Between you and me, I think it's because they don't want to see a three-legged fox running around their rich golf course," Kelly stated.

I pondered that for a moment.

"This fox wasn't hit by a golf ball, was it?"

Silence. I continued.

"I think that one of the rich assholes took a whack at the curious little fox, probably at the tee-off area," I continued. "They most likely meant to scare it away but instead smashed the leg." I delayed a moment. "It was witnessed by several people, perhaps even one of the players' wives. Rather than create a big scene, perhaps even have someone press charges for animal cruelty or, worse yet, risk getting kicked out of the country club, Mr. Whacker immediately atoned and offered to pay whatever it costs to make things right. He had friends in high places and his lawyer made some calls, and Officer Kelly Pinkett came to the rescue. . . . How am I doing so far?"

Kelly hadn't said a word. Finally, she acknowledged, "You're not far off."

"So when you told them I was able to save the fox but that I had to amputate the leg," I continued, "of course it couldn't be released back on the course, because it would be a constant reminder of what happened!"

"Bingo." Kelly hesitated. "But you didn't hear it from me."

There was a long silence. "Well, it's too late."

"What do you mean?"

"I've already gone to the paper with the story."

"*What?!*" she almost screamed.

"Not the real story, but the tale of the injured fox, the Good Samaritan who rescued it and offered to pay for its care, and the kindhearted veterinarian who donated his skills to save its life. The reporter already knows that the fox will be returned, in all of its three-legged glory, back to the same golf course!"

"You didn't! Please tell me you didn't." I could almost hear the panic in her voice.

"The reporter even gave it a name: he called it 'Fore the fox.' That's a nice alliteration, don't ya think?" I was really on a roll now.

"I'm screwed." Her voice lowered. "I hope you know that."

I was on the phone all the next morning with the local supervisor for the CDFG as per Officer Pinkett's request. I also ended up calling the local animal control, the director of the country club, and even the golfer who said he would pay for the fox's care.

Mostly I got the same response: "Why couldn't you fix it?" The rich guy even went so far as to tell me about his friend whose dog had broken its leg and his veterinarian had patched him up. If I couldn't fix the fox, I should have sent it to someone with more training.

Explaining the reasoning behind my decision to all the different parties, and in a couple of instances to the same person multiple times, I became a broken record: This was *not* a dog. It may have looked like a dog, but it was a wild fox!

Fortunately, by the end of the day, I was able to wordsmith my way to quelling all concerns about the ability of the fox to adapt back to the wild. I convinced them that being a tripod would actually help bring awareness to the good deed that was done.

"If I released a repaired fox to the course, it might make the country club newsletter the first month it's back. Observing from the sidelines, it will look like any other fox on the course, and in a matter of weeks nobody would know the difference and the whole incident would be forgotten.

"Now, with the tripod 'Fore,' *everybody* will recognize the fox every time they see it, for as long as it's alive, and it will be a celebrity—your new mascot! Imagine the stories that will evolve about how it was injured and then cared for by an animal-loving club member? You can even erect a plaque in the clubhouse documenting the story."

It worked.

I called Kelly and told her the good news.

"After yesterday's phone call, I was going to arrest you for having the bald eagle feathers on your bulletin board," she said. I could once again sense the famous Kelly smile over the phone. "But now I may just look the other way."

After the marathon of phone calls and patient appointments, I finally made it home and started packing for my next lecture trip, which was now just a few days away. With an attendance sometimes exceeding eighty-five hundred people, the Western Veterinary Conference, held annually in Las Vegas, was the largest veterinary continuing education event in the world. This was my first invitation to lecture there, and it was quite an honor.

Fore the fox was continuing to do well per Dave. He had really taken it personally to make sure that Fore was going to be a successful rehabilitation. The plan was to release the fox back to the country club golf course on the Friday after I returned from the conference. Since Dave had been the only one to support me when I made the decision to amputate, I wanted to make sure that he came along for Fore's reintroduction to the wild.

♦ ♦ ♦

I stopped by work to check on my patients on the way to the airport. The large python was continuing to improve. In fact, he was so strong now that I made it mandatory to have at least three people handling the beast. I called René and Lana, the Hollywood producers, to check on Iggy. They reported that the twisted lizard was almost completely straight now and doing well.

Finally, I checked in with Dave and the fox: all looked promising for its release when I returned.

The short flight to Vegas passed quickly. Thankfully I had a seatmate who slept the entire forty-five minutes. The conference was in the legendary Las Vegas Hilton, former Sin City home of Elvis Presley. I was pleasantly surprised by the elegant suite that was provided to me as an invited lecturer.

Monday and Tuesday were busy with lecturing. I finished my eighth hour and was heading back to my room, totally exhausted from standing and talking all day long, when a tall, impeccably dressed gentleman stopped me just outside of the conference room.

"Dr. Mader, I'm Ray Kersey." He handed me his business card. It read "Ray Kersey, W.B. Saunders, A Division of Harcourt Brace & Company, Philadelphia." W.B. Saunders was the largest medical textbook publishing company in the world. "You've had a long two days. May I buy you a drink?"

We did the impossible and found a quiet corner of the casino, and Mr. Kersey treated me to a welcomed ice-cold Diet Coke. "Every time I stopped by your lecture room it was standing room only. I've been waiting to talk with you since yesterday, but you're always surrounded by your fans and I didn't want to interrupt. It's nice to finally meet you." He raised his glass to toast.

"Likewise." I clinked my cola with his tonic water. "What can I do for you?"

"It was the same—standing room only—when I watched you at the North American Conference last month." Ray sat back in his chair. "My job at W.B. Saunders is to recruit new authors. It's clear that you know your stuff, and you have a huge following. I think you'd be a big success as an author."

"I'm honored." I wasn't expecting this. It wasn't uncommon for company reps to approach me and ask if I'd like to try their product, with the ultimate hopes of getting me to endorse it. But that a company as large as W.B. Saunders would want me to write a book?

"We'll give you an advance on the royalties, and whatever support you need."

"When would you need it finished?" I was already doing the mental gymnastics, trying to figure out when I would have time to write it. With the veterinary specialty boards coming up in a few months, there was no way I could begin to think about starting before August.

"It usually takes most authors about two years to write a text." Ray took a sip of his tonic water. "How about fall of '94?"

"That may be tough." I explained about my upcoming exam and that it was my number one priority. "I realistically don't think that I could have it finished until fall of '95 with all that is going on right now."

Ray bowed his head, touching his fingers to his lips in thought, then looked up. "You know, that would be fine." The smile returned. "Having you specialty-boarded makes the book even more impressive." He leaned across the cocktail table and extended his hand. "Let's do it!"

◆ ◆ ◆

I was the one sleeping on the short flight back to LAX this time, I was so exhausted, After landing I walked past several shops on my way to baggage claim. Suddenly something in my peripheral vision caught my attention.

Not quite sure why, I stopped and went back to a newsstand. The story on the top fold of the front page of the local newspaper read "Fore the Fox returns to the country club greens." Half the space was devoted to a color photo of Cliff crouching over a pet carrier and releasing the three-legged fox to freedom with its mouth open and tongue lolling to the side as it dashed out. The fox was also clearly missing a front leg.

"It was a tough decision," the paper quoted Cliff, "and it wasn't popular, but I decided that it was best to amputate the leg and get the fox back out in the wild as soon as possible. I could have fixed the original break, but recovery would have taken weeks to months. I did what I thought was best for the fox."

The article went on to describe the fox's odyssey, from injury to treatment to its relatively quick release. It painted a rosy picture of the generous Good Samaritan at the country club who offered to pay for the fox's care and the heroic efforts of Dr. Cliff Nordic and his team at the Noah's Ark Veterinary Hospital.

There were random quotes from the country club president, the Good Samaritan, Officer Kelly Pinkett, and various club members discussing how important it was to have "Fore" back home on their course. Even Dave had his moment in the spotlight.

"Hey," a gruff voice called out from behind the counter. "This ain't the public library. You wanna read it, you gotta buy it!"

I'd become so livid as I read the news article that I'd almost forgotten it was the day before Valentine's Day. Fortunately, a greeting card stand filled with red-hearted cards and gifts was situated alongside the newspaper rack. Once my seething rage had settled some, I grabbed a card and some candy from the airport shop.

Ellen and I hadn't had any time off together since Willy and I started the hospital over three years earlier. We had been looking to take a trip and finally found a scuba diving vacation to Honduras that seemed like an ideal getaway. I cut out an advertisement from a scuba magazine, slid it inside the card I bought at the airport, and left it and the sweets on the breakfast table with some fresh cut flowers for my lovely, absent Valentine. I hadn't been home in time to see her the previous night before she left for work, and she wasn't back this morning before I left for work, but at least she would know I was thinking about her when she did get home from her overnight shift.

When I arrived at the hospital, my first stop was at the wildlife ward and the empty fox cage. Not sure how I might respond when I saw Cliff, I made an extra effort to take several deep breaths before going inside. Instantly I got the feeling that everybody was afraid to talk to me: the technicians all looked away, as if expecting some sort of gunfight. Regardless, I greeted the staff with a somewhat forced "Good morning" and made my way through the hospital to the conference room. As usual, I was the first to arrive.

The team finally showed up and we had rounds as usual, the doctors filling me in on what happened while I was away. Except about the fox. After rounds were over, I asked Cliff if he could take a minute to talk.

"I've got a ton to do, boss. Can we catch up later?" He looked down at some papers he was organizing and reorganizing. "Welcome back, by the way."

"No." I kept my eyes on him. "This will only take a minute." I motioned to the chair he was standing next to. "Please sit down." I was blunt: "Why did you release the fox?"

"Dave felt it was ready to go." Still no eye contact.

"The plan was for me to release it today."

"Yeah, but Dave said—"

"Dave's not the doctor. He doesn't make these decisions." Cliff did not respond. "I also read the news article. You were quoted as saying 'It was a tough decision, and it wasn't popular. I did what I thought was best for the fox.'" I stood up and looked at him intently.

"That whole quote's a lie, Cliff. You and the rest of the staff were adamant that the fox should be euthanized. You said that it would never live if the leg was amputated!"

"I never said that!" He was finally looking at me, his voice raised an octave. "I was 100 percent behind you!"

"Doctors, we need you up front, *stat*!" Lisa screamed over the intercom in the conference room.

"We're not finished," I warned as I headed to the waiting room.

Mr. Rockwell was there with his young Asian wife and their seven Pomeranians. The former pro football player towered over his wife by at least a foot and a half. He was holding four dogs, Mrs. Rockwell had one in her arms, and two were scampering around her legs on leashes. All were barking, yipping, and jumping around—a true frenzy of fur.

The giant was nearly in tears when I arrived. "I think I may have just killed all my dogs, Doc. Please!"

That was perplexing. All the dogs were actively—almost hyperactively—barking. "What are you talking about? What happened?" I took Lucy, the battery-eating dog whose life we had saved a few months back.

"It's my fault!" Mrs. Rockwell spoke up in a heavy Japanese accent.

"Please, just tell me what happened." By now almost the entire staff was up front, everyone grabbing a dog.

"I left a box of chocolates on the table," Mrs. Rockwell confessed.

"I heard a commotion and I went into the kitchen, and all the dogs were up on the table eating the candies." Mr. Rockwell bent over and kissed the black-and-white fuzz ball dwarfed in his large hands.

"How much do you think they ate?" I looked at the eyes of the one I was holding. The dog was panting heavily, shaking, its eyes dilated from the chocolate buzz and flickering side to side.

"It was a two-pound box, Doc." He looked worried, pale. "It was almost gone!"

I did the mental calculations while I listened. Chocolate can be highly toxic if eaten in large quantities. A ten-pound dog only needs to eat about three to four pieces of dark chocolate to become poisoned. Each of these dogs weighed in that neighborhood. Assuming they had each eaten an equal share, most likely they were all at risk.

"Can you pump their stomachs?"

"No, but I can make them vomit." I handed the dog I was holding to Tanya and then grabbed one of the others from Mr. Rockwell. "How long ago did this happen?

"I came right over." He kissed the two dogs left in his arms. "Are they going to die?" His wife was crying.

"Not on my watch." I farmed out the remaining two dogs to Robert and Maria.

The crew took all seven barking dogs to the treatment area. By this time they were all beginning to show signs of toxicity: spastic barking, trembling, and now projectile diarrhea. "Okay," I commanded Stacey, "you're in charge of coordinating the treatments. I want one person assigned to each dog. Get a temperature and heart rate on each one every fifteen minutes." I pointed around the room. "Each person must stay with their assigned dog the entire time."

We spread out to different tables and counters. Some of the group sat down on the floor. Stacey went around with the thermometer taking temperatures and getting weights on each dog, recording the vitals on their charts.

I went around the room and gave each dog a dose of apomorphine, a medication used to induce vomiting. Stacey kept a record of the amount and the time given.

Maria had gathered seven kitty-litter pans and handed them out, one for each dog. Within about two minutes each dog began to salivate, then dry heave, then explode with copious amounts of warm, mucus-covered, dark chocolate vomit.

The scent in the room quickly changed from aseptic medical to outhouse chocolate. Dogs were heaving and puking all around. Gag, choke, splash, cough. The odor of pervasive vomit mixed with diarrhea was becoming unbearable. Not more than five minutes into this scene of continuous retching, we had our first human casualty. Maria suddenly let go of her charge and dashed over to the treatment sink, hurling her egg burrito breakfast into the stainless bowl.

Maria's upchuck had a snowball effect. Fred, Tanya, and then Cliff followed. Heaving, gagging, and grunting. The occasional loud flatulence, whether from dog or person, trumpeted out between other primal noises.

The once fluffy, well-groomed Pomeranians now looked like mudsoaked, wet mopheads. The good news was that all the dogs had spewed out copious amounts of chocolate. Since measuring the amount was not possible, I had the human survivors who remained keep track of the dogs' body temperatures. One by one the dogs were taken to the grooming area and washed off.

After being bathed, each dog received activated charcoal and subcutaneous fluids to compensate for the vomiting. Once cleaned, they were paired with another pup per Mr. Rockwell's instructions and placed in cages so we could keep a constant check on their vital signs. It was a long, arduous day of constant monitoring and anxiety. Fortunately, all seven dogs recovered.

I know one thing for sure—this was one Valentine's Day neither the Rockwells nor our staff would ever forget.

◆ ◆ ◆

My last patient of the day was Iggy, the Hollywood iguana. If she hadn't been accompanied by the duo of René and Lana, I would not have recognized her. Her body was perfectly straight, and she was walking completely normally. She had come in to have the stitches from her recent surgery removed.

"She is doing so fantastic, Doctor!" Lana came over and gave me a very personal full-body hug. The intensity of her perfume brought back memories of our first meeting.

"Yes, thank you, Dr. Mader." René pumped my hand once Lana and I had disengaged, holding on for what seemed a bit longer than necessary. Was this some type of alpha male gesture?

"Did she shed?" I asked, gently lifting Iggy's front legs off the table so I could better see her belly scar.

"Yes, Doctor." Lana was smiling more than I had ever seen. "Twice since the surgery!"

"Ah." I set the lizard back down. "I don't need to remove her stitches today!" I looked up at the two confused owners. "Mother Nature did it for me." I smiled triumphantly. "When she shed, all the stitches fell out naturally with the old skin." I rubbed Iggy's smooth belly. "The perfect sign that everything is healed."

Another big hug from Lana.

"Please, Doctor," René said, handing me his business card. "You have been so kind to us—"

"And Iggy!" Lana interrupted.

"You have been so kind to us, please let us treat you and your wife to dinner at one of the finer restaurants in Hollywood." He pointed a finger at me as if giving me his approval. "Call me any time!"

◆ ◆ ◆

After the previous morning's puke party, things got hectic, and I never had a chance to meet with Cliff and finish our discussion about the fox. Dave came in later in the afternoon, nearly in tears, and apologized over and over. He said that Dr. Nordic had asked, only once, how Fore was doing, that Dave had told him "great," and the next thing he knew, Officer Kelly Pinkett had arrived with her carrier and picked up the fox. It was only because he had begged Cliff that he was allowed to go along for the release.

After Iggy left and I finished writing in my records, I had some quiet time so I called Kelly and talked with her about what had happened. She too had been surprised that I was not the one who would be at the release. She said the request for the release came from both Dr. Nordic and the director of the country club.

It turned out that Cliff's father was a member of the club, and the board of directors thought it would be great if the young veterinarian son of one of its own longtime members was the one doing the fox release for the press. As soon as Kelly told me that, it all came together.

To say I was peeved would be an understatement. I had stuck my neck out and spent half a day on the phone with all the principals getting them to buy in to my plan. Had something bad happened to the fox (or should something bad happen in the future), I would have been the one who took the blame.

Once again, as when this had all started two weeks ago, I found myself sitting in my upstairs office, staring off into the distance. The sun was falling in the late-afternoon sky to the west, so the snowcapped San Gabriel Mountains, which I find so cathartic in times of stress, were barely visible through the veil of smog, clouds, and waning light out my window to the east. I would focus on my mission: what I did for the animals. In truth, it didn't matter who released Fore. The important thing was that he got a second chance.

◆ ◆ ◆

"Are you Dr. Doug Mader?" the kid asked between chomping on his chewing gum. He was wearing a college-type backpack and had a skateboard under his arm. He looked to be in his late teens or early twenties.

"Yes." I didn't recognize the young man wearing a Cal State San Louis Obispo hoodie standing just outside the front door of my office.

"Cool." He set the skateboard down and twisted out of his pack. He unzipped the top and removed a legal-sized manila envelope. "Consider yourself served." He handed me the package, then took off down the sidewalk on his skateboard before I could even mutter a word.

The kid totally blindsided me. My first reaction when he handed me the envelope was that I must have really pissed someone off. I couldn't think of any clients who were upset with me. Perhaps I was being sued for amputating the leg on Fore the fox by some animal rights group?

My disbelief only grew when I opened the letter. Written in all its abstruse legalese was a summons to appear in civil court as an expert witness in the case of "Iggy v. Dr. Remsdell." The plaintiffs, Iggy's owners Lana and René, were suing the defendant, Dr. Remsdell, for $3 million. The cause of action: loss of consortium.

I immediately called our attorney, Matt Leonard.

"You're kidding!" Matt laughed when I told him about the summons. "Really? Do you know what happened?

"Never mind that." I didn't think being served was funny. "What the hell is this? Am I in some kind of trouble?"

"'Loss of consortium' is a legal term that refers to the deprivation of the benefits of a family relationship due to injuries caused by a tortfeasor."

"Well, that makes it super clear. In simple English, please."

"Basically the lawsuit is saying that the husband can't get laid by his wife, and he's blaming the defendant, Dr. Remsdell, for it."

"Go on," I prodded.

"Seems that Dr. Remsdell must have done something so horrible that it caused psychological stress in the wife, and now she can no longer perform or function in her marital capacity."

"And you can sue someone over this? For three million bucks?"

"It's the USA."

◆ ◆ ◆

"I'm really starting to like snakes," Tanya stated proudly after finishing her morning treatments of the large python.

It had been almost two months since the python came in on Christmas morning. With all our supportive care the monster serpent had gained fifteen pounds, but it had yet to take a meal on its own. As soon as we got it to eat, it could be discharged back to Texas. Tanya had been in constant contact with the mother and young daughter. The pigtailed, red-haired little girl had sent several hand-drawn get-well cards to the snake over the past two months, and the technicians had them taped to the front of its cage.

My first client of the day was Pat Peters, the neutrois philosophy professor at the state college. She had come in with a new pet, a three-foot-long black-and-white tegu lizard from Argentina. These lizards had become all the rage with their large, muscular bodies, pit bull-like heads, and striking striped pattern. On top of this, they were known as easy keepers and were readily tamed, making them atypically responsive for a reptile. These pluses added up to a unique pet with a high cool factor, especially for college students, who can easily keep one in a university dorm room.

"What an impressive specimen!" I was truly in awe. I had only seen a few tegu, and this one was particularly handsome.

"Thank you, Doctor." Pat was always polite. She had become friends with Robert and requested that he be in the room whenever she came in with one of her charges. Tanya was standing to his side.

"Unlike most other reptiles," I noted as I did my examination, my comments really meant for Tanya, "it's not possible to tell the gender of a tegu just by looking at it."

"Oh, good!" Pat responded. "I didn't want to know."

I looked at her and smiled. The joke went right over Tanya's head. "Why did you name it Thor, then?"

"I didn't." She sighed. "That's what it was called when I got it."

"I'm curious."

"It was one of those things." She reached over and took the saurian from me. In doing so, she placed the front legs and head on her shoulder, holding it like a human baby. "I had a student who was failing. His parents said that he had to get rid of his lizard and start concentrating on the books or they would stop funding his education." She stroked the tegu's shiny scales. It looked so relaxed on her shoulder. Pat's scraggly beard touched the top of its back.

"When I heard the story I offered to give it a temporary home until he got himself back in good graces with his parents and his grades picked up. He's a good boy."

"How can I help you and Thor today?" I reached out and pet the lizard. The scales were like smooth half pearls covering the skin.

"I'm worried. Thor hasn't eaten since I got him."

"What are you feeding him?"

"I've tried everything: broccoli, shredded carrots, beets, cubed watermelon, even grapes."

"That's your problem, Pat." I gently lifted Thor off her shoulder and set it on the table between us. I used my left hand to pinch its nose so it couldn't breathe, my right thumb and forefinger to grasp the fold of skin under the chin. In doing so, it readily opened its impressive jaws, revealing a hundred or more extremely sharp teeth. "Those are the teeth of a carnivore."

Pat bent over for a closer look. I checked to make sure that Tanya and Robert saw what I was talking about before I let go of the mouth and it snapped closed.

"I knew that he ate mice, but I wanted to give him a vegetarian diet." Pat looked concerned as she stroked the lizard's head and neck. "I'm a vegetarian, and I can't stand the thought of him eating mice."

"But, Pat, that's his normal, natural diet."

She continued to pet him for some time and then in a quiet voice asked, "Are there any alternatives?"

"They will eat raw eggs, with the shell."

"That's still an animal product. I have a philosophical objection to feeding any animals or animal products."

"Pat, I understand that you have that right regarding your own diet." I looked at my two helpers. This was going to turn into a debate that would have no proper ending. "But these lizards are carnivores. That is what they eat. Evolutionarily, they are not designed to live on a vegetarian diet."

"I hear what you say, Doctor, and please, don't think I'm trying to disrespect you or be argumentative, but I just cannot feed animal protein to this lizard." It looked as if she wanted to cry. "I only eat a vegetarian diet, and likewise, my dog and cat are vegetarians. They are just fine."

I had to silently disagree. Cats are carnivores and don't do well on a vegetarian diet. One look at her cat told you that. However, this was not the time to take up that discussion.

"Pat, you come to me supposedly because I know what I'm doing and am reasonably good at it." I looked right at her, waiting for eye contact before finishing my statement. "By feeding a vegetarian diet to this animal that you so generously adopted, you're doing it a disservice."

"I *do* respect your opinion, Doctor." She really seemed beside herself at this point. "It's just that I can't do it. I can't feed little mice to Thor."

"I understand." I was trying to come up with some alternative. "Will you at least give it some canned cat food? That way you don't have to feed it actual mice."

"No, I can't." Pat looked hard at her lizard, obviously in deep thought. "I know what goes into the cat food." She wiped her eyes with an old kerchief from her front pocket. "I just can't do that." She picked up the lizard and put it back on her shoulder.

"Okay, Pat." I was disappointed. I respect Pat. She's a very educated woman and has strong opinions, but I also hoped that she would be smart enough to realize that her personal beliefs were detrimental to the lizard. "Perhaps this isn't the right pet for you." I put on my unhappy face. "Please think about what you're doing."

• • •

It was officially rainy season, and the rainfall didn't stop all day. With the colder temperatures and miserable conditions, business was slow.

Our hospital was on the lower side of the street as well as on its downward slope along a slight hill, so when it rained, even moderately, all the runoff not only flowed down from the crest of the hill but also from across the road. As a result, the gutter on our side of the street would flood during heavy rains; the water would crest the curb and come up onto the sidewalk. On days like today, clients were not able to park along the curb, and with no off-street parking it was difficult for people to get in or out of the office.

The day was just about done and the rain had lessened a bit. I had no more appointments, so I decided to take a minute and run over to the local store. When I returned I parked a couple of blocks from the building, as usual, and walked back along the flooded sidewalk.

The sky was mean, the clouds a swirling kaleidoscope of different shades of gray. The sun was nowhere to be seen, but it was definitely getting late. The temperature was in the low forties, a damp cold not unusual for this time of year in Southern California.

The chilly rain stung my squinting eyes as I walked back to the office. Head bowed and through half closed lids, I saw Harriett the hooker standing at her corner post in front of the hospital. It struck me as odd to see a hooker under an umbrella.

I noticed one of my clients exit the building, tiptoe along the flooded walkway holding a cat carrier in one hand, a large bag of food under the other arm, and her high-stepping poodle leash strapped around her wrist.

Suddenly, Harriett splashed her way over from the corner and covered the client with the umbrella. She then lifted the soaked little dog up from the gutter runoff and walked with the client down the street to her car, helped her and her dog inside, loaded her pet supplies, then made sure the door was shut before waving goodbye. The client gave a courtesy honk and drove off.

The rain was relentless all night. Several of the morning's clients had either cancelled or just not shown up. The dark skies and damp cold made for a depressing start to the day.

"This guy is a real loser," Stacey commented as she handed me the chart for my next patient.

"Stacey! He can hear you." I shot her a disapproving look.

"I don't care. He's an asshole." She essentially tossed the chart at me and walked away.

"How much to fix his broken leg?" he asked when I entered the examination room.

No introduction, nothing, just *how much?*

"I'm Dr. Mader." I extended my hand over an obviously young, beautiful brown-and-white pointer curled up on the exam table.

He ignored my hand and repeated, "How much?" I waited for a moment, then pulled back my hand. I could see that the dog had a badly broken front leg. It was going to need a metal plate to fix it properly.

"I'd like to get some X-rays to see how bad the break is. Then I can give you an exact price."

"How much?" He was insistent. I now realized what Stacey was referring to.

"That depends on what we need to do." I tried to stay collected. I really didn't appreciate clients who tried to rattle me. "Depending on whether we just put it in a cast, or have to do surgery, it could be anywhere from eighty to five hundred dollars."

I'm not sure of it, but I think he spit on the floor.

"How much to kill it?" He shook his head. The little dog looked at me with pathetic eyes.

"This is not a serious injury." I was stern. "A broken leg is easily fixed."

"How much to kill it?" He stared me down. He had the eyes of a man with no tolerance, and I got the feeling that he could snap, in a violent way, at any moment.

"How about I adopt your dog, fix it, pay for it myself, and then find it a home?"

"It's just a stupid dog." He picked the dog up. It yelped in pain as he manhandled it.

"Hey, why don't you just leave it with me?" Why was he so abusive to the poor little dog? "I'll take full responsibility for it." I reached out and tried to take the dog from the man.

"A bullet's only seventeen cents! It's my dog!" He twisted away from me. "I can do what I want." Before I could respond he headed to the exit.

The man stormed out without paying for the exam. Mai Tai screamed at him as he passed. "Shut the fuck up, stupid bird!" were his last words as the door slammed behind him.

I stepped up to the receptionist's office to explain what had just transpired to Lisa and Stacey. Just as I started to recall the conversation with the man, we were jolted by an ear-piercing crack of what sounded like thunder directly overhead.

I ran out in the pouring rain. Parked at the curb at the side of the building in a handicapped parking space was a dark-green, beat-up F-150. Standing next to the truck was the dog's owner. He was soaked, his wet hair matted to the side of a sardonic grin.

He was holding a handgun.

I went closer to the vehicle to get a better look. Lying on its side in the bed of the truck was the young dog, shot through the head. Its eyes, blood red and angry, bulged up and out, as if looking at its owner for the last time. The mouth was agape, the near side of its head sunken, a small round, dark hole just behind the temple. Brain tissue was splattered like trunk paint across the bed of his pick-up. The gushing rain flushed a darker blood from under the tailgate onto the street below.

The dog's owner stared me down with an evil look. Smoking gun in hand, he stated coldly, "See? Just seventeen cents."

My eyes darted back and forth between the dog and the man. My heart was pounding in my chest and my ears were ringing. Finally, I fixed my glare on the asshole.

I walked up to him. If he hadn't had that gun I think I would have killed him. I wanted so badly to hurt him like he had hurt that poor dog.

Standing in the downpour, he lifted the pistol, pointed it at my face, and smiled. "Bang!" He leered at me as the single word came out. Then, quickly, he pulled the gun back, blew on the tip of the barrel as if clearing the smoke, turned, slipped into his cab, and drove off.

My pen didn't write well on my wet hand, but I managed to scribble his license plate number on my palm.

MARCH

Raoul at the Ferret Club

Raoul Hernandez, our new student from Colorado State, arrived one Monday afternoon. I usually pick up the students from the airport, but my grandmother had passed away the previous night and I was busy dealing with family issues.

I was in a mental fog for much of the day and didn't have a lot of direct interaction with Raoul. I did what I had to do at work, then went home and took Wok for a long walk, telling him all about our family's ninety-six-year-old matriarch.

Tuesday was my half day. I finished my morning appointments, then took Raoul up the street to Lili's Country Kitchen for lunch. I wanted to get to know him better since I hadn't had the mindset to spend time with him on his first day. Midway through Lili's famous teriyaki burger, complete with a ring of canned pineapple garnishing the sweet Asian sauce, Lili came over to say hi and asked if I'd heard the news about Rodney King.

"No." I looked up. I had eaten there so many times that Lili and I had become good friends. On most days she was the greeter, waitress, cook, and cashier. "This is Raoul, our new student." I motioned to the handsome young Latino sitting across from me.

"Nice to meet you," Lili extended her hand. "There are no black people!"

"What?" I was confused by the non sequitur.

"Rodney King! There are no black people." Lili was tiny, a scratch over five feet tall. She had a round face and short, cropped black hair, wore thick horn-rimmed glasses, and spoke with choppy, broken English. She threw up her hands as if exasperated that I didn't understand. "On the jury! No black people on the Rodney King jury!"

Oh, now it made sense. She knew everything. If you wanted to know about anything happening in our neighborhood or city, you just asked Lili.

"They got one Filipino, one Hispanic, like you," she pointed at Raoul, "and *ten whites*." This time she pointed at me. "Six men, six women."

I just looked at her, not sure what to say.

"It's gonna be bad." She looked so serious. "No way Rodney King's gonna get a fair trial." Actually she was referring to the four police officers on trial, accused of excessive force and beating Rodney King the night he was pulled over. Rodney King was not on trial, as he was never charged with any crime. "If those cops get off there's gonna be riots everywhere, this city's gonna burn, people gonna die! Black people don't like us!"

By "us," Lili was referring to Koreans. About a year ago, a fifteen-year-old black girl had gone into a Korean liquor store to pick up some orange juice. The store clerk, fifty-one-year-old Soon Ja Du, whose family owned the liquor store, believed the girl was trying to steal the juice. There was a confrontation, and ultimately, Soon Ja Du shot the girl in the back of the head.

The jury found Soon Ja Du guilty of voluntary manslaughter and sentenced her to a maximum of sixteen years in prison. However, the white judge in the case overruled the verdict, cancelled the prison sentence, and instead gave Soon Ja Du a $500 fine, five years' probation, and four hundred hours of community service. The black community was outraged and lawyers immediately filed an appeal, which was still pending.

"God, I hope not." My appetite was suddenly gone. "I hope the cops don't get off for what they did." My mind immediately flashed back to the video images of the horrible, senseless beating of the unarmed man.

"I'm gonna get me a gun!" Lili sounded more like Clint Eastwood's Dirty Harry than an affable five-foot-tall chef.

◆ ◆ ◆

The hospital was out of bird food. Just a short walk down the street past the China Girl strip club, after the Rip Off Upholstery sweat shop, and a few steps beyond Casa Sanchez, the "Can your stomach can handle it?" Mexican joint, was a pet shop, Birds of a Feather.

"Morning, Jeanne." I flashed one of my best smiles. Multiple wrought iron cages inhabited by a variety of jungle birds filled the small store, leaving barely any room for the narrow isles leading to the proprietor's counter. With all those big beaks, I was surprised some patron hadn't been bitten while careening through the maze.

"Hey, Dr. Mader," Jeanne welcomed.

"Wow, you've got lots of nice new birds in." I was looking at a green-winged macaw chick, maybe sixteen weeks old. Its brilliant red, green, and blue feathers had not quite grown in yet, making it look a bit ratty to the uninitiated. These incredible birds imprint on the person doing the feeding and become bonded for life—which can be seventy-five plus years. They cost thousands of dollars.

"We just got that one in. I've been hand-rearing it at home. It's ready to find an owner—you interested?"

"I think my wife would die for one, but it's a bit out of my budget." I smiled, thinking that Ellen really would love a baby bird. However, these large macaws needed a lot of attention, and we both were so rarely home, it just wouldn't be fair.

"You let me know when you're ready. I'll give you a special price."

"Appreciate that." I reached a finger through the bars and rubbed the red feathers on the chick's head. It leaned forward, pushing back against my finger, like a kitten looking for love.

"Let me know. I think that little one's going to go fast."

• • •

While I was working on some charts one morning, Fred approached with a big smile on his face. "I know you're busy, Dr. Mader, but I've got some great news for you." He had a late-'80s Magnum P.I. moustache that he deliberately wore long to try to hide a crooked top incisor, the Achilles' heel of this ladies' man's self-esteem.

"What have you got? I could use some good news right now."

"The snake ate!" I must have looked stumped—my mind was elsewhere. "The Texas python. *It finally ate on its own!*"

"No way!" The snake had been here almost two and a half months and had not eaten for at least three months prior to that. "That's fantastic! What did it eat?"

"That's the funny part." Fred sat down at the conference table next to me. I hadn't seen him this happy in a long time. "Greg offered the snake a large rat. It sniffed at it but wouldn't eat. Greg said that was the most interest in food he'd seen from the snake since we got it." Fred continued. "As it turned out, Greg had picked up some Kentucky Fried Chicken for dinner earlier in the night, and so he had the idea to wipe the grease from inside the KFC bucket all over the rat. When he threw it back into the cage, the python scarfed it down!"

"Oh my God!" I cracked up. "That's hilarious!" I gave Fred a high five. "I think we need to publish that technique. Why don't you be the hero and give the Texans a call with the great news. If the snake keeps it down, eats again, and then passes stool, I'll feel good about sending it home."

• • •

Lisa had booked me off the entire afternoon so I would be available for the deposition in the Iggy "loss of consortium" case. The plaintiffs, René and

Lana, had their attorney come down from Hollywood with his stenographer to take my statement in our conference room. The lawyer questioned me for several hours about how the first veterinarian handled the Iggy case:

"Why did he take the blood while the iguana was on its back?"

"Why did you take the blood with the iguana standing upright?"

"Why do you think the iguana got all twisted up after the other doctor took the blood sample?"

"Why didn't the other doctor know that Iggy was a female?"

"Why didn't the other doctor know that Iggy was pregnant?"

"Why didn't the other doctor recommend calcium?"

"Why didn't the other doctor recommend surgery to fix the problem?"

He asked me the same questions multiple times and in multiple ways, trying to get me to say something damning about the other veterinarian. I always gave him the same answer: "The other veterinarian did nothing wrong."

"Did the other doctor's counsel already contact you?" I could tell Iggy's attorney was frustrated with me. "Are you getting paid by them?"

"No, and *no*!" I was getting tired of this. I didn't know the other veterinarian well personally, but he had a good reputation. Through the grapevine I'd heard that there had been an argument between René and the doctor, who must have said something to really upset René. Unfortunately for the doc, René had the money to push back, and he was doing it with a $3 million lawsuit.

The deposition was worse than any day at work. Rather than go straight home after work, I took the short drive down to the shore and went to my favorite sushi restaurant. I sat at the glass counter and was looking through the sneeze guard at all the sumptuous fresh fish, nursing a Diet Coke, and nibbling on some edamame when Goro, the head sushi chef, placed a tokkuri, the little ceramic carafe that serves the sake, in front of me. "A gift from admirer," Goro said in his broken English, and then bowed in traditional Japanese style.

"*Domo arigato*," I answered, thanking him in Japanese. Across the dimly lit room, partially obscured by the colorful Japanese paper lanterns hanging from the ceiling, was a stunning blond sitting at the opposite end of the sushi bar. She was wearing large hoop earrings that peaked out from shoulder-length, shag-cut hair and accented her immaculate, tanned complexion, long lashes, and alluring lips. I watched as she picked up a cherry, appeared to ponder it for a moment, and then sensuously slipped it into her mouth.

I glanced over at Goro and subtly flicked my gaze in the beautiful woman's direction. He smiled, nodded, and then went back to crafting a perfectly formed spicy tuna roll wrapped with an ultrathin layer of avocado. The vision of this stunning woman made me immediately forget my bad day, the lawyer, deposition, broken bones, and all the other struggles of professional life in the nonhuman health-care field.

I took a sip of the chilled, unfiltered sake. It was the good stuff. My eyes closed, I held the liquid in my mouth savoring the taste. For that brief moment the real world was light-years away.

"Are you going to share?"

The sweet voice broke my trance. I opened my eyes. The blond was sitting next to me, holding an empty sake cup next to her frosted peach lips. Without taking my eyes off hers, I lifted the tokkuri.

"*Dozo?*"

"*Domo.*" She knew the routine.

I filled her cup, careful not to spill any of the expensive wine.

In traditional style we interlocked arms, my right with her left, elevated the sake to the sky, and toasted, "*Kanpai!*" The move was so smooth it seemed practiced. There were smiles on both sides as we tipped back the cups.

"Are you alone?" She took another sip, then unlocked arms.

"Not anymore." I smiled.

I noticed that she wasn't wearing a ring. I never wear mine. Not that I want to pretend that I'm single, but I'd be constantly taking it off for surgery and would probably misplace it. More importantly, I can't afford the chance that a large dog might bite my hand. If I had a ring on, it could easily cost me a finger.

"Lose your wedding ring?" I nodded toward her left hand.

"What makes you think I'm married?" The blond smiled, teasing.

I pointed to the tan line on her ring finger using the pinkie of my hand holding the sake. "Your husband's one lucky guy."

"I think so." She buried her whimsical smile in another sip of her sake. The peach lipstick left a small imprint on the cup.

"May I treat you to dinner since you were so kind to treat me to this fine sake?"

"On one condition."

"What's that?"

I could feel the warmth of her lips close to my ear as she leaned in to whisper.

"If I can treat you to dessert . . ."

◆ ◆ ◆

Life can be so unfair. After Thursday's late night of sake and sushi and more with my beautiful wife that I so rarely get to see, I did not want to get up and go to work yesterday morning. Ellen, lucky her, got to sleep in.

We so rarely had the same night off together. We had planned on meeting at the sushi house after I got off work, and we actually got to enjoy a great meal, some wonderful spirits, and quality time like a real married couple. After dinner we went for a stroll past the shops near the shore, then ventured out on the beach under a waxing moon, hand in hand, walking along the waves crashing on the sand.

It was mid-March, and the weather was brisk, but the sake in our bloodstreams kept us warm as we ambled along until the late hours of the night, barely passing another soul on the nearly deserted beach. We talked about the scuba trip to Honduras in May, both deciding that we each worked too hard not to take some time off and smell the proverbial flowers. The plan would be for me to make the Central America trip my last hurrah for the spring, then when I returned to the United States I'd start my hardcore studying for the specialty boards. Ellen agreed that it sounded like a great idea.

This morning's rounds were a welcome shot in the arm. The giant snake had not defecated yet, but it did eat another large rat the previous night, this time without having to be scented with fried chicken grease.

Halfway through this morning's appointments I got a call from Jeanne at Birds of a Feather, the pet shop down the street.

"Dr. Mader." I could tell instantly by the tone in her voice that something was wrong. "You remember that beautiful little green-winged macaw chick that you were looking at?"

I did. I had even talked about it with Ellen the night before during our date night. We had both decided that Wok, Sidney, and the fish were all we could handle at this time.

"I've got horrible news." She paused. My first thought was that it was sick. "Somebody just stole it!"

"Oh my God!" I felt like someone had doused me with a bucket of cold water. "Are you all right? How'd it happen? What can I do? Do you need me to come over?"

"No." I could hear her sniffling over the phone. I knew the store had experienced some recent financial problems and that this was a major blow. "But I'd like you to contact your veterinary friends, anyone you know with birds, the bird club, and anyone else you think of and let them know to keep an eye out for it."

"Of course." Sadly, I suspected that the expensive bird was already halfway to San Francisco or San Diego. "I'll get some calls out right away." I paused for a moment. "How did it happen?" I asked again.

"I'm pretty sure it was some gangbangers. A couple came in, flying colors; the guy had his pants halfway down his ass. His girl came up to my counter and started arguing with me about the price of some bird toys." She took a breath. "I couldn't see what the guy was doing. You know how crowded the front of the store is."

"Yeah." I remembered my visit last week. The macaw chick was in a cage near the front entrance. It was nearly impossible to see the checkout counter past all the cages.

"I heard the bell on the front door open and close while I was talking to the girl. Just seconds afterward she suddenly yelled, 'Whatever, bitch!' and walked out. I was so upset that I didn't even notice the chick was gone until I went to do my midday feeds."

"Did you call the police?"

"No." She paused. "I'm afraid."

"They don't have anything against you, Jeanne. They just wanted the bird."

"But if I call the police, they'll come back for revenge. You know how it works."

"Call the police." I was about to hang up, then added, "Anything else comes up, call me and I'll be right over."

• • •

Halfway through morning rounds, Lisa interrupted the discussion—something that was generally considered taboo unless it was an emergency.

"I'm sorry to bug you, Dr. Mader," Lisa leaned in through the doorway and handed me a note. "But there's someone on the phone that says she is from *Good Morning America* and would like to talk to you."

"You better take that, boss. Sounds important." Cliff smarted.

"Ooh, you're famous," Stacey chimed in.

I excused myself and went to an extension around the corner, away from the peanut gallery.

"Good morning, Dr. Mader! Thank you so much for coming to the phone. I hope I'm not interrupting." A cheery female voice greeted me.

"Not at all," I lied. "How can I help you?"

The woman introduced herself as being from ABC's *Good Morning America* and said they were doing a story on the ferret underworld in California. She said, "I understand that you are one of the few veterinarians who will treat these animals, and actually advertise in your yellow pages that you do so."

"All true." I wasn't sure who this was or what she wanted. Anybody could say they were from a TV show.

"We would very much like to interview you. We're going to go to one of the underground Ferret Club meetings and then, if possible, would like to get you on camera to discuss ferrets as pets, from a veterinarian's perspective."

"I don't see why that would be a problem." It was illegal to own a ferret in California but not illegal to talk about them. Any chance I could get to educate the public about ferrets and how they interact with humans would be worth the time.

"Oh, wonderful!" The woman seemed a bit too exuberant, but I suspected that came with her job. "We know that the meeting is Friday night, but we won't know where until an hour before it starts."

"I know the drill." We both laughed. "I look forward to meeting you."

The first rule of the Ferret Club was that you never talk about the Ferret Club. The club was a clandestine group that met in the shadows of the inner city. It was illegal to own ferrets in California, but there were no laws that said you couldn't get together with others and talk about the weaselly-looking critters. You just couldn't talk about the club outside the meetings.

The second rule of the Ferret Club was that you *never* brought a ferret to a club meeting. If you showed up with one you were immediately kicked out of the club and sent packing. Ferret owners were all paranoid. They were petrified that a CDFG undercover officer would follow them home after a meeting and barge into their house, confiscating and ultimately killing all of their pet ferrets. Officer Kelly assured me that this had never happened or ever would.

Rumor had it that some members were so radical that if they found out that another member had broken one of the cardinal rules, they would place an anonymous call to the CDFG to report the individual.

Meetings, always at a different location every month, were convoked by a phone tree. There were about a dozen or so places where they gathered, never at the same place twice in a row. One person, usually one of the board members, would decide when and where the meeting would be held. Approximately ninety minutes before the starting time, the phone tree would launch. The master-at-arms would call four people on their list; then these people would do the same and the process would continue until all members were reached, with the process usually completed in a span of about fifteen minutes. Since this was the norm, all members would be by their phones ready and waiting for the call, so it was very efficient.

Any new members had to be vetted by the "security council" from the club to make sure that they weren't infiltrated by outsiders or, heaven forbid, the CDFG.

I had to laugh about all the cloak-and-dagger. Officer Pinkett said that the CDFG was very aware of the meetings and that they did have an agent that attended every month—only nobody knew who it was.

I had been to the meetings a number of times as a guest speaker. The ferret owners and the whole concept of the underground club were a bit over-the-top for me, so I generally didn't attend their meetings on a regular basis, as I did with the Herpetological Society.

After the phone call I rejoined the morning rounds just as they were finishing up.

The other breaking news was that the big reticulated python finally defecated. Now it was not only eating on its own, passing stool, and slithering around like a normal snake, but it had gained nearly twenty pounds since it arrived in a comatose state on Christmas morning. Raoul

liked all the exotics we cared for at the hospital, but his favorites were
the reptiles. He particularly relished working with the large reticulated
python and had been calling the owners almost daily. With today's great
poop news, it was time to send the snake back to Texas. Raoul arranged
for the mom and daughter to pick up the now healthy monster snake in
ten days. They were so excited they could keep alive their late husband's/
father's legacy: a true once-in-a-lifetime Christmas present. Anyone who
doesn't think reptiles can be good pets just needs to take the time to get
to know one.

After the python's three months at NAVH, the staff had all grown fond
of it, and we had mixed feelings about seeing it go home. The lesson to
be learned from this case was that if it is a reptile, *never give up*! They are
amazingly resilient, and if given the chance, they survive. After all, they are
living reminders of the dinosaur era.

♦ ♦ ♦

California has probably the strictest rules of any state in the country when
it comes to owning exotic pets. Why had I picked this state for practicing
exotic animal medicine when I could have chosen a state like Texas where
almost anything was legal to own?

Wolf hybrids, the current exotic animal craze, were a cross between
a domestic dog, usually a husky, malamute, or similar, and a wild wolf.
According to California law it was illegal to own a wolf hybrid if it was a
50 percent or greater cross. For instance, if a domestic Siberian husky bred
with a wild wolf, the puppies would be 50-50 domestic-wild. Owning such
a cross was illegal. However, if you then took that 50-50 cross and bred
it back to another domestic dog, it would then be 75-25 domestic-wild,
which would be legal.

It was also mandatory in California that all canines, including hybrids,
be vaccinated against rabies. That said, it was illegal for veterinarians to vaccinate the 50-50 hybrids. So it was not uncommon for an owner to come in

with their "wolf hybrid" and ask for a rabies vaccination but claim that they were less than 50 percent wolf so they could get the necessary paperwork to make them legal.

A wild wolf has a distinct look and demeanor. Even if it was found as an abandoned pup in the wild and raised in a home with people and other dogs, it never behaved like a typical domestic dog. It couldn't, because, genetically, it wasn't domesticated. The bottle-fed pups may appear tame, but the wild gene was still there. You can see it in their eyes.

My first client of the day came in with two enormous wolf hybrids. She needed rabies vaccines and certificates so she could get them licensed. As soon as I laid eyes on them, with their long snouts, tiny, pointed ears, and wary eyes, I knew that they were not less than 50 percent hybrids. Based on size and comportment, I guessed they had to be at least 50-50, or possibly more.

After my usual pleasantries I asked the owner if she had proof that these were less than 50 percent, as required.

"They're only 25 percent!" She was indignant, in a way that screamed deceit.

"I'm sorry, but I have a hard time believing that."

"Are you calling me a liar?" The woman was almost aggressive.

"No, ma'am. But I could get fined or have my license suspended if I vaccinate a 50-50. I have to be very careful."

"Well, I can *assure* you that they are 75-25." She held both hybrids tight on short leashes. The larger male was tugging at her, trying to get to me. Raoul stood back in the corner.

"Again, I'm sorry. I can't just accept your word. If I vaccinate one of these animals and it bites someone and you don't have written proof of its lineage, I'm in big trouble with the State Veterinary Board."

The big hybrid growled.

"I've never!" The woman's attitude amped up another level. "I've never been called a liar."

"I'm *not* calling you a liar. I'm just asking for written proof so that I am protected. That's all."

"I don't have any breeding records, but I know where they came from, and I can assure you that they are not 50-50."

"Okay, I'll make you a deal." I was not about to be hoodwinked. "You let me get a blood sample, and if they come back less than 50-50, not only will I do the rabies vaccines for you, I'll do them for free."

She clearly had not expected this. "This is bullshit." She yanked on both leashes. "I don't have to prove myself to you." With that she pushed past Raoul and me and headed toward the exit. As the wolves brushed by, the larger of the two turned and snapped. Fortunately, I saw it coming and yanked my hand away, but not quickly enough, and the animal's incisors pinched the skin on the side of my palm.

"Now look what you've done!" The woman yelled at me at the top of her lungs, as if the dog's aggressive behavior was my fault. Before I realized what had happened she was out the door.

Sure enough, the bite broke the skin on my hand. Fortunately, the wound was no more than a scratch, but I was bleeding nonetheless. The fact that they were here for rabies meant that they most likely had not been vaccinated and there was an outside chance I could be exposed.

The likelihood was minimal, but I told Lisa to contact Animal Control, regardless. I had no intention of going to the hospital. I'd have Stacey or Fred clean my wound. But I wanted to file a complaint against her to make a point.

Robert was standing in the hallway when this all went down and witnessed the bite.

"I called Professor Pat Peters." He seemed unaffected by the whole scene with the wolves. "Her tegu hasn't eaten since she was here." As usual, his expression was flat.

"Would you mind calling her back and telling her that she really needs to bring the lizard in for an exam?" I wrapped my hand in a damp cloth that

Stacey handed me. "They aren't like snakes. They can't go more than a few days without eating."

"Will do." He turned away, stopped for a moment, then turned back to face me. "Did you know it's a full moon tonight?" He paused. "And you just got bit by a wolf."

I shrugged.

"You could turn into a werewolf." And with that, Robert gave me one of the eeriest looks I have ever seen.

• • •

The phone rang at 6:17 p.m. "6337 East Mono Lake Road," the caller stated, then hung up.

"That's our cue," I informed Raoul as I replaced the handset on the cradle.

"Are you sure it's okay for me to go?"

"No." I looked at him, shaking my head. Raoul was one of those people who are always so eager to please that it was easy to poke fun at him. "But let's give it a try. Worst-case scenario, you'll just have to wait in the car." He had a really great attitude, and I enjoyed him as a student.

I was not familiar with the address, so we had to look it up on a map. Not surprisingly, it was in a shady part of town. We drove down a graffiti-blemished alley to the back of an old warehouse. Dozens of cars lined the narrow road. Near the back, parked next to the rusted roll-up door, was a brightly colored news van. "KABC Los Angeles—Channel 7" was emblazoned on the side panels, and it had a large satellite dish on an extension arm attached to the roof.

So much for being inconspicuous.

An older woman and a young man were attending the side door to take names and check people in.

"Hey, Doc Mader!" a young Hispanic man greeted us. "Who you got here?"

"This is my senior student, Raoul, from the Rocky Mountain State—where ferrets are legal."

"*¡Con mucho gusto!*" the door guard rattled off, and the two started conversing in Spanish.

"I guess that means they're going to let you in?" I asked ironically.

"*Si. ¡No problema!*" he laughed.

The building was an old storage facility, easily twenty thousand square feet. The cavernous room with its high, bare ceiling and massive open space dwarfed what was a relatively sparse crowd of maybe forty or so people. In the center of the room someone had set up rows of folding chairs, and in the front was a gray-checkerboard card table with some paperwork scattered about. Several people were milling around and watching as a perfectly coiffed newswoman was interviewing a lady wearing a T-shirt imprinted with a picture of a ferret head and the caption "Ferrets are Family." A hirsute assistant wearing a black leather vest and a backward *Good Morning America* cap was capturing the action with a shoulder-mounted camera. A second woman walked around the room with a smaller camcorder collecting B roll and stopping occasionally to ask a random question to the assembled.

I waited patiently as the news reporter finished her interview and then introduced Raoul and myself. It was the reporter who had called me. "I'm so glad you made it," she said as she introduced me to the cameraman and the other reporter.

"We're just going to follow the meeting and, when it's over, take a few minutes to interview some of the members and you, if that's okay?"

"Sure." I smiled. "I'm on your clock."

The woman in the ferret shirt, who was president of the club, welcomed us and started out the meeting by stating its goal (to make ferrets legal in California) and the rules (you don't talk about Ferret Club).

She then introduced the *GMA* team and also welcomed Raoul and me as special guests. "If you have any ferret vet questions, make sure you ask Dr. Mader before he slips out!"

Thanks. As if I were there to offer free vet advice.

The meeting seemed to go on and on as people brought up the same concerns they had brought up at every Ferret Club meeting I'd ever attended.

"When are they going to be legalized?"

"What if I buy my ferret outa state? Can I bring it into California?"

"What happens if it gets sick? Can I take it to the vet? Will they turn me in?"

"What's best to feed a ferret?"

"Can my friend who has ferrets come to visit with them? Since she doesn't live here, they're not California ferrets."

"I have kits for sale!" (A kit is a baby ferret.)

"Ooh, how much?"

"I wanna see!"

After the inane questions came the horror stories.

"My friend's neighbor's cousin had the CDFG take her ferret right out of her house. They broke its neck, right there on her porch!"

That one got the attention of the newswoman.

"I had a friend whose daughter got bitten. Then they went to the ER, but the doctor wouldn't treat her when they found out it was a ferret bite."

"My husband was told by the IRS that if he kept ferrets in the house they would audit his taxes!"

The stories got more and more apocryphal as the meeting wore on. Some of it struck me as showboating for the cameras. Finally, the president called the meeting to an end. People milled about, hoping to get on camera. The roving camcorder lady walked around the room taking cameos of just about everybody. I wasn't sure if she was doing that just to appease them or to actually document their presence (for some future legal reason?).

Two plus hours after we arrived it was just the president, the two gatekeepers, the *GMA* crew, Raoul, and I who were left in the cavernous building. The cameraman set up a large light and placed a hidden microphone under my collar. They sat me in a chair with nothing but dark space in the background—perhaps a dramatic effect to show the emptiness of the building.

"I won't be on camera. I'll be standing next to it. When you talk, talk as if you're speaking directly to the camera, not to me," the reporter told me and pointed to the man with the video recorder. I nodded. "Do you mind if we give you a prop?"

"No." I was wondering what she would use. Just as I was about to ask, the president of the club came out of the darkness holding a cat carrier. Inside was a beautiful sable ferret.

Wow. She was breaking the second rule of the Ferret Club.

For the next fifteen minutes I held and petted the contraband ferret. The reporter asked me dozens of questions, many rephrased versions of the same, in an attempt to get me to say something extra juicy.

I had learned years earlier how to speak in sound bites. That way, an editor or producer couldn't take parts of a longer sentence, cut them, and then piece them together to end up with a statement completely differently than what I'd intended. Cognizant of the contradictory opinions about the creatures, I tried to be careful to give a balanced evaluation of the pluses and minuses of keeping ferrets as pets.

When the interviews were finished and the *GMA* crew was packing up its gear, the club president admonished, "Listen up—*nobody* tell *anybody* that we had a ferret here!"

Only ten million viewers would know that secret.

◆ ◆ ◆

One week after Jeanne from Birds of a Feather called to tell me that her green-winged macaw chick was stolen, I found myself on the phone with her once again. "Dr. Mader." I could barely hear her. "They're here."

"Who, Jeanne? Who's here?"

"The bangers that stole my bird! They're here, in the shop." Her voice got only slightly louder and clearly more anxious. "*Right now. And they have the chick with them!*"

"Are you sure it's the same bird?"

"*Really?* I raised it from a hatchling. *Of course it's the same bird!*" If it's possible to yell and whisper at the same time, she was. "I don't think it's the same bangers, though. It's two guys. No girl. Both wearing colors."

"Call the police. Stall them."

"No way! I'm not calling the police by myself. They scare the shit outa me."

"Where's your husband?"

"That coward took off out the back door as soon as he saw the gangstas."

"I still think you should call the cops, then stall the bangers until they arrive."

"You said I could call you if I needed anything and you'd be right over!"

She had a point. "Okay." I paused briefly and tried to come up with a plan. "Do you feel comfortable stalling them until I get there? I'll leave right now."

"Please hurry!"

I yanked off my NAVH scrub top, put on a dark, plain hoodie that I kept in the closet, and scurried out, yelling to Lisa as I passed the reception desk that I'd be back ASAP.

Within minutes of Jeanne's call I was at the store. Just as I was about to enter, the pair with the bird came walking out.

Oh my God, I had to think fast.

"Wow! Did you get a new bird?" I walked right up to the banger pair.

"Yo, man." A man sporting gold grills on his teeth held up the young chick. I noticed that it had grown a lot of new baby feathers since I first saw it. Had I not known the background, I don't think that I would have recognized it as the same bird.

"It's my sista's bird. She wantsta sell it." He was holding the chick in one hand and made some hand signal with the other—two fingers pointing down, the thumb up.

I reached out to pet the bird. It pushed its head against my fingers just like it did the first day when it was still in the cage. "God, yeah! My wife would love it." I reached out to pick it up, but the guy pulled it back.

"Hey, no touchin'! Dis a 'spensive bird!" The guy's partner, who looked even more menacing, stood well over six feet tall and was muscled like a football player. He stepped closer, more or less between the bird man and me.

"How much you want for it?" I refused to stop petting the bird, although I anticipated him pushing my hand away at any minute.

"Fifteen large."

"Holy shit!" I stepped back. "That's a lot for a red bird." I needed to stall. "She's got a lot of red birds in there." I motioned toward the store. "Besides, look at its feathers." I pointed to the multitude of new pinfeathers growing in all over the body. That was totally normal for a chick, but I was hoping he didn't know that. "It looks like it's got mange or something!"

"Fuck if you doan' want it." They started to walk off.

"Hey, wait." I followed. The big man stepped between us again like a well-trained blocker for the NFL. "I know my wife would love it."

"Fifteen."

"Okay. Okay." I shuffled. "I can do that."

He smiled. "Cash." His gold teeth flashed.

"I can't do that. I don't carry that kind of coin on me. I can give you a check?" I didn't have a check, and I knew that there was no way he'd take one, but I was trying to drag out the negotiation as long as possible.

They started walking again. I looked back at the pet shop and wondered if Jeanne had called the cops. Jeanne was peering out the front window from between two big, wrought iron cages. I didn't know how much longer I could hold off the birdnappers.

"Can you give me thirty minutes? Please?" I stepped back in front of the bird guy to stop him from walking. "I just need to run to the ATM if you want cash. I can get it and meet you back here?" I phrased the statement as a question.

"Cash? Fifteen?" They looked at each other. "Yeah, thirty minutes, no mo."

"'K. I'll be back in thirty. Meet you in the store, 'cause I gotta get some bird food too."

The birdman nodded in the banger way, flicking the head in a brief backward twitch.

They left around the corner, and I took off in the opposite direction. I knew that would confuse Jeanne, but I wanted to give them the impression that I was, in fact, in a hurry to get to the ATM.

As soon as I got back to NAVH, I called Jeanne and told her what had happened. Then I called Roy, my police friend from the herpetology club, and he called two of his undercover cop friends with the gang unit.

Since it was Saturday we had a lot of cash in our hospital safe since there were no deposits on the weekend. I grabbed $1,500 in large bills.

"What the heck are you doing?" Willy saw me take the money.

"No time to explain." I stuffed the money in a plain white envelope. "I'll do my best to bring it back." I looked at him with a bit of panic in my eyes. "If I don't, it'll mean that I'm probably dead."

Money in hand, I made it back to the pet store in less than fifteen minutes. About five minutes after I got there, a man and woman came in together, split apart once inside, each looking around as if shopping for something. After realizing there were no others in the store, the man eventually moseyed in my direction.

"Dr. Mader?" he whispered.

I nodded.

He discreetly lifted the bottom of his jacket and flashed a police badge. I noticed a semiautomatic pistol holstered just behind it.

"When they come in, engage them like you're going to buy the bird," he instructed without looking at me. "Did you bring the money?"

"Yeah." I was wondering what they'd do if I didn't have it. I knew that Jeanne didn't keep that kind of cash around.

"Okay. It's important that we get him taking the money. Since these aren't the ones who actually stole the bird, we can't arrest them for grand theft." He paused, looking around to make sure no one else had entered.

"But we *can* get them for possessing and selling stolen property." He turned his back but continued to talk. "These guys are little bitches. If you bust them, they won't take the fall but roll on whomever they got the bird from in the first place."

Wow. I had been hoping that I could just give a subtle nod when the bangers came into the store: I hadn't realized I was going to have to play such an integral role.

We waited another ten, fifteen, thirty minutes. A dad and his daughter came in to buy some canary seed and a cuttlebone. Jeanne was pleasant but clearly in a hurry to get them out before anything happened. I knew that the cops would not want them in the store when the bangers returned.

"You sure they are going to show up?" The female cop finally came over and spoke to me.

"That was the plan." I pulled the fat envelope with the cash from the pouch of my hoodie and showed it to her. "I was to go get the money and meet them back here in thirty minutes."

"They got spooked." The detective laughed at herself. "Get it? Spooked?"

And they say prejudice doesn't exist in the LA police department.

"We need to give them more time." Jeanne finally spoke up. I could see she was a bundle of nerves. She couldn't stop fidgeting. "I gotta get my bird back."

"Unfortunately, we can't wait all day." The male cop spoke up. "She's right—they probably got alarmed for some reason and decided to take the bird elsewhere."

"Jeanne, if they're hot to unload this bird today, why don't you call the other pet stores in the area. They may be making the rounds."

"Good idea." The female cop agreed.

Suddenly the male cop startled, pulled his coat back, and grabbed the pager off his belt. "Oh shit," he blurted out, looking at the screen. "It's a 911. Gotta run." With no further explanation, he darted out of the store.

"I'll stick around a few more minutes," the female cop offered. It was almost an hour past our scheduled meeting time. I couldn't blame her. Many far worse crimes were happening at any given moment in the big city, and I knew they were only here because my cop friend Roy had called them.

Just as we were about to pull the plug, the front door bell jingled. Only the bird guy, not his enormous partner, came in. He was holding the red chick in his hand.

"Hey, man!" I went over to him. "What took you so long?"

"You got the money?"

"Yeah." I pulled the envelope out of my pouch and handed it to him. Aside from being scared out of my wits, I was really hoping I'd get that money back.

As he grabbed the envelope, I took the bird. But before he could look inside, the cop came up behind him, gun drawn, and commanded, "Hands up and down on your knees."

The banger turned just in time to see the business end of a 9mm positioned about six inches from his face. Without a word or a struggle the gangsta complied, knelt down, and raised his hands, holding the envelope high.

I seized the moment and grabbed the cash before anything happened to it—like being confiscated as evidence. The fledgling was safe in my other hand.

The banger looked up at me from his knees with evil eyes, snarling, flashing his grill, with his head cocked to the side. "Muthafucka!"

I thought it odd that the stolen bird ended up back in the same store, so I called Roy to ask about it and he gave me the whole story. Apparently the initial guy and girl had stolen the bird for drug money, but nobody local would buy it, and the couple didn't know what to do. The guy was just going to kill it, but the girl felt bad for the chick. At first she had planned to take the bird back, then thought better of it and gave it to another friend.

That person also tried to sell the bird but again couldn't find a buyer. The bird got passed around a few more times, so that finally with so many degrees of separation, the two guys who finally ended up with it had no idea where it had come from. One of them got the bright idea to try to sell it to a pet store and happened to go back to the store from which it was stolen. I just hoped the guy I tried to buy the bird from didn't remember me when he got out of jail.

• • •

It was a big day: the Christmas snake was going home!

The big question for me was what to charge the owner for over three months of hospitalization. It had received multiple IV jugular catheters, gallons upon gallons of IV fluids, several bottles of antibiotics and vitamins, countless tube feedings, a half dozen rats, and one large rabbit for dinner, not to mention all the staff time involved. This was not like a small cat that could be handled easily by just one technician. The huge snake, especially as it got stronger, required at least two to three technicians every time it was taken from the cage. I couldn't even begin to calculate the total person hours that had been invested in its care.

I suspected that the owners did not have much money. If the snake had been a dog or cat staying that long and receiving that much intensive care, the veterinary bill would have been several thousand dollars. Although this was definitely one of those feel-good cases and I wanted to help them out financially, Willy was all over me about making sure we got paid for our services.

After a lot of thought I decided to charge her a total of $1,500 for everything: the Christmas morning emergency visit and all the hospitalization and treatments. I figured that would just barely cover our actual costs of supplies. It was bad business, but the part of me that values the human-pet bond was driving my decision. Willy would just have to deal with it.

I swear that the snake recognized the little girl. We pulled all eighteen feet of the serpent out of the cage while the redheaded child sat cross-legged on the floor of the treatment room. The python immediately started tongue flicking and slithered directly over to her. The constrictor lifted its head, and when it came face to face with her freckles, its tongue went crazy. The little girl reached out, tears in her eyes, and gave it a big hug.

Mom, the staff, and I all stood around and enjoyed the moment. Watching the mother observe her daughter's joy, I knew once again that I had picked the right profession.

"I suppose we need to settle up the bill." She turned toward me, wiping happy tears from her eyes.

"Sure." I motioned for her to follow me. We went into the conference room for some privacy. I had three months of charges printed out on several sheets of paper. My plan was to review all the fees, point out the actual total, then let her know the final figure reflecting the super-large discount I had factored in.

"I don't need to see all of this." She was direct but very pleasant. "Please just tell me what I owe. I know you all did a tremendous amount of work."

"Your snake was here for ninety-five days." I skipped right to the summary as requested. "I've given you a discount. The final total is $1,500, for everything."

"Oh my God!" Her mouth dropped open, and she covered it with her fingers.

I had been afraid of this. I suspected that she was going to have to make payments. Why hadn't I kept her appraised, at least weekly, on the status of her charges? That was my responsibility.

"That's all?" She looked at me, then threw her arms around my neck, crying. Happy tears. "I was imagining, like, at least $5,000 or more."

"Like I said, I factored in a big discount. It's my Christmas present to you and your daughter."

"I certainly wasn't expecting discounts. You gave up your Christmas to take care of us. You are so generous!" She released the hug and stepped back. "I got a quarter-million-dollar life insurance settlement from my husband's accident. I was fully prepared to pay whatever the cost necessary to bring our snake back home."

♦ ♦ ♦

Pat Peters brought in Thor, the black-and-white tegu lizard, for me to see how it was faring on its vegetarian diet. Of course, Robert was in the exam room when she arrived. Raoul was also there, excited to see such a cool lizard.

"Are they always this skinny?" Raoul whispered.

The tegu had not eaten since I had last seen it, five weeks ago. I weighed the lizard in front of Pat on a small, portable scale. It had lost 25 percent of its body weight. I didn't need to say anything. This woman's IQ was probably 100 points higher than mine.

"I was worried about that," Pat said, clearly regretful.

"Yeah." I lifted the emaciated lizard off the scale. It was weak from inanition, not the same feisty beast I had first met. "You've tried your way, Pat. In fairness to this lizard, it really needs to be given a proper diet or it will die. Soon."

"I'm resolute about not feeding it live prey," she stated as a matter of record. "I am a vegetarian. I don't believe in eating animals."

"Fine, Pat." I had to take a stand in defense of the tegu. "I respect that you don't want to eat animals. That's a choice you're free to make." I rubbed the limp lizard's head and neck. "But these guys never got that choice. God, or whoever you believe to be the decision maker, *created* them as meat eaters. Period." I watched her shuffle her feet, looking down at the floor. "As a philosopher, I know you understand that concept."

Pat nodded. There was an awkward pregnant pause while she pondered the dilemma.

"As I said, I am resolute about not feeding it live prey." She looked at me as if this edict was final. "But at the same time, I am also acquiescing by acknowledging that my beliefs put this creature in peril."

I know that philosophical debate was Pat's raison d'être. However, I wondered if before now she had ever been forced to actually have one of these soul-searching discussions with herself.

"When I adopted Thor from the student, I took it upon myself to provide for it." She paused. "Like a marriage. I made a commitment to this lizard, as far as I am concerned, for life."

I was really not sure where she was going.

"I think the best thing, since I will never go back on my word, is if you keep it here and feed it."

I had not anticipated this conclusion.

"As I said, I cannot in good faith feed it live prey, but I accept that is what it needs to be healthy, and I talked to Robert, and he said he would feed it if I left it here with you."

"I am not completely sure if I am understanding you, Pat? Do you want to bring it by on the days that it needs to eat, Robert will feed it, and then you will take it back home?"

"No. I have a problem living with something in my house that eats meat. I'd like to permanently board it here and pay you all to take care of it."

What an unexpected resolution. After losing my shirt on the charges for the big snake, I needed to make sure that, if this was what she really wanted to do, I charged her appropriately for the long-term room and board.

"Can't you give it back to the boy you rescued it from?"

"I'm afraid not." She shook her head. "The last I heard, his parents had made him move back home. I think he's out of the picture."

I had one last question. "Pat, why don't you just adopt it out to someone who will give it a proper home? These lizards are really popular. I can take it with me to the next herpetology meeting, and I can guarantee you that I'll find it an excellent home." That, to me, seemed like the best solution. I wasn't too keen on keeping that large lizard here, living in a hospital cage, for the rest of its life. An animal that large and robust needed appropriate housing to be content.

"You don't understand, Doctor." She looked at me. "I made a commitment to this lizard that I would care for it for the rest of its life. It is *my* responsibility. I can't just pawn it off on someone else because it is inconvenient or its lifestyle goes against everything I stand for. I want to keep it here, with you and Robert."

Greta Can't Get a Break

My new student, Greta Altenhoffer, from a veterinary school in Germany, was not scheduled to arrive until the weekend, so I was without an extern for the next few days.

"Dr. Mader." Lisa pulled me aside as soon as I finished my morning surgeries. "I need to talk with you about Lori."

"What now?" I knew that Lisa and the other receptionists had been having problems with Lori for the past few weeks.

"I think she's high."

"What?" It was absolutely forbidden for any employee to come to work after they had been drinking or doing any type of drugs. "Why would you say that?"

"She got back from lunch all twitchy." Lisa pointed to her upper lip. "And she's constantly wiping her nose." Lisa made the motion.

"Maybe she's got a cold?" Wishful thinking.

"I think she's snorting."

"Was Fred involved?" I would be devastated if he was.

"No. They haven't been together for a few months now."

Stacey pulled me away from my conversation with Lisa and handed me the chart for a rat that was scratching itself raw. It was a new client, but the rat's symptoms reminded me of those of Mickey the mouse, the little mouse that had scratched its own ear off. That case hadn't ended so well.

The beautiful black-and-white rat, commonly called a Gunn rat, was as sweet as could be but was miserable because it couldn't stop scratching. It was covered from head to tail with excoriations. Fresh and dried blood was smeared throughout its normally smooth fur. As with Mickey, this was another bad case of mites.

I assured the owners that I could help their pet if I could keep the rat for the night and give it a tranquilizer and medication to kill the mites and help it stop scratching. They were happy with that plan, and I walked them to reception for checkout. Lori was at the front desk, so I waited and watched her with the transaction. She seemed a little off, but not high, as Lisa had suggested.

One of the owners gave the rat a kiss on its forehead before handing it to me. "Take good care of our little boy!"

"You want me to take it in the back, Dr. Mader?" Lori offered.

"Sure, thank you." I passed the rat over to Lori and went directly to my next patient.

I had barely started my exam when Lisa came barging into the room.

"Dr. Mader, we need you, *stat*!" she said, panic and fear in her eyes.

I followed her back to treatment. Robert had Pat Peters's tegu on the exam table, and Stacey was holding the Gunn rat under running water in the sink.

"What's going on?" I looked around. Nobody was making eye contact with me. Lori was in the corner, crying.

"Lori put the rat in the cage with the tegu!" Maria fessed up.

"Thank God I was here, or this rat would have been toast!" Stacey exclaimed. Blood was streaming off the side of the rat from a gash in its cheek.

"Just put pressure on it, Stacey." I reached into a glass container and pulled out some fresh gauze.

"Stacey saw Lori toss the rat in the cage," Robert chimed in. "She yelled at her to stop, but it was too late."

Our exotics cages all had glass fronts so that the technicians and doctors could monitor the sick patients without having to open doors. There was no excuse for Lori to have put the rat in the same cage with the lizard.

"How did you get the tegu to let the rat go?"

"Stacey sprayed rubbing alcohol into the tegu's mouth," Robert said as he wiped the lizard's face with a paper towel. "As soon as she did that it spit the rat out."

Stacey was busy cleaning the rat. Her quick thinking had literally saved the rat's life, and us from getting sued or, worse, having our veterinary licenses suspended.

I quickly sedated and assessed the petrified rat. Thank God the lizard bite wound, although bloody, was not serious. In fact, if I hadn't already examined the rat, I would not have been able to distinguish the lizard bite from the self-mutilation caused by the rat's own scratching.

Once I saw that everything was under control, I asked Lori and her immediate supervisor, Lisa, to sit down for a talk. I was hoping Willy would be there, but he hadn't returned from lunch yet, and what I had to tell Lori could not wait.

◆ ◆ ◆

It was a good thing I had Wok. He was always there for me, even when my wife wasn't. When I got home that night I had no appetite for dinner. I went for a much more aggressive run than normal, then took Wok out for his prance in the park shortly after dark. After Wok made his mandatory rounds marking his territory, my best friend joined me on our bench.

I told him what had happened to the rat and how lucky we were that Stacey had come to the rescue. The ethical question was this: since there was no permanent harm to the rat, should I tell the owners what had happened? That a possibly coked-out receptionist had carelessly tossed their beloved pet rat in with a starving carnivorous lizard ten times its size? That their rat had been literally seconds away from being shredded alive?

Should I charge them for any of the services we performed? For the bath, pain medications, antibiotics, etc., we'd administered? We would have done it all anyway to treat the bad skin, and they were expecting to pay for it, so in actuality there was no extra charge on account of the lizard incident. If I didn't tell them anything, they would never know, because their rat was going to get better due to our treatments for the mites and damaged skin.

It seemed to be a no-brainer. There was no reason to freak out the owners and tell them what happened, right? Sadly, I know veterinarians who would have done just that—kept it a secret. But I was not one of them.

Once again, I barely slept at all. I got to work especially early to check on the rat, although I knew that if there had been a problem Greg would have called me. To my astonishment, the rat looked better than I expected. The fur was clean, there was no more dried blood, and the emollient shampoo had removed the ugly scabs. The little rat was happily munching on a sunflower seed and didn't scratch once the entire time I stood in front of the glass cage.

I waited until 8:00 a.m. and then called the owners with the news that the rat was doing well and was ready to come home. Needless to say, they were thrilled. I planned to tell them what happened with the lizard when they picked the pet up. There would be no charge for their visit.

◆ ◆ ◆

They say that everybody gets their fifteen minutes of fame. Mine was about to debut. Everybody arrived at work early to watch the *Good Morning America* segment featuring the underground Ferret Club. There were some sleepy eyes in the conference room at this premature hour, but I was able to counter the sunrise lassitude with a box of fresh doughnuts.

It took a while before the story aired, since it wasn't "hard news," but finally the reporter was on camera talking about the clandestine group that meets in the bowels of Los Angeles. The piece started out showing two cute little ferrets playing, rough and tumble, on a carpeted floor in someone's house. I assumed it was probably the home of the Ferret Club's president, although they didn't say where the footage was taken.

Cut to the reporter, sitting behind a desk, who then went into a brief history about the outlawing of pet ferrets in California. Segue to video taken from inside the TV van as it drove down the dark alleyway to the back door of the warehouse, again without showing anything that would give away the location.

There followed footage of the president, then some testimonials from the audience, including some horror stories about the CDFG killing ferrets right in front of the owners.

Finally, they showed my interview. As much as I had tried to speak in sound bites, they managed to twist things around, editing the order of their questions and my answers so as to alter my intent and create their own narrative.

I was introduced as Dr. Doug Mader, "veterinarian to the underground ferret world." They neglected to mention that although owning ferrets in California was illegal, treating them was not.

Among the questions I had been asked in various ways during my fifteen-minute interview was whether I thought that ferrets made good pets.

Some of my sound bite responses had been:

"Ferrets can be great pets for the right person."

"Ferrets are quite interactive with people."

"Ferrets have been known to have a dark side."

"Ferrets can be playful and friendly, but they have been known to bite."

"Children should never be left alone with a ferret."

"There have been a number of reports of sleeping babies being bitten by ferrets."

Those answers seemed pretty straightforward, and I felt I had been honest about the behavior and suitability of ferrets as pets. Unfortunately, that was not how I came across after the edits. The final segment went something like this:

Reporter: "Dr. Mader, do you think ferrets are safe pets for children?"

Me: "Ferrets can be great pets."

Reporter: "Why do you think that children are so attracted to ferrets?"

Me: "Ferrets can be playful and friendly."

Reporter: "So then you are saying that it is okay for a child to have a pet ferret?"

Me: "For the right person."

End of interview. Nothing was discussed about ferret health care, which was the reason I was supposedly brought in to share my expertise in the first place.

The final segment of the broadcast was an interview with a precociously eloquent eight-year-old dressed in her schoolgirl uniform. It began with the girl showing one of her hands to the cameraperson. She was missing three fingers.

"I was just an infant when it happened," she explained. "I was still asleep when, with only the stealth that a natural hunting animal could possess, the ferret got into my crib and attacked me." The camera pulled back from the hand shot to show her face, horribly disfigured: her left ear, left eyebrow, and a large portion of her nose chewed off.

"The forensic experts suspect that the ferret started by eating away at my face; then out of reflex I must have tried to protect myself with my hands, and that's when the aggressive carnivore started on my fingers." The articulate little girl calmly relayed the story.

Everybody watched on in horror.

Moments before, I had been quoted saying, "Ferrets can be great pets."

◆ ◆ ◆

Officer Kelly Pinkett brought in a golden eagle that had been shot by a poacher and needed emergency surgery. The golden eagle, like the bald eagle, is a federally protected bird. The wildlife officials stop at nothing to safeguard them and want only the best care if they are injured.

After the bird recovered from the anesthesia, I called Officer Kelly with an update.

"So did you end up amputating the wing so we could release it in a couple of days?" Kelly teased. "Seriously though—while I've got you on the phone, I've got some other news that you'll like to hear."

"What's that?"

"It seems that you were right about Fore the fox and all PR it generated for the golf course, as much as I hate to admit it."

"What are you talking about?"

"The country club is putting a big spin on this whole three-legged-fox thing. It seems they have an entire 'Fore the fox' marketing scheme now: golf hats with a picture of a three-legged Fore the fox on the front, three-legged fox key chains, bumper stickers, and a whole lot more!"

"That just goes to show that you really should listen to me more often."

"Really? You always have the best advice?"

"Really!"

"By the way," Kelly continued, "that was some interview on national television!" I could hear her laugh. "'*Ferrets can be great pets.*' I should have you arrested!"

"Smart-ass." There weren't many law enforcement officials I could joke with like that.

After stopping in at work, I took Greta with me to the research facility where I performed monthly health checks on the primates. The German student seemed quite interested in and fascinated by everything, but she did not seem as energetic as she had the first two days of her externship. I was worried that the whole "research on animals" concept might be concerning her, as the rules and regulations are so different in this country than they are in Europe.

She assured me that she was good with what she saw and even impressed with how well the animals were all taken care of. When I asked why she seemed so quiet, she said that the jet lag had caught up with her and she was feeling a little under the weather.

• • •

Morning rounds started as usual, with the exception that there was no student. We waited a few minutes for Greta, but the agenda was full so we had to get started without her. By midmorning Greta still had not shown up in the clinic, and I was beginning to worry, so I had Lisa go upstairs to her apartment. The report was not so good. Per Lisa, Greta had the flu and was running a temperature of 103 degrees.

I had to give a lecture to the Southern California Veterinary Medical Association after work. Greta felt too sick to come along, so I went alone. Dusk had arrived by the time I hurried out the front door. To my surprise, Harriett the hooker was already at her post on the corner.

"My, my, Doctor! Don't you look fine." Harriett turned my way when she saw me exit the hospital. I typically wear a business suit when I present professional lectures.

"G'evening, Harriett. How are you doing tonight?"

"You gotta date with the missus?" She walked over, sizing me up and down as she approached.

"Nope." I smiled.

She was on the prowl. I've been propositioned by hookers many times over the years, but I never thought that I'd have a hooker friend. Harriett had been working from my corner for the past six months, and I saw her on a regular basis. We chatted on occasion, so I guess she qualified, loosely, as a friend. Our initial interaction had started out a bit edgy, but she had kept her word and not only stopped harassing my clients but was actually helpful to some.

"I don't think I can ever 'member seeing you lookin' so yummy." She walked over and slowly ran her hands up the front of my jacket.

"Now, Harriett," I said, gently taking her hands and removing them from my lapel, "I've gotta be going, not, well . . . you know."

"That's funny!" She stepped back and held her stomach. "Ooh, Dr. Doug. You are a funny doctor!"

"Happy to make you smile, Harriett." For some reason, I felt I had to give her a hug. "I've really got to get on the road."

◆ ◆ ◆

"Your next clients are just the cutest, Dr. Mader!" Lisa was clearly in a good mood.

Greta and I entered the exam room, and sure enough, there was a young mother with a very young daughter, the latter holding a very young kitten. The little girl looked to be about seven or eight, and the kitten perhaps seven or eight weeks. I introduced Greta and myself.

"We just adopted this kitten from the shelter." The mom looked at the daughter, who was busy petting the purring kitten sitting in her lap. "Can you tell the nice doctor his name?"

"His name is Frisky." The happy-faced little girl looked up through thick, red-rimmed prism glasses, the kind that children wear when they're born cross-eyed. Her brown hair was braided into pigtails that were tied off with a bright red bow at each end. The orange-and-white kitten had a matching red collar with a tiny silver bell.

"What a perfect name!" Lisa was right. Too cute.

"I'm worried about the spots on his ears." The mom pointed to several angry red circles on the backside of both of the kitten's tiny pink ears. "They just started to show up in the last few days."

The kitten had one of those diseases that you could literally diagnose from across the room. "I'm afraid your kitten has a disease called ringworm. It's not actually a worm, even though it looks like there is a little round worm living in a circle just under the skin. It's a fungus that kittens catch at the shelter. It's treatable, but it can also infect people."

Just then Stacey opened the door and handed me a Wood's lamp, a flashlight-like device that emits light in the same spectrum as blacklights used on psychedelic posters. "We can confirm the ringworm by shining this special lamp on it. If the skin glows green, it's positive."

Greta switched the lights off. I turned the Wood's lamp on, and sure enough the lesions on the kitten's ears glowed bright green. I made sure that the mom, daughter, and Greta all saw the reaction to the lamp.

Greta turned the lights back on.

"Frisky has ringworm." I looked at the pair. For a moment there was an awkward pause. Then the mother turned and spoke quietly to the young girl.

"Go ahead." The mom whispered. "It's okay."

The little girl refused to look up. Instead, she just kept petting the kitten and aggressively shook her head back and forth. "Honey, he's a doctor. Show him."

The little girl looked at her mom, then slowly handed her the kitten. Once her hands were free, she lifted her skirt up to expose her underwear. There were several red, inflamed circular lesions on the skin of her upper inner thighs where she had been holding the kitten.

Without saying a word I handed the Wood's lamp to Greta. She turned off the room light again and pointed the lamp at the child's lap. Sure enough, the entire groin region glowed bright green like the kitten.

"Before you turn it off . . . " The mom spoke out from the dark. The next thing I knew she had lifted her shirt and removed her bra. I could see several glowing lesions between her breasts from across the table. Greta stepped between us, deliberately blocking my view to give the mother some privacy, and shined the lamp on her as well, accenting what we already anticipated.

Greta waited for the woman to get dressed again before turning the room light back on.

"Well," I said, keeping it simple, "it's no surprise you all have ringworm. Like I said, it's highly contagious."

"Can we treat it, Doctor? My daughter just loves the kitten."

"Absolutely! I was going to warn you that you and your family have to be careful not to catch it, but it's too late for that. I can tell you how to treat the kitten, but I'd also like you to immediately go see your family physician so you all can be treated."

The mom put her hand on the daughter's head, stroking her hair. "See, sweetie; it's going to be okay."

"You should know it can take as long as six to eight weeks for the ringworm to resolve. In the meantime, anyone else in your family, if they don't have it, may get it." Again, before I could get out the next sentence, Stacey opened the door and handed Greta some NAVH printouts on "Pets, People, and Ringworm" that I had written up for clients.

After the duo left with their kitten, I turned to Greta. "I'm so glad you were there. That could have been very awkward."

"Me too," she answered. "But not for the same reason as you! I've never seen it before. That was very special."

"You'd better go wash your hands, even if you didn't touch the kitten. You should also go change into some fresh clothes and toss those directly into the wash."

"Okay, but what about you? You were touching the kitten all over."

"Good point. Once you get ringworm you develop resistance to it. That's why you rarely ever see adult cats and dogs with it. I had a bad case of it a few years ago, so now I can touch it and not have to worry."

◆ ◆ ◆

My first appointment of the day was with an old cat named Cutter. Matthew Hellman was only five years old when he found Cutter, who was then a kitten. The kitten was so young that its eyes were barely open. Matt said that his mother taught him how to care for such a young cat. Sadly, Matt's mother had died several years ago. Aside from Matt's cousin Scott, who also lived here in the city, Cutter was the only family he had. Matt was twenty-two, so I figured Cutter had to be at least seventeen.

Matt didn't have a lot of money, so routine veterinary care was never part of his budget. That did not mean that Matt loved Cutter any less, however. As I listened to Matt's story I realized there was a special bond between them. I wanted to do whatever was needed to help.

Cutter was skinny and dehydrated and, according to Matt, had been urinating all over the house—something he'd never done before. The few cat diseases that cause those symptoms are relatively easy to diagnose but can be difficult and sometimes expensive to treat. Unfortunately, the laboratory analyses confirmed that the older cat was in kidney failure—an inevitable death sentence.

Matt was devastated. He slumped down on the stool in the exam room and buried his face. "What if I had brought him in sooner?" he cried. Matt had early male-pattern hair loss, and what little hair he had left was turning gray, thinning, and frizzed out to the sides. It appeared that he hadn't shaved in several days, and all in all, he looked rough. His physical appearance no doubt mirrored what he was feeling on the inside. I noticed that as we talked Matt was fondling a small crucifix on a choker around his neck.

"It wouldn't have mattered. Sadly, cats develop kidney failure just like humans. It was nothing you did or could have done differently."

"Is there anything we can do for him?"

"Matt," I said, not wanting to give him false hope, "if Cutter were a human he would be placed on dialysis, a machine that replaces his kidneys. This would be for life, or, if the conditions were right, until he could get a kidney transplant."

"Can you do that?" he asked with a look of desperation. I could tell he would do anything for his cat.

"Unfortunately, no." I really didn't want to go in this direction. "The only place that does that is the veterinary school at UC Davis, near Sacramento."

"I'll do it." He stood up, like he was ready to run out the door at that very moment.

"Matt, Cutter would not qualify for a new kidney." I knew that would totally crush him, but he had asked. "He is too old. They only do kidney transplants on young cats, in much stronger condition. Cutter would never survive the surgery."

"But you said he could have dialysis and then get a kidney!"

"Matt, I said he would need dialysis for life, or if the conditions were right, he could get a transplant."

"Are you sure?"

I was. Kidney transplants were still in their infancy in veterinary medicine. They were complicated and very costly, in the range of $10,000 and up.

"How much longer?" His voice dropped as he sank back onto the stool.

"No way of telling. But I've had cats live for several months or longer with aggressive in-home nursing."

"I'll do whatever . . ."

"I know you can do it, that you'll be there for him no matter what."

"I'll never give up on him. Just tell me what I need to do."

"For now, we have to get him through this acute crisis." I grabbed a tissue from the container in the pass-through window and handed it to Matt to dry his eyes.

"I can start Cutter on IV fluids to flush his system. It's a little like dialysis in humans. If, and that's a big *if*, we can get his kidney blood values to come back to normal, or even come down somewhat, then you *may* be able take him home and I can teach you how to give fluids under the skin, which *may* help slow the progression of the disease."

"Okay, Doctor." He stood up again, showing some renewed hope. "Do whatever you need to do. He's been by my side my whole life. I'll never give up on him."

◆ ◆ ◆

I've been called predictable and boring, but I can't help it if I like Lili's teriyaki burgers. So yes, I go to her Country Kitchen a lot.

I brought Greta with me. She was also enjoying a teriyaki burger on my recommendation when Lili waddled over to our table. "There's gonna be trouble. You should leave now if you no live here." The older cook waggled her stubby index finger at the young German girl.

"What are you talking about?" I loved that Lili always seemed to know what was going on around town, but I didn't like what she had just said.

"Soon Ja Du!"

"What?" The name rang a bell.

"Soon Ja Du! The Korean liquor store owner that killed the black girl o'er the orange juice. The appeal to make her have a tougher sentence got denied! Jus' now!" Lili was clearly exasperated. "The blacks no like us Koreans. There's gonna be trouble!"

Once again Lili pointed directly at Greta. "You betta leave soon. This place is gonna burn to da ground!"

♦ ♦ ♦

I arrived at work early only to find the lights in treatment off.

"We blow a fuse?" I asked as I walked toward the darkened room. When I turned the corner, I was surprised to see Stacey shining the Wood's lamp on Greta's face. Double silver dollar–sized, interlocking rings, shaped like a figure eight, were glowing bright green down the left side of Greta's nose.

She had ringworm. On her face. That really sucked.

"Five to seven days," I said and flipped the lights on as Greta hid her face with her hand, "is about the average incubation time for signs of infection to show up."

"How long is it going to last?" Stacey was grossed out.

"Just like in pets, it can last four to six weeks." I took the Wood's lamp from Stacey and wiped it down with disinfectant. I turned to Greta. "Why don't you go talk to Lisa about going to see a doctor for a prescription."

"Can't you just give her something from here?" Stacey was washing her hands from her fingertips to her armpits.

"Only if you want me to lose my license." I gave her a sour look.

As an afterthought I called my doctor friend, Kristin Sullivan, and she, on my word, called in a ringworm prescription for Greta to the local pharmacy.

The day was busy with new clients, rechecks, and a treatment for the eagle. Cutter, the cat in renal failure, was doing better. Matt, the owner, came to visit, and I explained that even though Cutter's blood tests had improved slightly with the IV fluids, the kidney disease was advanced. However, if Cutter's blood values continued to respond favorably, we might be able to send him home tomorrow. Matt was thrilled.

It took some convincing, but I got Greta to agree to go with me to the herpetological meeting. After the meeting Roy, the snake-loving police officer, stopped me in the exit hallway. "Hey, Doc. Got a minute?"

"Sure, Roy." I introduced him to Greta. "What's up?"

"The Rodney King jury went to deliberation this morning." He spoke softly. "There's word on the street that if the cops get off, there's going to be big trouble."

Echoes of Lili.

"Like what kind of trouble?"

"Like, bad shit's gonna hit the fan." He hadn't looked this serious even on the day he found the dead guy in my front yard. "You're not in the best part of town. I would be really, really careful if I were you. And if you don't have a gun, get one. Make sure your hospital is ready. This place is going to go to hell."

I had never seen Roy look so grim.

♦ ♦ ♦

Cutter was looking like a new cat. Although his kidney blood values were still elevated, he was feeling much better than when he presented. The IV fluids did their job. He was eating, drinking, and acting like a normal cat. I felt he was doing well enough to go home. His owner, Matt, didn't have much money, so I wanted to get Cutter discharged as soon as possible to help keep the costs down.

I had Matt bring Cutter back to recheck his blood first thing the following Monday morning. Unfortunately, as I'd feared, without the daily IV fluids, the old cat had taken a dramatic turn for the worse. I talked it over with Matt, and even though money was tight, he agreed to keep Cutter with us a few more days for more IV fluid treatments. Hopefully we could get the blood values down and then customize a fluid therapy protocol he could manage at home. That the old cat had decompensated so quickly once off the IV fluids was a bad sign.

"I'll be back for you, ol' boy. You hang in there." Matt ever so gently bent down and kissed the old cat on his furry forehead.

"This was my mom's." He fingered an antique-looking crucifix hanging around his neck. "She taught me how to care for Cutter when he was a kitten. I know that she's watching over him."

• • •

"They're rioting!" Greg announced as he rushed into the treatment room. His face was ghostly pale. It was only 6:00 p.m. Greg usually didn't show up for the start of night shift until 7:00.

"What?" I was preoccupied with Cutter. The old cat's IV catheter had failed, and since he was so dehydrated, even the deft Stacey was unable to get a new one into the vein in his other leg.

"They're rioting!" Greg screamed again. He looked around at the busy room, panic in his eyes.

"The cops that beat Rodney King got off! Rioters are pulling people out of their cars and killing them. Right now, in LA!" Greg wore an expression of sheer terror.

Just like that there was deafening silence. Everybody stopped what they were doing and stared at Greg. "They're showing it on TV! It's all live!"

At once we all dropped whatever we were working on and scrambled to the conference room to watch the broadcast.

A Los Angeles News Service helicopter was hovering over the intersection of Florence and Normandie avenues in South Central Los Angeles. The live feed showed total chaos on the streets below. Hundreds of individuals were swarming the area. The cameraman focused on a riotous crowd looting a corner liquor store.

As cars attempted to drive through the intersection they were ambushed by mobs and assaulted with rocks, bricks, garbage cans, sticks, or anything else that could be hurled. If a car stopped, or crashed, it would be attacked by gangs. Throngs of angry protestors mobbed the vehicle, jumping on the hood and roof and smashing the windows. The drivers were in the wrong place at the wrong time. In the midst of this chaos the police were notably absent. You could hear the voice of the pilot pleading, "Where are the cops? Where are the cops?"

The staff watched in horror as the drama unfolded live. I forced myself away from the images of the escalating violence and slipped out of the room to call Ellen. It was time for her to go to work, and I was petrified of the thought that she had to drive through town and then work in the ER all night. It was surely going to be hell.

No answer at home. I called her mobile phone and got an automated response: "All cellular networks are busy at the moment. Please try your call again later." I imagined her cell phone service provider was overwhelmed.

Scared and worried, I went back into the conference room. Everyone watched in silent terror as the chopper camera showed a white-panel truck being surrounded by an angry mob. An army of protestors smashed the windshield and side panels, forcing open the door, yanking the driver out, and throwing him to the road. Immediately a half dozen men started beating the hapless man with their fists and kicking him in the head. An attacker left the circle of thugs and took a fire extinguisher from the cab of the truck, then returned and repeatedly bashed the man's head until he slumped unconscious to the pavement. An expanding halo of blood was visible all the way from the helicopter.

It was gut-wrenching to watch.

Suddenly the camera's focus panned in a different direction. A large semitruck with a red cab and two silver trailers entered, then stopped, in the middle of the intersection, just feet away from the disabled white truck.

Several men immediately ambushed the driver of the new big rig, smashing his windows with rocks. Two men climbed the side steps of the cab, forced open the driver's side door, then threw the trucker to the ground. A third attacker joined in, jumping on the driver's neck and pinning him down while a pack started beating on him just as they had the previous truck driver.

The man's white T-shirt turned blood red with the unrelenting assault. First came the fists and feet; then rocks were flung at the downed victim. As the driver attempted to get up on his knees, another aggressor smashed the back of his head with a large white canister, knocking him back to the bloodied asphalt. While he was down, another mugger took a hammer and struck him on his head and back.

Like a dying animal in a feeding frenzy, every time the prey tried to get up, he was kicked back down. When he refused to give up, someone took a brick and slammed it into the back of his head. For ever so brief a moment you could see the white glistening of his skull bone before it flushed red. That final blow knocked him unconscious, face down, blood gushing from the torn scalp and pouring onto the street.

The triumphant attackers circled their victim, standing over his body while staring up at the helicopter and flashing gang signs. One man spat on the victim repeatedly while another ransacked his pockets.

The camera from the chopper panned out, showing a newcomer standing just feet from this horrifying scene, filming the attack with a large video recorder mounted on his shoulder. He did nothing to help the unconscious man on the ground.

As the savagery continued, a motorcyclist pulled up alongside the big rig and started shooting the fuel tanks on the opposite side of the red cab with a shotgun, clearly trying to trigger an explosion.

The macabre scenes repeated themselves in an endless nightmare as driver after driver was dragged from their vehicle and beaten to a bloody pulp while hundreds of onlookers cheered.

Several minutes later, the camera from the news copter panned back to the downed driver of the red semi. He had miraculously risen, on his own, and was staggering, blinded by blood, toward the cab of his truck. Out of nowhere a black man approached the dazed and confused driver, grabbed him by his bloody shoulders, and guided him to the door of his cab. He then helped the injured man in, pushed him to the opposite side, got in the front seat himself, and drove the truck away.

We all watched in amazement as this man risked his own life to save that of the trucker. A tiny scintilla of compassion in the midst of this senseless slaughter.

"Guys," I interrupted the silence. "We need to come up with a plan for tonight." All of this live drama was just a few neighborhoods away. It might soon move into our area. "Let's get all the patients situated."

Since NAVH was a hospital, people would know that we had drugs and medical supplies inside. In a crisis, we would be a prime target. Greg, Stacey, Fred, Maria, Robert, Lisa, Gene, and Greta were all sitting at or standing around the table. Willy and Dr. Furtano had already left before the news of the riots. Cliff was standing in the back of the room next to Greta, who looked like she was about to go into shock. Not a word was spoken.

If ever I needed to be a leader, now was the time.

"Robert, Maria, get the garden hoses and put one inside each exit door". I pointed, gesturing for them to get moving. "Greg, Stacey, fill every container that you can find with water and bring them inside. Fred, fill all the sinks with water, and go upstairs to the apartments and do the same there."

We didn't have time or the materials to board up the large plate glass windows. "Lisa and Gene, get some packing tape and do the best you can to tape the insides of each front window, first in a big X, and then in concentric circles starting at the outer perimeter of the window and working in to the middle." My thought was that if the windows were broken, at least they wouldn't shatter and fall apart if they were taped this way. And hopefully if enough glass stayed in place it would deter people from entering.

"Greta," I addressed my petrified student, my mind flashing back to Lili's finger-wagging warning: *You should leave now if you no live here.* "When are you supposed to leave? When is your last day?"

She looked at me like a deer stuck in headlights. Cliff reached over and put an arm around her.

"Greta?"

"I was supposed to leave Saturday." She could barely get the words out.

"Okay. Don't worry—" I stated.

"Come stay with me," Cliff interrupted. "I live just a few blocks away."

"That's a great idea. Thanks, Cliff." I was truly impressed. Greta looked up at the young doctor and nodded silently.

"Can you two do me a favor and find all the fire extinguishers and put them near the exits?"

After a frenzied few minutes the staff once again mustered in the conference room. Night was falling, and the scene on the streets was playing out under the harsh floodlights of the news copter, the rioters performing for the camera with the streets of Los Angeles as their stage.

The intersection of Florence and Normandie was the epicenter of the violence. You would think that by then people would have known not to go anywhere near the area, but that wasn't the case. Cars and trucks were still trying to drive through. Why hadn't the police set up barricades to keep people away?

Fires were beginning to burn all around the city. Using picture-in-picture technology, many news stations now had roving reporters on the streets with handheld cameras showing the action from different locations in smaller insets on the screen. Back at Florence and Normandie, one of the camera crews broadcast as a mob forced a pickup truck to a stop, pulled the driver out, and beat him savagely. I had to look away. Around the room the tension was palpable. Greta was crying.

"Okay, everyone. I think we all need to get to our homes while it is still light and somewhat safe to be on the road." They all looked at me like I was crazy. "Seriously, the riots seem to be concentrated to the business districts; they haven't expanded out to residential streets yet. Now's the time to go home. You're all going to be fine." No one responded. "If anyone wants to stay here, you're welcome, but I don't recommend it." I was thinking about Lili's Country Kitchen and all the other Korean shops in our neighborhood. They were sure to be targets. "If anyone wants to come home with me, you're welcome to stay at my house."

No takers.

"Thanks, Dr. D," Greg finally responded, "but I'll stay here and watch the place. If it starts to get hot, I'll call you." The color had returned to his face, but I could tell he was terrified.

"You don't have to do that, Greg. Nothing's worth you risking your life. Come home with me." I thought about what I had just said. Willy and I had built this hospital with our hearts and soul, and every last penny we could beg or borrow. "We have insurance if the place burns down."

On the television screen a news copter flying over the 405 freeway was showing dozens of palm trees burning alongside the overpasses. "Okay, everybody, get your stuff and we'll walk out together. We'll go as a group."

I turned to Greg. "Call me immediately if anything comes up." I reached over and gave him a hug, whispering, "And if you decide to come to my house, I can come get you."

We left through the back wildlife gate on the side street, staying in a tight pack as planned, until everybody had reached their car and driven off. Finally, I got into the car with Cliff and Greta, who drove me one block over and dropped me off where I had parked.

On the way to my car I noticed that the bouncer was leaning at his usual post against the doorjamb of the China Girl strip club, as if nothing were happening. As far as I could see, our street, the California corridor, was quiet, but on the horizon just to the north you could see the glow of several fires.

The short drive home to my neighborhood was uneventful. Cars were traveling in both directions in no particular hurry. I saw no evidence of unrest along the streets. I pulled up in front of my house. It looked totally normal. Ellen's car was not there. She was at work. There was something fundamentally comforting about the serenity of seeing my home in its undisturbed condition.

As soon as I entered, Wok met me at the front door with his leash in his mouth, tail wagging in overdrive. "I guess you haven't been watching the news?" I bent down and gave him a big hug. Sidney waltzed into the entrance hallway and shouted a loud "feed me" meow. The fish were swimming frantically at the corner of their tank, waiting for their flakes.

"Not tonight." I ran my hand over Wok's furry head. He gave me a very sad look. I immediately turned on the television, and the news was reshowing the merciless pummeling of the driver of the red truck. They had found out his name—Reginald Denny—and announced that he had been taken by the Good Samaritan to one of the local hospitals. He was in a coma but mercifully still alive.

While the news was playing in the background I fed all the pets, then tried calling Ellen at work, but the phone in the ER just rang and rang and rang.

I called Greg, and he said everything was quiet. He had gone up to the roof and could see the fires in South Central. He also reported that Lili's husband and a few other neighboring business owners had stationed heavily armed sentries as guards on their rooftops. That was actually comforting to hear. I didn't have a gun but now wished I had listened to Roy.

Finally, I called Willy. He was home watching the television with a friend. He lived in an upscale, gated community several miles south of the practice. He wasn't concerned about trouble in his area, but naturally he was worried about the hospital.

It had been impossible to sleep. Between being glued to the events unfolding live on television and worrying about Noah's Ark and Ellen, I just couldn't settle down. Wok and Sidney curled up on the couch next to me as we watched the unfolding nightmare.

♦ ♦ ♦

The first call came in just before 6:00 a.m., startling Wok, Sidney, and me from the couch. The television was still on, volume barely audible, images of burning buildings filling the screen.

"Are you okay?" Ellen sounded exhausted.

"Fine." I rubbed my eyes, thankful to hear her voice. "I've been trying to call you all night." I looked outside. The sun was peeking over the trees in the backyard. I could see Dewe, my desert tortoise, out for a crepuscular graze on the back lawn. It looked so normal.

"Yeah, the ringing has been nonstop, and so has the floor. It finally got to the point where we just had to ignore the phones completely."

"Are you seeing a lot of fallout?"

"Oh my God." Ellen voice was weak. "Like someone opened the flood-gates. Beatings, burns, gunshots. Even a rape. It's a war zone."

"Are you safe?"

"Yeah, sorta." She paused. That didn't make me feel too confident. "There are no cops anywhere. They're all out at the command centers. But we called in all the rent-a-cops we could, and they're standing guard at the doors." She let out an uncomfortable laugh. "None of them have guns. Nobody but the victims and one family member is allowed in the hospital, so there are hundreds of people outside in the parking lot. It's like a mini riot out there." She continued with her description of the trauma center scene.

"Sounds like chaos."

"They need me to stay." A frustrated pause. "Just wanted to let you know that I won't be coming home any time soon."

"That sucks." I thought about it for a moment. "But you're probably safer there than trying to drive home."

"Yeah, I'll try to grab an hour of sleep in the overnight room with some of the others." Another pause. "Everything at the hospital okay?"

"So far. I haven't gotten any reports of problems overnight."

"Gotta go. Call you later." I could hear the urgency in her weary voice.

"Be safe, love you," I managed to slip in before she hung up.

Before I could even let go of the receiver, the phone rang again. I assumed it was Ellen again. "Did you forget to say 'Love you too!'?"

"Dr. Mader, it's Greg." There was obvious distress in his voice. "Stacey's been stabbed!"

"*What?*" My first thought was, *Stacey, not again!*

"She was on her way into work. As she was walking down the sidewalk a gang pulled up in a car and threw something at her. Whatever it was stabbed her through the forearm like a spear!" Greg screamed into the phone.

"Is she all right? How bad? Where is she?"

"She's at Community. Dr. Nordic is with her. He says she's going to be okay."

"All right." I looked around the house for a moment and realized I was still wearing the same clothes I'd come home in just hours before. "I'll be right in."

As quickly as possible I fed everybody, threw on a fresh scrub top, then headed into work. I thought about going straight to the Community hospital to check on Stacey but remembered what Ellen said. Though it was a different facility, most likely their security protocols were similar, and if Cliff was with her, I doubted they would have let me in. I knew I would be needed more at NAVH.

As I drove down the diagonal across the city toward work, KLOS's morning DJs, Mark and Brian, were pleading for people to stay home, off the streets and, for God's sake, be safe.

When I drove past the community hospital I noticed Cliff's car in the parking lot out front. At the bottom of the hill I turned onto the corridor toward my hospital and was immediately struck by the thick layer of smoke blanketing the city off to the north.

The street was virtually empty except for an occasional car passing in the opposite direction. Rather than go directly to NAVH, I decided to drive past it and check on Lili's restaurant at the opposite end of the block. Fortunately, her place was not damaged. I decided to take a chance and continue the drive another two blocks past McDonald's, the line in the sand that we told our students to never cross. To my shock and horror, several stores and buildings lay in ruins, smoldering unchecked from torchings the previous night.

This was mere blocks from my hospital. A cold chill ran down my spine. I immediately checked to make sure my doors were locked, did a U-ey in the middle of the street, and booked it back to work. The front of our building and the plate glass windows were intact. There were even flowers in the planters. For all intents and purposes, it was just like any other day—until you looked at the sidewalk and saw that it was once again splattered with Stacey's blood.

It was still early, and the front door was locked, as it should be, so I walked around the back of the hospital and entered through wildlife. As I turned the corner of the building, the first thing that struck me was the new graffiti all down the side of the wall: maybe from the same gang that stabbed Stacey?

To my surprise almost my entire crew was already in. Everybody was on pins and needles, and Stacey's stabbing didn't help matters. Many of my employees lived alone. The general feeling was that there was safety in numbers, and they'd rather be here than by themselves.

Trying to act normal, I gave a "Good morning" to everyone and asked how they were. I got mostly weary, stressed, and fatigued grunts in response. I grabbed my camera and went out front and took several photos of the bloody sidewalk and the new graffiti. I knew the cops would not have time to deal with it now, but down the road the documentation might come in handy. With that, I grabbed the five-gallon bucket of paint and quickly rolled over the spray-painted graffiti tags. Every few strokes I glanced over my shoulder to see if anyone was approaching.

Willy drove a white convertible Corvette. Not the smartest car to be driving on the streets right now. It looked to be a quiet day, so I called him and told him that he didn't need to come in. I also had Lisa call Dr. Furtano and tell her to stay home.

Maria came into the conference room, where several of us had gathered to watch the news. After she sat down she pulled a pistol out of her waistband and set it on the table next to Lisa's coffee mug.

We all looked at her. There was something perverse about a near-term pregnant woman carrying a gun below her expanding belly. What a contrast—one a sign of new life, the other, death.

"What?" Maria frowned.

"Is it loaded?" I asked. I hate guns.

"Yeah, it's loaded! That's the point, isn't it?" She lifted the gun, pulled back the slide, and displayed a hollow point 9mm round in the chamber.

"Is that a Beretta?" Lisa asked. She reached into her purse and pulled out a similar-looking handgun, satin black with a crosshatched grip.

"Yeah, the mini." Maria tipped the bullet out of the chamber, checked the safety, and handed the gun to Lisa. "It's a chick's gun."

"I got the Glock 26. I like it because it has"—she popped out the clip, pulled the slide emptying the chamber, then handed it to Maria—"ten plus one."

The girls admired each other's weapons.

Just then Cliff, Greta, and Stacey walked in. Stacey's arm was bandaged from the wrist to the elbow and supported in a sling around her neck. Her shirt and pants were bloodied. She looked rough, and I immediately got up and gave her my seat.

Cliff pulled a large revolver out of his waistband and set it on the table. My God! I had no idea my staff was so well armed.

"They gave her some good drugs," Cliff told the room. "I tried to take her home, but she wanted to come back to work."

"I'm not goin' home by myself," Stacey snarled. "I'll just crash upstairs if that's okay." Stacey was pale, quiet. This stabbing seemed to have scared her more than the last one.

She had seen this one coming. After she got through telling everybody her first-person version of what had happened, Greta helped Stacey upstairs and let her sleep in her apartment.

Dave came in shortly after eight and checked on the eagle. Things were all good on that front, but he had heard rioters up and down his street all night and hardly slept. I told him to go home and be with his wife, that we would call him if he was needed.

I went up front to chat with Lisa. There were no appointments on the books. We told everybody to go home and be safe, but nobody wanted to leave. Instead, they camped out in the conference room and watched the television. Several had brought food from home.

The previous night's activity seemed to have largely died down with the dawn. LA mayor Tom Bradley had called for a curfew shortly after midnight. We figured that the gang that attacked Stacey was on their way home from a night of rioting.

However, by midmorning the violence returned with a vengeance. Looting and arson exploded across Los Angeles County, with anarchy expanding into the neighborhoods of Central Los Angeles and affluent Hollywood. More violence spread in all directions, engulfing Hawthorne, Compton, Inglewood, and Long Beach.

The news stations had multiple helicopters in the sky and an army of reporters on the street. One thing was clear: the police presence was still minimal, sending a message to rioters and looters that they had free reign to do whatever they wanted. Residents of Los Angeles's Koreatown felt abandoned by police and formed their own militia. A live broadcast showed a gun battle between a group of armed looters and Korean shop-keepers armed with M1 carbines, shotguns, and handguns. After several tense minutes of gunfire, the looters backed off.

Arson was so widespread that the firefighters were not able to respond to all the calls. Several firemen had been shot or shot at overnight. Without the police presence to protect the fire squads, they stopped responding and just let the structures burn to the ground.

The only call that came in all morning was from Matt Hellman checking on Cutter. He said that he had wanted to come get him the previous night but was not able to make the drive to the hospital. That morning when he woke up he had found that his car had been torched, so he was trying to get ahold of his cousin so he could catch a ride to come visit his cat.

I told him that Cutter was stable, still on the IV fluids and eating well, but with all that was going on we did not get a chance to repeat any of the blood tests. Matt said he'd be in as soon as he could find a way to get to the hospital. I told him not to take any chances and that we would call him if anything changed.

By late afternoon some two thousand troops from the California Army National Guard arrived to help restore peace to the streets. It seemed as though there was finally some hope.

Throughout the day I stopped in at the conference room and checked on the news reports. Most of the staff members were either asleep on the floor or riveted to the television. It was just more of the same: mass looting all over the county and beyond. From parking lots reporters were broadcasting live videos of people walking out of the smashed storefronts of Kmarts, supermarkets, gun stores, and NAPA Auto Parts branches with shopping carts full of merchandise.

"Don't you realize what you're doing is wrong?" A reporter pushed the microphone into the face of a young mother lugging two full carts from the Super Kmart, three young children by her side. "It ain't wrong." The mother was all smiles. "It's all free!"

"Hey, boss!" Cliff came up behind me while I stood, mesmerized by the drama unfolding on the screen.

"Yeah?"

"You're supposed to be leaving tomorrow."

I looked at him and realized he was right. Ellen and I were supposed to leave for our Honduras trip the next night.

"Well, that's not looking so good right now." As soon as the words came out of my mouth, I realized how selfish they sounded.

"Hey, maybe by tomorrow night it'll be settled down enough that you can still leave."

"Yeah, maybe." I rubbed my hand over my face, pausing to put pressure on my eyes in an effort to quell a mounting headache.

"We need to get Greta outa here as well. If it's safe, maybe we can bring her with us to the airport when—er, *if* we go."

I had Greta call her airline and change her reservation. In the meantime, I called Willy with an afternoon update. We discussed my trip and whether or not I should stay. He was convinced that things would settle down now that the National Guard was here and that I should plan on going.

Shortly after the call, Lili came by to tell me that her "Korean family" had arranged protection for our block and that she would have them keep an eye on our hospital too. She said that many of her friends and relatives who lived closer to the epicenter of the unrest had lost everything they owned. Their stores and shops had been looted and burned, but she wasn't going to let that happen on our street! Her men would take shifts standing armed guard on the rooftops all night.

By late afternoon it was clear that things in NAVH were stable. The only two medical cases were Cutter and the eagle. While it was still light out and seemingly calm on the local streets, I decided to head home and check on my house and my fur family, and get things ready in case I was able to leave tomorrow night. I would make the final decision as late in the day as possible, based on news reports and the happenings in the NAVH neighborhood.

Just before I left, Cliff pulled me aside.

"If I recall, I believe that Cutter's owner's girlfriend is black?"

"Yeah, why?"

"'Cause I've been watching the news. The reporters keep showing these burned-out neighborhoods where store after store is torched to the ground. Then, suddenly, there will be a shop totally fine, no damage."

"Your point?" I really needed to leave.

"All of the shops that weren't vandalized had big signs in the windows that said, 'Black Owned.'"

"Willy and I aren't black."

"Yeah, boss. That's my point. We can put a sign in the window that says 'Black-Owned Pets Inside.'" Cliff motioned fervently to the front windows.

I thought about it for a moment. It wasn't a lie. "Okay. I think that's a good idea. Do it."

I passed two, maybe three cars on my way home. The deeper I got into the residential neighborhood, the more normal things seemed, just eerily quiet—not a single person out and about. Just as I turned off the diagonal onto my side street, I noticed a black man walking down the road carrying a gas can. My neighborhood was predominantly white, and the sight of this man, with a gas can, appeared so out of place.

There was something about his expression as I approached that made me stop the car. The second I came to a halt in front of him, he turned to run.

"Hey, wait!" I called out the window. "Are you all right? Do you need help?" I started to inch forward so I could keep up with the man as he retreated. He finally froze, dropped the can, and held his hands up in the air. He was older, salt-and-pepper hair, gray beard, conservatively dressed, and clearly petrified.

"I know what this looks like—a black man in a white neighborhood with a gas can." His voice was tremulous, submissive.

"Hey, you look like someone who could use some help." I stopped the car when I got close, opened my door, and got out. "I'm Doug." I extended my hand. "What's your name?" I smiled, hoping to calm the stranger.

"Reggie, Reggie Lester." He slowly lowered his hands and cautiously shook mine.

"I was trying to take my family outa town, to our auntie's, to get away from here, and we run outa gas." He pointed to a nonspecific location down the road. "I wen' over to da gas station but dey was closed."

"I have some gas at my house, Mr. Lester. Come with me. I'll take you to go get it. There's no reason for you to be running around here alone." I gestured for him to get in my passenger door.

He looked at me, clearly weighing his options—run around as a black man lost in a white neighborhood with an empty gas can, or take a chance with a white man who was a total stranger.

"Come on. I just live down the street." I needed to help this man before someone not so nice came by. "I understand if you don't trust me. If you prefer, I'll leave you here, go get the gas, and come *right back* and take you to your family."

"You sure it's okay?" He was understandably conflicted.

"Of course." I waved him into my car. "Let's go so we can get your family on the road."

He slid into my passenger seat, clutching his gas can tightly to his chest. I quickly drove the last couple of blocks to my house and parked the car out front in the street.

"Be right back."

I raced around the side gate and into the backyard. Wok started barking like crazy when he saw me. I gave him a quick pat on the head, ducked into my shed, and grabbed a full five-gallon can of petrol.

"This should get you wherever you are going." I held up the can as I put it in the back hatch. "Where's your car?"

"'Bout a mile dat way." Reggie pointed back toward the city. He had walked quite a way carrying the empty gas can. He was fortunate he hadn't been accosted.

We made some small talk as I drove him to his car and family, mostly concerning the craziness all around. In short order we pulled up alongside an older model Chevrolet Caprice parked under the dwindling shade of a large oak.

The car looked empty. *What had happened to his family?* I wondered. Then suddenly three heads, one larger and two smaller, peeked up from the rear seat. They had been hiding.

Reggie and I went over to his car, and he introduced me to the young woman as his daughter and her two children. I could see the relief in their eyes when their granddaddy got out of the stranger's car. I emptied my can into his tank while the kids looked on through the window.

"I can pay you for this, sir." Reggie pulled out his wallet.

"No way, my friend. You put that away." I gave his hand one last shake. "Now go, get your family out of here, and be safe."

Wok was waiting for me inside the door when I got back home. To my surprise, in the few minutes that I was away helping Reggie, Ellen had also arrived home.

"I'll bet you are exhausted." I hugged her tight, not wanting to ever let go. Wok sat by our side, looking up lovingly, his curly tail wagging full speed.

"Yeah, it's been rough." We sat on the couch and she proceeded to tell me about her experience from the perspective of a person living a nightmare from the middle of Hell.

KNBC was broadcasting on the tube, mostly showing repeat after repeat of the same beatings, burnings, and lootings. I pretty much tuned it out unless I heard something new.

Suddenly, news anchor Jess Marlow came on air with an important announcement: "Today Mayor Bradley is urging us all to stay home, stay off the streets, and watch the series finale of *The Cosby Show*. Mayor Bradley believes that we all need this time as a cooling-off period. If major events dictate, be assured that we will return to live air immediately."

And with that, the deteriorating world as brought to us all by NBC left the chaos of the mean streets and cut to the one-hour finale of *The Cosby Show*.

Don't Mess with Sophie

Ellen's acquired work biorhythm had her up in the middle of the night when most normal people were sleeping. Somewhere around 3:00 a.m. she emerged from the bedroom, clearly restless, and joined Wok, Sidney, and me on the couch. I had been channel surfing, hoping to find an iota of reassurance that this lunacy would soon end. The curfew mandated by Mayor Bradley was a joke, as the looting and burning continued, even at that hour of the morning. National Guard troops had more than doubled and were now patrolling the streets in Humvees. With luck, the increased presence would cease the lawlessness.

Ellen did not get called back in and was now officially on vacation. The plan was for us to leave for Honduras later in the day. I decided to head into work shortly after sunrise to see how Greg was holding up. He had been a real trooper throughout this ordeal.

At the top of the hill just before my hospital I slowed, checking to make sure that the streets below were empty. Convinced it was safe, I stopped at the crest so I could overlook greater Los Angeles. With the sun rising behind me, it was still dark enough that I was able to see the orange glows from hundreds of fires burning across the horizon. I opened my window. The air was acrid with smoke.

I drove past the hospital as I had yesterday morning and was comforted to see that it was not damaged. A large cardboard sign hung in the front window: "BLACK-OWNED PETS INSIDE." Farther down, I saw that Lili's restaurant was unscathed. An older Korean man, resting what looked like a 12-gauge shotgun on his shoulder, was smoking a cigarette on the restaurant's front patio. Just past McDonald's even more buildings were burned, and the Kmart was completely trashed, the front windows shattered and the wreckage strewn all over the parking lot. A few individuals were picking through piles of boxes near the entrance.

I'd seen enough.

Back at work it looked more like a normal morning. Greg was in the treatment room administering Cutter his medications. He said that during the night he had heard only a few gunshots in the street. Cutter was stable, but it dawned on me that Matt had never come by yesterday after he called.

The TV droned on in the conference room, as it had continuously for the last thirty-six hours. The room was empty, so I took a seat at the table and watched while I waited for others to show up for rounds—largely a formality, since we only had two patients in the hospital.

Staff filtered in, exhausted and stressed: Willy and Dr. Furtano, Stacey, arm wrapped and in a sling, Fred, and Greta.

The morning schedule was slow. A few clients came in for supplies like food, but there were no regular appointments. I still hadn't decided whether or not to go on my trip. In reality, things were so slow that I certainly was not needed. If we could safely get to the airport and the flights were leaving, then I should go. I called the airlines, and they told me that if flights were departing, I could not cancel or get a refund. I decided I would make a decision by late afternoon.

Shortly after lunch Lisa paged upstairs to my office.

"Dr. Mader, you might want to come down to the conference room. Rodney King is about to give a news conference."

We all watched the live broadcast of Rodney King standing in front of his attorney's office in downtown Los Angeles. King, wearing a conservative suit and tie and surrounded by reporters, friends, family, and security, tearfully pleaded for people to "just get along" and said, "Can we stop making it horrible for the older people and the kids?"

Perhaps the end of this madness was in sight, I thought, and I decided to make my trip a go.

Greta was able to change her ticket home to Munich and leave with us. The plan was for Cliff to bring her to my house around 8:00 p.m. Originally, Cliff was going to drive us to the airport for our midnight flight to Central America. However, there was still a dusk-to-dawn curfew in place, and we felt it was too dangerous for him not only to drive us to the airport, which took us past the heart of the unrest, but even more so for him to drive back alone.

I called a private transportation company that was willing to send an unmarked van to pick us up for a premium fee. Getting out safely would be worth the extra cost.

The television was on when Cliff and Greta showed up to our house. News helicopters flying over the city showed structures ablaze as far as the camera could record. There had been reports that airplanes landing at Los Angeles International Airport were being shot at, so air traffic control had to switch landing and takeoff patterns so that flights both arrived and departed over the ocean.

A few minutes later a black twelve-passenger Chevy van pulled up out front. There was nothing written on the side of the van making it obvious that it was a commercial vehicle, but it was windowed all around, meaning everybody inside was easily visible.

We stuffed our dive gear into the back along with Greta's suitcases and then climbed into the front two rows, with me in the front passenger seat. Our driver's name was Janet. I offered her perfunctory introductions.

"Thanks for coming to get us."

She was middle-aged and wore jeans, a black T-shirt, and a khaki corduroy vest like construction workers wear. Her face looked drawn and tired.

"I won't say 'my pleasure.'" She flashed a welcoming but clearly fatigued smile. "You're my twelfth trip to LAX in the last forty-eight hours."

"No way! You've been driving through all of this?"

"Yeah," Janet pulled away from the curb. "I'm one of just a few drivers willing to make the drive into LA."

"I hope you are getting combat pay."

She gave me a sideways look with a partial grin.

"Aren't you afraid?"

"I saw a lot worse in the Gulf War." Janet stared straight ahead with a flat expression.

I was impressed. "Still, aren't you worried about getting attacked?"

She looked back over her shoulders to see if the rear passengers were looking. "I pity the fools that try." Janet reached under her seat and pulled out a semiautomatic just far enough for me to see, then slid it back into its holster.

With the curfew there were hardly any cars on the road as we cruised up the 405 at over 90 miles per hour.

"No cops." Janet noticed me looking at the speedometer.

I nodded my head in agreement.

We exited west off the freeway onto Century Boulevard, the final stretch to the airport. Janet didn't stop at the bottom of the off-ramp for the red light but merely slowed to make sure there was no cross traffic. The last mile and a half looked like hell. There were no lights on in any of the buildings, random fires were burning unchecked, gangs were milling about the street, storefronts were smashed, and debris was all over the road.

Janet deftly careened between people and rubble, alternating her speed from careful to hauling ass, depending on the looks she got from the street groups. I prayed silently that she would not get a flat, as I was sure that type of trap had been used to stop others.

I glanced back at Ellen. She maintained a stoic face as she watched the scenes passing by. I was certain she had seen much worse in the ER. Greta, however, was terrified, her eyes wide and blurry. Ellen was holding her hand as we traveled toward the airport—the only structure with lights, clearly emergency powered.

An impressive police presence guarded the entrance to the airport, mandating us to stop and show our tickets before we could enter the departure area.

The silence continued as we unloaded our bags. Fortunately, we were all departing from the international terminal in the center of the airport complex, so we didn't have to leave Greta yet.

I had prepaid the shuttle fee with a credit card on the phone, but before Janet left I gave her a $100 tip.

"Thank you." I gave her a hug.

"Safe travels." She laughed, then added, "I'm sure you'll be safer wherever you're going."

Inside the terminal was total chaos. Numerous flights had been cancelled or delayed, either because they could not land or were not allowed to take off. We walked Greta over to her airline counter and got her checked in, said our goodbyes, and then went to get our boarding passes.

◆ ◆ ◆

¡Fuego en las Calles! "Fire in the Streets!" read the headline in the newspaper when we touched down over twenty hours later in Tegucigalpa, the capital of Honduras. Our connect-the-dots journey took us from LAX to Guatemala, then El Salvador, and finally Honduras. In every country we were asked about the riots. "Why are you destroying your own city? Americans are *loco*!"

The time away should have been the catharsis I desperately needed. Problem was, I had no way to contact my office, and they had no way to contact me. There was no television or access to world events. The only newspaper was two days old, so I had no idea what was happening back home and could not unwind.

••••

We made the trip back to LAX in less than fifteen hours. As soon as the plane landed, I sent a page to Janet to pick us up at baggage claim as prearranged. By the time we made it through customs, our gear was already circling the carousel.

As promised, Janet was waiting with her van curbside when Ellen and I exited baggage claim. "Welcome back!" Janet greeted us with a genuine smile.

"No bullet holes," I joked, looking at her van. "Good to see you made it." It was like seeing an old friend.

We loaded up the gear and headed back the same way we had come, this time in daylight. The sidewalks and storefronts along Century Boulevard looked even more devastated than I remembered.

On the ride home, Janet rattled off some startling statistics: over sixty dead, two thousand injured, eleven thousand arrested, and more than thirty-seven hundred buildings torched. About half of the arson and looting was to Korean-owned businesses. I worried about Lili and prayed that her restaurant was not one of them.

Wok went nuts when we walked in the door. As soon as I brought my bags inside, Ellen and I took him for a long walk. Back home, I gave Willy a call to let him know we had arrived safely. He told me that everything was fine, the hospital was undamaged, all employees were uninjured, Stacey was healing, and neither Lili's restaurant nor anywhere else on our block had suffered any damage. The only sad news was that Greg had given his two-week notice: he had been accepted to graduate school and wanted to take some time off before starting his master's program. Greg was one of our rock stars and would be sorely missed.

On the flip side, Willy reported, he had interviewed two different technicians to replace Greg, both named Alex. He had offered the night job to one of them, who would move into the apartment the weekend Greg left.

Finally, the student of the month, a Sophie Rubenstein from one of the Caribbean schools, was due to arrive tomorrow. Her university had not wanted her to travel until the civil unrest had ended. I doubt Sophie would have had any problems even if she had started in the middle of the riots. She was one tough lady. Besides her obvious physical prowess, Sophie was a second-career student who had served in the armed forces. Her tour of duty in Iraq had been with the military police, so she was no stranger to violence. More than that, after leaving the military, she had had a short stint as a professional boxer.

It was good to be back at work and especially good to see that essentially everything was back to normal. Maria had her baby two days after the riots settled down—a healthy eight-pound, nine-ounce boy. Stacey's sutures had been removed, leaving a huge scar across the front of her forearm; otherwise, she seemed no worse for the wear.

There were several cases in the hospital, including Cutter, the kidney failure cat, and the eagle that Officer Pinkett had brought in. According to Dave, the large bird was on track to be released in about three weeks.

I was surprised that Cutter was still here. I asked why, and Lisa told me that his owner, Matt Hellman, had never come to pick him up. She had tried calling every day but only ever got the answering machine. Unfortunately, Cutter was not doing well and might not last long.

It was a tough situation. The old cat was in failing health and costing us a lot of money every day to keep alive. Willy was beginning to get worried that we would never see a dime and wanted to start legal proceedings so that we could euthanize the cat if Matt never turned up to claim him or pay the veterinary bill. He instructed Lisa to send a certified letter advising "Mr. Hellman" that he had a balance due and that if he didn't pick up and pay the amount on the invoice within seven days, the cat would be considered abandoned.

My day was fully booked. Some clients had insisted on seeing me, even if it meant that their pet had to wait several days for me to return. At some point during the midafternoon Lisa grabbed me between appointments. "Dr. Mader, there's a gentleman up front who would like to talk to you. He's not a client but said it's important if you have time."

"Who is he?" I looked at my watch. Time was slipping away, and I was getting further and further behind.

"I don't know, but he came in last week, and when I told him you weren't in, he said he would come back."

"Okay. Please tell my next appointment that I'll be just a few minutes."

I walked up front. My first thought was that it was probably another process server with a subpoena—Officer Kelly had told me to expect one for the eagle case.

It turned out to be someone whom I would have never expected: "Mr. Lester!" It was Reggie Lester, the grandfather who had run out of gas in my neighborhood the second day of the riots.

"Hello, Dr. Mader." He was all smiles as he walked over and shook my hand. "This is a beautiful hospital you have here."

"Thank you." I was flabbergasted that he had come to see me. He was wearing recently laundered blue mechanic's overalls and carrying a brown paper bag. "What brings you in?"

"My daughter baked you some bread." He held up the bag, folded down at the top, and graciously offered it to me. "We all just wanted to thank you for your kindness."

I thanked him. I was really touched. "This is totally unnecessary. I was happy that I was able to help."

"Doctor, you really have no idea what your brave and kind actions meant to me and my family." He had such a sincere smile.

"Mr. Lester, I have a feeling that if the roles were reversed, you'd have done the same for me. But how did you know where to find me?"

"When you stopped to help me, you were wearing your doctor clothes." He pointed to my scrub top. Across the breast pocket was written "Noah's Ark Veterinary Hospital."

◆ ◆ ◆

I made a deal with Willy: I was going to take off every Tuesday and Thursday afternoon and every other Saturday to study for my specialty boards. Three months and counting to the big day.

That didn't work out so well. As I was about to walk out the door to go home and study as planned, Mr. Rockwell showed up, once again in a total crisis mode with one of his Pomeranians. The little puffball had accidentally jumped out of his arms, hit the floor, and broken its front left leg. So rather than spending my first Tuesday study hall with my textbook on gastroenterology, I spent it in the surgery room with Fred, a metal bone plate, several stainless steel screws, and a little black Pomeranian named Bitsy.

• • •

I finished my morning surgeries and was upstairs in my office completing my charts and getting ready to leave when Lisa paged me.

"Dr. Mader, uh . . ." Lisa paused. "I think you really need to get down here right away."

"What do you need?" I didn't want a repeat of Tuesday.

"I'm not sure." She was almost whispering. "All I can tell you is that there's some guy here that needs to talk to a doctor."

"What guy? Did he say what he wanted?" I was getting irritated. The deal was I would take Tuesday and Thursday afternoons off. Why couldn't Willy or someone else talk to this guy?

"He didn't say much else. But he was holding a certified letter." A short pause. "Please!" Lisa pleaded.

Reluctantly, I headed downstairs to the conference room. I turned the corner and stopped cold when I saw the stranger at the table. He was a younger man, probably in his early twenties, sitting hunched over the table in the conference room. In front of him on the table was the certified letter Lisa was referring to, easily identifiable by its green sticker.

The man was wearing a ratty gray T-shirt over soiled black jeans and unlaced, badly worn boots. His hair was slicked back over a scab-covered ear. He had several days' stubble on his face and was picking at a large wound on his left forearm. I took a swallow and entered the conference room. "I'm Dr. Mader."

"Matt spoke so highly of you." The subdued stranger looked up with a bloodshot, unfocused eye on the side of his face with the injured ear. I noted that he was missing several teeth. Cracks and healing scars accented his lips. His tone was distant, hollow.

"Matt?" Looking at the condition of this man, I suspected he had been in a bit of trouble and therefore had been sent by our attorney, Matt Leonard. But he had used the past tense, which made no sense. "How do you know Matt?"

"I got this." The man pushed the letter across the table. It had come from our office and bore the name "Matt Hellman" clearly on the address label. "I was at his apartment. I had to sign for it." The wounds on his forearm were oozing. The fingers touching the wrinkled envelope had dried blood under the nails and caked around the ragged cuticles. "I opened it." He wiped the back of his hand down his face, grimacing when he crossed over his eye. "I don't have much money, but I came to try and pay it for him."

A cold chill shot through my body. "I'm sorry, sir—I didn't get your name." I had a feeling that he wanted to cry but did not have the emotional energy left to do so.

"Scott." He reached his hand across the table.

I reached out to make the connection, and when I touched his hand it all came back to me. "You're his cousin?" It was more of a question than a statement.

He nodded.

"Where's Matt? I recall him speaking of you as well."

The man looked across the table. His good eye was watery, and it was almost as if it was looking through me, while the other eye was involuntarily staring down at the table, exposing an angry red sclera. "He's dead."

I wanted to say something, but no words came out. A zillion thoughts ran through my head. That's why we had not heard back from Matt. I remembered his last phone call, the Thursday before I left, the second day of the riots. Matt had said that his car had been burned and he was looking for a ride so he could come see Cutter.

"What happened?" I choked it out.

It took him a minute before he had the energy to speak, but then he told me the entire nightmare. Matt had called Scott asking for a ride to come visit Cutter. Scott did not have a car, only a motorcycle, but agreed to drive him across town to NAVH. It was the middle of the afternoon, so they felt it would be safe. As they were heading down the California Corridor, about a half mile from our office, several gang members stepped out into the road and hurled a car tire at them.

The tire struck Scott on the side of the head, knocking them off the motorcycle. The bike slid on its side to a stop, but before they could get up, the gang was on them. One of the bangers pulled out a gun and shot Matt through the forehead, execution-style, killing him instantly.

They then shot at Scott three times at point-blank range, but the gun had jammed. Scott remembered the gang laughing, spitting on him, and then kicking him until he passed out. The next thing he knew it was several days later and he was in the hospital.

I looked at the letter and felt incredibly guilty. This man and his cousin had attempted to come visit their dying cat in my hospital. In doing so, they were ambushed, one killed and the other tortured.

And I was out having fun on vacation.

But hey, you still have to pay your bill.

"Don't worry about this." I reached out and slid the envelope off the table. My comment seemed inappropriate, but I had no idea what else to say. Scott bowed his head. He looked defeated.

"Cutter is struggling but still alive." I touched his hand again. "Do you want to see him?"

Scott looked up and tried to smile. Only the right side of his face responded. "Yes, please."

"Wait here." I got up and walked out, patting his shoulder as I passed by. I felt my eyes well up as I made my way to the hospital ward. Everybody was standing in the treatment room, waiting for the story. Stacey was holding Cutter. She had disconnected him from his IV fluids and had him wrapped up in a blanket, ready for me to bring him to Scott. Cutter had lost so much weight that I was surprised he was still alive.

I brought the bundled old cat to the conference room and, kneeling down next to Scott, gently handed Cutter over. "You're a good man, Scott. I am so sorry for all you've been through."

Scott buried his face into Cutter and immediately started to sob. I stood up, took a step back, and looked away, unable to control my own tears. I was just a foot away from the TV on the shelf in the corner of the room. Just two weeks ago we had all sat around in horror watching as human monsters ravaged innocent people on that very screen, killing many of them. Matt and Scott were two of those innocent people. The dead and beaten weren't just nameless faces on the TV. They were real. One was sitting right here.

"He's dying, isn't he?" Scott wiped phlegm from under his nose with the back of his hand.

"Yes," I turned back to look at Matt's cousin and squatted down to be at his level. I stroked the ungroomed fur on the back of Cutter's head while Scott clutched him to his chest. The cat lay motionless in the blanket, its eyes sunken, cheeks gaunt. Its breath carried the smell of death.

"The only reason he's still alive is because we have him on the IVs."

"I don't want him . . . Matt wouldn't want him . . . to suffer." He choked back tears until he could no longer hold them in.

I pulled a chair over so I could sit next to the physically and mentally broken man. I put one hand on his shoulder, caressing the fur on the back of Cutter's neck with my other. "Are you asking me to end his suffering?"

Matt's cousin looked up through tears and nodded. Cutter hadn't responded even in the slightest to Scott's voice or touch.

"I'll give you a moment to say goodbye."

As I stepped out of the room Stacey was standing in the hallway.

"Here." She handed me a syringe filled with pink fluid. The syringe of death. I noticed that she was crying as she quickly turned away.

I quietly reentered the room and sat next to Scott. Cutter's breathing had slowed considerably in the few moments I had stepped out. I gently placed my stethoscope on the thin cat's chest and could hear the heartbeat slowing.

I surreptitiously slipped the euthanasia syringe into my pocket. It wasn't going to be needed. He didn't need my help to cross the Rainbow Bridge. He had waited for Matt to come back like he promised. But somehow I felt that Cutter now knew that Matt never would and was ready to join his owner on the other side.

I sat quietly next to Scott and Cutter. No words. Scott, his head bent forward, snuggling with Cutter, gently rocking back and forth, like a mother coddling her child.

I watched as Cutter's breathing continued to slow, from breaths per minute to minutes per breath.

Finally Cutter took one last, audible gasp and went limp.

"He's gone, isn't he?" Scott whispered, not looking up.

"Yes." I placed a hand on Scott's shoulder, leaned forward, and kissed Cutter on the top of his head.

Scott reached his hand into his front pocket, pulled something out, and handed it to me. "Can you please bury this with him?"

It was Matt's crucifix.

• • •

I did not sleep that night.

After I saw Scott off and took care of Cutter's remains, I left work and went for an ill-advised, dangerous road trip. I found myself cruising down the Corridor, deep into the woods where Hansel and Gretel were warned never to venture. For some twisted, illogical reason I needed to see the place where Matt was murdered.

There was still abundant post-riot debris scattered along the streets and sidewalks. Based on Scott's recollection of the nightmare, I had a pretty good idea where the attack occurred. I pulled my SUV over to the curb and got out. The pungent smell of burned buildings was pervasive. As I walked around I tried to imagine the horror the cousins must have experienced in Matt's last few minutes on this earth.

Scott had told me that it all happened in slow motion, even the tire flying out of the gangbanger's hands as it slammed into his head. The fall, the skid, the yelling, the slowly expanding flash and smoke from the gunshot as he yelled "Noooooooooo!" when they blew his cousin's brains all over the asphalt.

Scott had recalled that each time he got shot he could not feel it, that between bullets he kept wondering why he wasn't dead. He had no memory of how he got to the hospital.

And now, Cutter, his only link to Matt, was also gone.

I wiped away some tears. In my periphery I noticed some individuals watching me from across the street.

I closed my eyes and said a prayer for Matt, Scott, Cutter, and all the others who had suffered so needlessly from this madness.

Back at home I loaded Wok into my car and took him to the shore for a long walk. When we got to the end of the beach, we sat on the rock jetty watching the sun set in the distance while the perpetual motion of the waves pounded the sand at our feet.

One after another. No two the same. They did not stop. Even when the sun was long over the horizon and the white-crested waves were nothing but ghosts tickling the shore, the sound continued. The kinetic energy of life never stops.

Wok sat by my side. We didn't talk much.

◆ ◆ ◆

It was a sad day at NAVH: the last morning for me to come into work and say "G'morning!" to Greg. He had just worked his final night shift.

Greg had been with us since shortly after we started the hospital. Originally a client who'd brought in a sick snake, he and I had hit it off immediately, and shortly thereafter we offered him a job as a day technician. Then as we grew and expanded our nighttime care, we had him move into the apartment upstairs to take over our night shifts. He had been a rock since day one. He never called in sick, was totally reliable, and dedicated himself to the team and the animals.

At the same time, it was a happy day. We sent home Mr. Rockwell's Pomeranian, Bitsy, with a stainless steel bone plate in her injured leg. To show his appreciation, Mr. Rockwell and his wife brought in a huge platter of McDonald's food from one of his restaurants as lunch for the staff: Big Macs, double cheeseburgers, McChicken sandwiches, french fries, apple pies, and Ronald McDonald cookies.

◆ ◆ ◆

Alex, the new night technician we hired to replace Greg, arrived the following morning. The plan was for him to move into the apartment in the afternoon before starting his first night shift.

Alex had experience as a veterinary nurse, but his previous job in a veterinary hospital had been cut short when he quit to join the army and fight in Desert Storm. When the war ended, a lot of veterans came home looking for work. After Alex was discharged he spent some time with his family, did a bit of traveling, then finally decided to look for permanent employment.

Alex was hired while I was in Central America. I was in the reception area working on some paperwork when around noon there was a knock at the front door.

"Hi! I'm Alex." A midtwenties, well-groomed, athletically built black man wearing a dress suit and tie was standing at the entrance. He had one very large suitcase and a smaller box by his side, and wore a gold hoop earring in his right lobe.

"Welcome!" I shook his hand, then reached down and attempted to pick up his large bag. I wasn't expecting it to be so heavy; I could barely lift it.

"Here, let me get that." Alex smiled, taking the enormous bag effortlessly using his left arm. Not wanting to seem incapable, I grabbed the smaller box and welcomed him inside.

"As I said, welcome to Noah's Ark Veterinary Hospital. I know you know where your apartment is, but let me walk you upstairs."

We crested the steep stairs to the landing on the second level and were greeted by our student, Sophie.

"You must be my new neighbor!" Sophie announced, using her loud New Jersey voice, then reached out and immediately gave Alex a big hug.

"Hey, girlfriend!" Alex returned the gesture as if they'd been friends forever.

"You two know each other?"

"Nope!" Sophie stepped back, picked up his large bag like it was filled with feathers. "Just welcoming family."

◆ ◆ ◆

"G'morning!" I greeted Alex as I had done every morning with Greg over the past years. Alex was busy filling in patient records. It was a new day, a new chapter for NAVH.

"Morning, sir!" Alex paused from his charting and greeted me with a big smile. He was wearing pastel pink scrub pants and a matching top.

"This isn't the military," I joked. "You don't need to 'sir' me."

"Morning, Doctor!" He stood at attention and saluted.

Goofball. I liked him already.

The next day: "Morning, Doctor!" Alex stood at attention and saluted when I entered the treatment room.

"Morning, Alex." I saluted back, smiling. This apparently was going to be a daily routine.

"You got a call!" Alex frantically waived a pink callback slip at me. "I want to go. I love horses!"

I had no idea what he was talking about. He handed me the call note. Per the time stamp it had just come in moments before I arrived.

And Alex was right—it was about a horse. Sara, a veterinary assistant who worked at an animal hospital across town, had called wanting to know if I could do a field visit to check on her horse. Apparently it had stepped on a nail, and she couldn't get in touch with her regular equine veterinarian.

Few of my colleagues knew that I had started my career wanting to be an equine surgeon, putting myself through horseshoeing school when I was fifteen and starting my own blacksmithing business. After the several surgeries and many months of rehabilitation therapy that followed the terrible car crash I'd had, I'd never regained the strength or confidence to return to horse work. Instead, I switched to small mammal and exotic animal medicine. Nevertheless, horse care still lingered in my DNA.

I had done no veterinary work on a horse since graduating, but doing a favor for a colleague was appealing, even if it meant missing another Thursday study hall. If what I found on her horse was outside my comfort zone, I would refer her to someone else.

Sophie and Alex joined me for the equine exam. We stopped by the animal hospital across town and picked up Sara, the horse's owner. She kept her steed in one of the many stables located along the greenbelt that paralleled the Los Angeles River. Although most of the equestrian centers along the river were nice little Edens, getting to them could be a challenge, as the majority of the neighborhoods that bordered the river were not the safest.

We drove through the heart of the city to get to the horse barn along the same route I took to go to the monthly herpetological meetings. In broad daylight we got to see just how bad the areas had gotten. In some neighborhoods the sidewalks were littered with old TVs, sofas, refrigerators, stereos, and other belongings. I found out later that many of the looters, when they got home with their new "free" stuff, put their old stuff out on the street.

Sara was in the front passenger seat providing directions. Alex was behind me, and Sophie was behind Sara. I was pleased at how well Alex and Sophie had hit it off in just the few days they had come to know each other. The similar experiences from their time in Iraq probably helped them form an immediate bond.

About five miles into our drive we stopped at an intersection. It was a beautiful late spring day and we all had our windows open, enjoying the breeze and fresh air. Suddenly we could feel the vibration, then hear the pounding base of a car stereo blasting as it approached from behind. An older-model dark-blue sedan pulled up alongside, music blaring out the windows. Reflexively I turned to look as the car stopped next to us at the light. As soon as I saw its occupants, I turned my gaze forward again. The car was filled with gangbangers, recognizable by colored bandanas. The pounding base of the rap music was deafening.

In my peripheral vision I could see the passenger was yelling at Alex.

"Wassup?" Alex hollered out his window at the car.

In an instant, the music stopped.

"Fuck you, faggot!" The banger yelled back, flipping Alex the middle finger.

The profanity sent a lightning charge through us all, and we turned and looked back and forth between Alex and the bangers.

"Fuck off, punk!" Alex yelled back, waving his fist.

At that the hoods erupted in yells and began flashing gang signs at Alex.

Before it could escalate further I made a quick, I'm certain illegal, right turn across the lane next to me, through the red light, and took off down the cross street as fast as possible.

"What the *hell* are you doing, Alex?" I screamed at him, looking directly at his face in the rearview mirror while trying to drive as fast as possible to get away. His face was pumped, eyes wide, jugular veins throbbing.

"Sophie and I risked our lives in Iraq defending this country. I don't need no punks like that giving me lip."

"That's right, Alex." Sophie puffed up. My real warriors, adrenaline fueling their inner soldier as they sat in the back seat, were showing their colors.

"That's bullshit," Alex declared.

"I hear what you're saying, but we don't need to invite trouble." I immediately thought about Matt Hellman and how he been ambushed.

Feeling confident we had lost the sedan after another few blocks, I made a series of turns back toward the stables. A mile or so down the original road we again stopped at a light.

"Oh shit," Sophie called out.

The gangster car pulled up alongside us once again. This time when I looked over at it, I saw that the passenger in the rear seat was pointing a gun at Alex.

I stomped the gas pedal and shot out into the intersection amid a torrent of honks and screeching tires.

"The stables are just a half mile up to the right!" Sara was yelling, looking over her shoulder.

The sedan had also pushed through the intersection, but fortunately I had disrupted traffic enough that the chaos of cars slowed their pursuit.

"I don't want them to follow us to your barn." I pushed on like Mario Andretti, one eye on the road in front of me, the other on the rearview mirror. "If they follow us in, we're trapped." I was swerving and honking with no intention of slowing.

"Fuckers are back!" Alex called out a warning. I looked in my rearview mirror and saw the grill of the sedan just about touching my rear window. I could clearly see the gun, now being held by the front passenger, pointing directly at us.

Several blocks ahead I noticed a police cruiser coming at us from the approaching lane. I immediately started to swerve and flash my headlights. The cop flew past us, slammed on his brakes, did a U-turn, and came racing back up from behind, lights flashing and sirens blaring.

I immediately started to slow, forcing the gun-toting bangers also to slow or hit us and giving the police a chance to catch up.

The next thing I knew, the cop car pulled alongside the sedan and forced them off the road, without giving any signals for us to pull over.

So we kept going. And going. In fact, we drove far past the turnoff for the stable just to make sure that we were not being followed. After making a series of maze-like maneuvers, we wove our way back to Sara's barn.

I pulled in and drove my SUV around the back of the building so that it was out of sight of the main road. I turned off the engine, and we all sat for a few minutes without saying a word.

"That was really stupid, Alex." I finally broke the silence.

"I don't need to take that shit from anybody, Doc."

"I understand, Alex, but you could have gotten us all killed."

"I wouldn't let that happen." He looked away. "I ain't afraid of those punks."

"We've seen worse than that in Iraq." Sophie came to his defense.

"Maybe, but there you had guns and you could shoot back."

After a tense moment of silence Alex pushed up the sleeve on his scrub top. "I got guns." Alex lifted his arm and flexed his sculpted bicep.

"So do I!" Sophie did the same. Her upper arm was almost the same size as Alex's arm. They looked at each other and laughed.

"Not funny."

Sara sat silently through all this. Fortunately, her horse only had a minor foot abscess and was easily treated with antibiotics, pain medicine, and a tetanus booster. The actual time spent with the horse was only a fraction of the time it had taken us to get there, hide, and then drive back under the cover of darkness.

◆ ◆ ◆

Dave was in first thing to check on the eagle. He had been taking it out every day to a nearby wildlife facility that had a large flight cage. The big bird was able to fly, navigate, and catch live prey. Dave felt it was ready for release, and if all went as planned, it would be done the following Tuesday when I got back from my internal medicine meeting in San Diego. Meanwhile Dave promised me he would *not* let Dr. Nordic release it while I was gone.

Come hell or high water, I was determined to get out of the office by one o'clock and go home for some studying, but first I had to talk with Alex about last week's encounter with the street gang. I told him that I had the utmost respect for his bravery and service to our country. However, this was not Iraq, and even though he was provoked, he needed to learn to walk away from that kind of trouble. He could have gotten us all killed. He apologized and promised it would not happen again.

◆ ◆ ◆

I experienced some serious brain squeeze at my veterinary internal medicine meeting in San Diego. I made it a point to get up early, attend the extra breakfast meetings, go to all the morning lectures, sit in on the industry-sponsored "lunch and learns," sit through all the afternoon sessions, grab a quick dinner, and then participate in the evening wet labs and discussion groups. All in all, it was about ten to twelve hours of the highest level of internal medicine education that anyone could ask for each day. I finally felt like I was on track for preparing for my specialty exams just two months away.

I called work during my brief dinner break to say goodbye to Sophie. It had been an abbreviated month with her, since she had started late due to the riots, and I had to leave a few days early for my medicine meeting.

I wanted to thank her for being a part of our team and for her contributions during her short stay. She was quite a character, and watching her and Alex together had been gratifying. I suspected that they would stay friends for life.

Talking with her, I learned some more about Alex as well. It was obvious that he was gay, but I had had no idea that Alex had applied for the night technician job twice—the first time dressed as a woman. That explained the message I got from Willy about two Alexes applying for the same job. He/she had come in as a woman named Alex and done the interview with Willy and Lisa. The woman Alex did not have a résumé and was passed over. When Alex applied the second time, he came in as a man wearing conservative-colored scrubs and told the two of them that he was "dressed and ready for work." It also helped that the male Alex did have quite an impressive résumé. When Lisa called the references, they all checked out. None mentioned Alex's alter ego.

Sophie further went on to tell me that Alex had also landed a job singing, as a woman, at Slurpee's, one of the most popular gay clubs down in the shore, on his nights off. Turned out, Alex was a chameleon: he was not only a handsome, brave soldier and talented animal nurse, he was also a sexy nightclub singer.

◆ ◆ ◆

The internal medicine meeting ended at noon to give everybody travel time. I had planned it so that on my drive back from San Diego I would stop at John Wayne Airport and pick up our next student, Elizabeth Stettler from Oklahoma State University.

I spotted a young woman wearing a backpack, standing at the carousel, and waiting for her bag. She looked to be in her early twenties, average height, slightly heavyset, with a roundish face and her hair pulled back into a braided ponytail. It wasn't the Western-cut blouse, the cowboy boots, or the large silver belt buckle that gave her away but the stethoscope around her neck.

"Are you a doctor?" I smiled as I approached.

"Yes." She looked totally caught off guard. "No!" Then reached up and touched her stethoscope as if she had forgotten she was wearing it. "Are you Dr. Mader?"

"Yep! Welcome to California." I helped her pull a very large, well-traveled Samsonite from the belt.

"Did you have to use that on your flight?" I motioned to her stethoscope.

"No," she said, blushing and taking it off. "I just figured it would help you find me."

"It worked." We headed out to my car. As it was Sunday afternoon, the traffic was unusually light. I explained to Beth, as she preferred to be called, how the practice was run and what was expected of her, but all she could do was ask about the riots, if they were over, and whether it was safe to be here.

I assured her that it was, and not only that, her apartment was next to our night technician's apartment, and he was an ex-soldier from the Iraqi war, so she was well protected and had nothing to be afraid of.

Somewhere in the middle of assuaging her paranoia about Southern California, I asked her about the old suitcase.

"Have you traveled much?"

"No, first time out of Oklahoma."

We got back to the hospital about four o'clock. I helped her upstairs to the apartment with her luggage and got her settled in. Just as I was about to leave, Alex showed up wearing a suit and tie, having just returned from Sunday church service.

When Beth met Alex, I saw a look of shock rush over her face. I don't know if it was the idea of a strange man—a strange black man—living so close, but I could tell instantly that she was uncomfortable.

"Beth, get yourself settled in, and I'll be back in a few hours to take you grocery shopping and to dinner. Sound like a plan?"

"Sure. Thanks." She quickly slipped into her room and shut the door. We could hear the deadbolt slide shut.

Alex and I looked at each other, eyes wide, and smiled. Just as I was about to turn and leave, Beth cracked her door open and asked, "Is there a phone I can use?"

"I can take you to one, honey." Alex waved her out of the room.

"'K. See you soon," I commented to both. I shook my head as I trotted down the steps.

About an hour later my pager went off. It was work.

"Uh, Dr. Mader, it's Alex."

"Yes, Alex?"

"Uh, Dr. Mader, I don't quite know how to tell you this."

"What, Alex?"

"It's your student." His voice pitch was high and trailing off toward the end of the sentence.

"What about my student, Alex?" I didn't like this game.

"Well, she's gone."

"What do you mean, 'gone'?"

"Gone. As in *gone*!"

"Like gone shopping gone?"

"No, like *outa here* gone!"

"How do you know that she is 'outa here' gone and not just gone for a walk down to the beach or something?"

"Because I heard a loud noise, and when I opened the door she was dragging that huge bag, bumpety-bump, down the stairs. I asked where she was going, and she said that she 'had to leave.' I followed her downstairs, outside, and watched her get into an airport shuttle."

"What did you do?"

"I didn't do anything!"

"She wouldn't just leave! What happened?"

"Well"—there was a bit of a pause—"I have to sing tonight. So while she was waiting for you to come get her, I thought I'd show her my new tangerine chiffon evening gown, the one that I wear on stage."

"Oh, Alex . . ." I could see where this was going.

"I knocked on her door to model it for her. She acted as if she liked it!"

"And then?"

"And then, the next thing I knew she was dragging her bag down the stairs."

The Rolling Tortoise

"**W**here's our new student?" Stacey queried as morning rounds kicked off.

"Come and gone." I rolled my eyes. "Don't ask."

I had called the dean at Oklahoma State University the previous afternoon and told him what happened with his student and how she now held the record of the shortest stay for a veterinary student extern at my hospital. Needless to say, he was embarrassed and very apologetic.

It was also a big day for Dave and NAVH. After almost two months of medical care, the golden eagle's release was scheduled for that afternoon. I realized that if I went on the release, I was going to lose yet another Tuesday afternoon's study time, but this was worth it.

By the time I finished all my charts and left work, it was long after dark. I was physically, but more importantly, mentally and emotionally exhausted after a nonstop day of intense client interactions. The experts call it "compassion fatigue." One day I love what I do, and the next I struggle to make it through the day.

I took Wok out for a long stroll, ending up in our favorite park. I took a seat while he reasserted his claim on the territory. As always, we finished the outing sitting together on the bench with a soul-searching review of the day's work. What an emotional rollercoaster it had been.

First patient: emergency. Dog hit by a car. Severe injuries. Dog died. Owner screamed at us because we couldn't save her pet. Emotion: failure.

First room of the day: old man with a dying cat, his last link to his deceased wife. Euthanasia. Emotion: sadness.

Four feet away, forty-five seconds later: an excited family with their new puppy. Emotion: jubilation.

Return to the first room: jerk owner with mildly injured, easily treatable kitten. Owner too cheap to pay for medical care. Owner wants to kill it. Emotion: anger.

Four feet away: loving couple with cancer-stricken family pet. Money no object, but unable to help the old dog. Euthanasia. Emotion: helplessness.

I leaned against Wok's broad shoulders. He was strong and always there for me. Emotion: love.

◆ ◆ ◆

As they say, karma is a bitch.

With the big test less than two months away, I should have stayed home studying. Instead it was the first night of summer softball season, and I just had to go play with Ellen's hospital team. We won the game, and it would have been wonderful except for the fact that I tore the meniscus in my knee by sliding into home base and ended up spending the night in Ellen's emergency room.

It seemed ironically appropriate that I was having surgery on the anniversary of my horrific auto accident twelve years earlier. Ever since, I've considered June 8 my new birthday, or as I liked to call it, my second chance day.

I went into the hospital at 6:00 a.m. to get my knee fixed and was home by 2:00 in the afternoon.

◆ ◆ ◆

My first two Saturday appointments were relatively easy wellness checks and vaccines. With Stacey helping I finished them in normal time. My final appointment of the morning was a mother-daughter pair who came in with their pet box turtle. The reason for the visit listed on the appointment slot: "swollen tail."

The middle-school-aged girl put her turtle on the table for me to examine. She said that it had had a swollen tail for the past week. Per her mother's instructions, she had been rubbing Bacitracin on it twice a day every day, but it had not gotten better. This morning they noticed that the swelling had gotten worse and the tissue was starting to crack and bleed. Not only that, their shelled pet had not eaten in the last couple of days.

Without even touching the patient I ascertained what was wrong, but I wanted to give it a complete physical so that I would not miss anything.

After finishing my exam I carefully turned the turtle over. Using warm water and soap, I cleaned the end of the damaged tail. When I was certain that I had the wounds clean, Stacey used some soft gauze to dry the area. Mom and daughter watched our every move with genuine concern. When finished, I placed the patient back on the exam table and explained what I had found.

"Well, first off, Shelly is actually a Shelby." I directed my comments to the daughter. "Shelly is a boy turtle, not a girl turtle."

"How do you know?" the daughter asked. "I thought it was a girl." Her look was so serious.

I once again lifted the turtle and gently turned it on its back.

"I know, because, this is his male part." I pointed to the swollen tissue at the base of the tail.

"Oh my God!" The mother covered her mouth with her hand, stifling a laugh.

"You mean that's his *penis*?" The teenager jumped back, hollering as she did. Her eyes were so big I thought they'd pop out of her head.

"Yes." I tried to hold back my laughter.

"Gross! I was touching it!"

◆ ◆ ◆

By the time I got home after work, my knee was pretty sore. Because I wanted to try to study, I didn't want to take anything stronger than naproxen, a nonnarcotic anti-inflammatory, commonly used for postoperative pain control.

My usual poor sleep had been even more uncomfortable than normal the previous night because my leg was so stiff, but I downed some more naproxen the next morning and chased it with a Diet Coke.

Wok was disappointed with me since I still couldn't take him to the park, but I think he understood. Instead, he took up his place next to the ugly recliner in my office and made sure that I got some serious studying done—which I did, for the next seven hours.

◆ ◆ ◆

"You'll never guess who your next client is." It was more of a statement than a question. Lisa handed me a thin chart, obviously for a new client, and motioned with her head toward the middle exam room.

Intrigued, I went to take a look as I grabbed the chart. All the exam rooms had glass pass-through windows between them. So I went into the empty room next to the center exam room and peered in to see who was waiting. It was Harriett, our corner hooker, in her usual garb, petting a scruffy, gray tabby kitten.

I hadn't seen her on the street since the riots and, quite frankly, had completely forgotten about her. With her left hand Harriett was teasing the kitten with a short piece of pink yarn, and with her right hand she was stroking the little cat's back. She looked at the kitten like a parent watching her child.

"I never pictured you as a cat person," I limped into the room, all smiles.

"I found him!" She picked up the tiny tabby and gave him a big kiss on the nose.

I examined the little kitten. It was covered with fleas, and its mucous membranes were pale as a ghost. I explained to Harriett that these were not uncommon findings in kittens and we should be able to get her new friend all fixed up. It was obvious that she was really in love with her kitten.

"Do whatever you need to do, Dr. Doug. Money is *no* object!" The word "no" came out in song and with a big toothless smile.

The adorable little kitten got a thorough tune-up, and Harriett was sent home with the necessary medications to help strengthen her new best friend. She was thrilled with our hospital and excited about coming back with John for his next set of kitten vaccinations.

"Every hooker needs a John," Harriett explained.

♦ ♦ ♦

Felix, a large California desert tortoise, was not walking upright on all four legs like a normal turtle. Rather, it pathetically pulled itself across the tile floor using only its front legs, dragging the rear legs limply behind like a person with a broken back. With each lurch forward it would let out a barely audible grunt, rest on its belly for a few seconds, then reach out with its two front feet and repeat the process.

"He's been like that for almost three months now," Bob Queensbury explained. His wife, Michelle, was sitting on the stool in the corner.

"As far as we can figure, we think he's about sixty to seventy years old. He belonged to my neighbor, who had him for about forty years, and we've had him about ten."

Desert tortoises, the most common turtle pet in California, have been documented to live more than one hundred years in captivity. Several of my clients own the charismatic reptiles, having been passed down from grandparents to parents to children. They don't reach full size until about twenty years of age, so Mr. Queensbury's estimate of sixty to seventy years added up.

"We have been going to another veterinarian since it started. And we've spent well over a thousand dollars so far, but there's been no improvement." I could see frustration on the owner's face.

"Can you tell me what's been done?"

"I'd rather not." He looked at me with an odd expression.

"Why not?"

"I'd kinda like you to start from scratch. I don't want to prejudice you with anything from the other guy." Bob shook his head in the negative. "He's supposed to be some super expert."

"Well, can you at least tell me if he did any X-rays or blood testing?"

"He never even *touched* my tortoise!" The man almost snapped at me.

I took a moment to digest what he said. "But he treated it?"

"Yeah, he gave it a shot and sent me on my way with some syringes in a baggie."

"What was in the syringes?"

The owner shrugged his shoulders. I wasn't sure if he didn't know or didn't want to tell me.

I picked up the old tortoise. I love these guys. Felix reminded me of my own desert tortoise, Dewe. I hoped he would live as long as Felix.

The first thing I noticed was that for his size Felix was very light—as in skinny. It was clear he had not been eating well. There was very little body fat, and the muscles of his back legs were atrophied from disuse, just as in human paraplegics. My mind flashed back to Mikey the monkey.

I examined the shell, the skin, legs, head, neck and face, the eyes, and then gently opened the mouth. All seemed to be in order.

After my external exam, I carefully tipped the tortoise so it was completely vertical, its nose pointing straight up in the air, and cautiously slipped my fingers under the shell in front of the back legs. In a healthy tortoise this can be dangerous if the tortoise suddenly pulls its legs into its shell the way they do when they want to hide. Some tortoises are so strong that your fingers can be crushed.

Felix, however, was unable to use its rear legs, so they just hung limp. As soon as I felt up inside its flanks with my fingers, I knew what the problem was. "May I take an X-ray?"

"I wish you would!" Mr. Queensbury seemed exasperated. "I asked the other doc to do that every time I went in for a recheck."

No sooner had he said yes than Stacey entered the room and picked up the tortoise. "Got it."

"I know what's wrong with Felix," I said as Stacey left the room with the tortoise. "I just want to get an X-ray so I can see the extent of the problem. Now, would you mind telling me what the other doctor diagnosed and how he was treating it?"

The Queensburys looked at each other. I realized that the wife had yet to speak.

"Tell him." Her arms were tightly crossed over her chest. Her body language spoke volumes.

"It was Dr. Ridley Woakes," the man said. "He diagnosed malathion poisoning. He thought that Felix got it from walking around our yard. We had sprayed for fleas." He waved his arm around the room as if he were using a fogger.

This seemed an odd diagnosis. Malathion is an organophosphate pesticide used to treat mosquitos, fleas, and other yard bugs. It is generally considered safe unless ingested in large quantities, which was highly unlikely if it was only used on outdoor grass. In addition, as soon as the sun hits the chemical, it's deactivated. So unless the tortoise got into the container, or it was poured directly on him, toxicity was not plausible.

Most importantly, malathion toxicity produces seizures, not flaccid paralysis, so I had serious doubts that malathion was the cause of Felix's leg problems. My thoughts were confirmed when Stacey brought Felix and his X-ray back into the room.

"Do you recall what the shot was that Woakes gave Felix?"

Mrs. Queensbury pulled out a file from her large purse and riffled through it. "Atropine." She looked up at me. "He said it was an antidote."

"Yeah, and he had us give one injection in his arms every day for the next two weeks." Mr. Queensbury pointed to a spot on Felix's front legs. "As you can see, it didn't work."

"Atropine is used as an antidote for malathion, but that's not Felix's current problem." I put the X-ray on the view box in the room. You could immediately see a large white object in the belly of the old tortoise. I had felt it during my exam, but now I could show the owners.

I pointed to the large rock-like structure in the tortoise's insides. "That's a bladder stone." I outlined the easily seen bright white object on the dark X-ray. "You can see how large it is. It fills up the entire abdomen."

They both walked up close to the viewer to get a better look.

"I am convinced that what is happening here is a condition called obturator paralysis." I pointed to where the edges of the bladder stone were impinging in the inside of the pelvis. "There are two big nerves, one each on either side of the inside of the pelvic bones. The stone is so large that it's pinching the nerves, paralyzing the rear legs."

The owners studied the X-ray.

"I'll be a fucked monkey!" Mr. Queensbury blurted out. "That son of a bitch never even so much as touched Felix." He turned toward me. "How long do you think that's been in there?"

"Stones can form overnight in tortoises, but it takes years to get to that size."

"So he's been treating him wrong this whole time?"

"Felix may have had a toxic reaction to malathion when you went to see the other doctor. I wasn't there, so I can't say." I never like to criticize or second-guess other veterinarians.

"That's a bunch of crap, and you know it." Mr. Queensbury was angry. I couldn't blame him, but I was not about to join in.

"Is there anything we can do to help him?" Mrs. Queensbury took a tissue from her bag and wiped her eyes.

"He's going to need surgery to remove the stone." I pointed to the X-ray. "If there's no permanent nerve damage, he *may* regain his ability to walk again." I stressed the *may*.

"Have you ever done this surgery?" The husband asked, more like challenged.

"Yeah," I said, thinking about all the West Coast Turtle and Tortoise Club animals that I had taken to surgery, "many times."

• • •

It was Friday night, and our softball team had a game. Because of my knee, I was banned from playing sports for at least eight weeks.

Wok and I drove to the park with Ellen. If I couldn't play, Wok and I could at least go and support the team.

Getting to the city ball fields was like driving to the Herpetology Society meetings: a long stretch through some sketchy parts of town. Once we were there, however, it seemed protected and safe. With all the bright lights focused on the field, you could not see the dangerous neighborhoods surrounding the park.

The game was close. In fact, the score was tied with just two innings left. Ellen got up to hit. She was an amazing athlete, and opposing teams always underestimated her strength and skills. As a result, they tended to pull their outfielders in. Inevitably, she would put one way over their heads.

Wok took notice and was actually watching her swing. As expected, they played her short, and she drove a liner into the outfield corner. Wok immediately started barking as the team broke into a raucous cheer. Ellen hoofed out a standing double by the time the outfielder was able to retrieve the ball.

Next up to bat was a police officer who worked graveyard security in the ER. He wasn't the brightest or the friendliest guy, but he was huge and powerful and was an asset to the team. The behemoth took it yard on the first swing, launching the ball way over the outfield fence and somewhere into the dark yonder of the apartment complex behind the park. After both he and Ellen touched home and the frenetic celebration was complete, I decided to take Wok and go find the ball.

I could tell Wok needed to pee, so I let him off his leash as we walked around the back of the outfield fence. That particular diamond abutted an alley that ran behind some apartment buildings and was just in the penumbra of the shadows of the park's big lights. As soon as Wok trotted off, his black coat vanished into the night.

The street was dark, making it difficult to see much of anything, especially a baseball. Based on the trajectory of the home run, I expected it to be on the opposite side of the alley, closer to the apartments.

As I crossed the street I could hear voices and see the glows from a cluster of cigarettes. I paid no attention to the people and kept looking under cars, along the gutter, and on the lawns for the ball.

"Dis whatcha lookin' for?" a harsh baritone voice from nowhere called out.

I turned to see a silhouette off to my left. There was just enough light to see the white ball in his hand but not the face of the person holding it or anyone around him.

"Yes, thank you." I started to walk over and get the ball.

"It's mine now."

"It belongs to the park. I saw the last batter knock it over the fence." I didn't want a confrontation, so I tried to maintain a polite exchange and continued to walk over to the stranger. The closer I got, the more uncomfortable I became with the situation.

"Like I said, homeboy, it's mine now!" He tossed it up and down with his free hand, the other holding a cigarette.

"Hey, I don't want any trouble." I was thinking that, given my knee, there was no way I would try to engage this guy, especially since there was just one of me and many of them.

"I'd just like to bring the ball back. Please?" I held out my hand.

"Why don'tcha come and get it?" He held the ball out, tempting me to come forward.

I paused for a moment. Was getting killed or beaten over a softball worth it? No, but it was the principle.

Just as I started to approach him, a flash of growling white teeth flew past me, jumped up, and grabbed the ball from his hand. The startled man jumped back, yelling "Shiiiiiiiiiit!" as he retreated.

Wok hit the ground and slammed on his brakes. He stared down the aggressor then circled back and stood guard by my side, softball in his mouth, lips curled back to expose what looked his sharp white teeth.

"Good boy!" I reached down and took the ball. Wok continued his snarl.

"Thanks, guys." I tossed the ball up and down with my hand like the stranger had done.

I patted Wok on his furry head, then backstepped about ten feet, keeping an eye on the glowing embers from the cigarettes to see if they were following. I paused long enough to assess their response, and when I was comfortable that I'd get out of there with my life, Wok and I turned, ball in hand, and headed back to the park.

"Have a good night!"

◆ ◆ ◆

Officer Kelly Pinkett brought in a peregrine falcon. These birds are famous for their incredible speed, having been clocked at over 200 mph during their hunting stoops, the lightning-fast nosedives they make when swooping down on prey.

Peregrines are one of the few wildlife species that have adapted well to the urban environment, taking advantage of big-city habitat encroachment. These high-diving raptors frequently made their nests on the tops of skyscrapers in the downtown area, and it was not uncommon to see them take doves and pigeons midair as they swooped down from the tops of the tall buildings.

The bird that Kelly brought in today was a young male that had gotten itself into a sticky situation. Apparently it had tried to snatch a rat that was stuck to a glue board on top of one of the downtown skyscrapers, and in the process of grabbing the rat it found itself mired in the gooey trap as well. Between the rat, the falcon, and the glue board, it looked like some bizarre game of Mother Nature's Twister.

Regular cooking oil can safely dissolve the trap glue, so it could be removed without damaging the bird's delicate skin. We didn't have any in the hospital, so Dave volunteered to go pick some up. The plan was for him to walk down the block to the store and get the oil, then stop at McDonald's and grab some lunch on the way back.

I had busied myself with records while waiting for Dave to return when all of sudden Lisa paged up to my desk in a panic.

"Dr. Mader, you need to get down here right away. Lili is here and needs to talk to you!"

That was odd. I wondered if there was some neighborhood unrest she was aware of. It had been quiet the last couple of weeks.

"*Dr. Mader!*" Lili scurried across the reception room as soon as I entered. She was wearing her Country Kitchen serving apron.

"Your guy just got arrested!" Her round face was red, eyes animated, arms flailing. "Right in front of my place!"

"What guy, Lili?" I walked over to her and grabbed her hands to calm her down.

"The guy! The guy with the gray hair and big moustache!"

"Dave? What happened?"

"I was serving some people on the patio, and I saw him walk by and waved to him. He waved back. He is so nice!" Lili cupped her hands over her heart.

"Go on . . ." By now, several other staff members had gathered around.

"All of a sudden two cop cars pulled up, cutting him off, right on the sidewalk, and yelled at him to get down on the ground. He looked so scared!" She went back into her histrionics.

"The cops had their guns pointed at him and were screaming at him to get down, get down." She repeatedly pushed her hands toward the ground demonstrating how the cops were acting.

"He put his hands on top his head and knelt down on the sidewalk like he was told. But den, dis cop came up behind him and kicked him in the back, knocking him face first into the sidewalk. He hit hard, blood all over the place." She gestured to her face.

We were all in shock listening to her account.

"Then, the same cop stepped on the back of his neck, holding him down while the other cops came over and handcuffed him." She cupped her hands together like in prayer, her mouth gaped like a big O as she finished her description.

"Did they take him away in the car?"

"Oh, yes! Two more cars came. They kept him on the ground for a long time, lying in his own blood, before they dragged him into the back seat of one of the cars."

I don't think any of us had taken a breath the entire time she was talking.

"Thank you, Lili." I bent over and hugged the little Korean cook. "Thank you for telling us. I'll find out what happened and let you know as soon as I hear anything."

"He was all bloody!" She pointed to her face with open hands once again. "His hair was stuck to the side of his face."

I ran upstairs and called our attorney, Matt. He said not to worry, he would go immediately to the police station downtown and find out what had happened and would call me back with the details.

I hung up in shock. Dave was such a sweet man. I couldn't imagine him doing anything that would warrant such a violent response by the police. And the way they treated him! My God! He had a metal plate in his head from a war wound. He must have been in horrible pain.

I couldn't just stand around waiting for Matt to call, so I had Lisa move all of my appointments to the other doctors and headed to the police station. When I arrived, the desk sergeant confirmed that Dave had been arrested, but would not tell me any details or let me see him. I tried to tell the sergeant about Dave's medical issues, but he didn't want to hear it.

While I was standing in the middle of the booking room, surrounded by gangbangers, addicts, and prostitutes, not sure what my next move would be, Matt came walking out of the holding cell area.

"Oh, am I glad to see you!" I reached out and gave Matt's hand a firm shake.

"It's not good right now, Doc." Matt's expression was clearly stressed. "They got him on resisting arrest and carrying a concealed weapon."

"That can't be. Dave would never do that." I was incredulous. "And that's not the account I got from Lili, who witnessed the whole thing."

Matt was unable to get a first appearance before the judge in order to get Dave's bail set until the following morning, so Dave would have to spend the night in jail.

"Go back to work, call his wife, and stay by your phone," Matt advised me. "He had to get a few stitches in his head, but he'll be okay."

I didn't know how Matt could stay so calm, but that's why Matt was a good attorney.

"Will do." I reached out and gave Matt a hug. "Dave's a good guy. I'll cover your costs. I don't want him assigned a public defender."

◆ ◆ ◆

I stood in the corner of the surgery room watching Fred and Stacey prep Felix, Bob and Michelle Queensbury's paralyzed desert tortoise, for his imminent procedure. The dramatic black-and-white X-ray showing the large bladder stone was affixed to the front of the illuminated light box on the wall behind them and cast a bluish fluorescent tint over the stainless steel surgery table. The ventilator rhythmically hissed with each breath, and the tortoise's front legs and lungs were moving in unison with the sound.

"Okay, Doc. We're ready." Fred applied the final spray of the antiseptic orange Betadine on the tortoise's belly while Stacey checked to see that the anesthetic level was appropriate for my initial cut through the hard shell. As expected, the large bladder stone was pinching off both obturator nerves, causing his paralysis.

As soon as I finished applying the clear epoxy patch, I left the room. Stacey and Fred were the best, and I knew that they would get Felix into the recovery room and awake in no time.

"I'm going to call the attorney to see how it went in bail court, then head over to Dave's," I announced as I exited the surgery suite. "Page me if anything comes up."

I'd never been to Dave's before. He lived down the Corridor, past the "safe zone" that I always warned my students about. I hadn't driven in this direction since my visit to the location where Matt, Cutter the cat's owner, was murdered during the riots. It had been two months since the unrest, and the scars of burned buildings and broken glass were pervasive.

I heard the unmistakable sound of unlatching locks after tapping on Dave's door.

"Oh man, I'm so sorry!" Dave broke into tears when he saw it was me. His face was puffy. His left eye was bruised black, blue, and red; his cheeks were swollen; and there was a line of stitches just over his brow, on the same side of his head as the metal plate in his skull. Dried blood caked his shirt just under his cheek and the front of his pants. He hadn't shaven and looked horrible. Kim, his wife, was standing behind him, eyes puffy, as I entered.

I did not say anything, just reached over and gave him a hug. Kim came over and joined in.

I took Wok to the park after work as usual. We sat on our favorite bench, and I told him about what had happened to Dave on Monday, his night in jail, and his court appearance Tuesday morning.

It turned out that the "concealed weapon" that he was carrying was the red-handled butterfly knife that he used for his magic tricks. This type of knife, however innocent its intended use, was illegal in California, and

Dave was breaking the law by having it in his possession.

Apparently, just before lunch, a bank down the block past McDonald's had been robbed. The perpetrator was wearing blue jeans and a white T-shirt and was seen running down the Corridor in the direction of NAVH about the time Dave was walking to the grocery store to buy the cooking oil.

Dave was also wearing blue jeans and a white T-shirt.

But that's where the similarities ended. The robber had been reported to be Hispanic, heavyset, and about six feet tall with short black hair. Dave was Caucasian, maybe 130 pounds when soaking wet, five feet eight, and had shoulder-length gray-brown hair.

Nevertheless, the cops took Dave down in a SWAT-like assault as soon as they spotted him. Never mind that Dave was walking toward, not running from, the bank. Never mind that Dave did not match the description of the bank robber or put up any resistance. He was still slammed to the ground, had his head stepped on, his face split open, and was thrown in jail.

Oh, but he did have a butterfly knife in his pocket.

Wok looked at me with sadness in his dog eyes. We didn't talk much the rest of the time at the park. Instead we just sat together on the bench, buddies that we were, secure and happy with each other's companionship.

♦ ♦ ♦

After feeding Dewe and Traci, I picked some fresh roses from the garden. As I was walking back inside, I looked down at my tortoises, happily munching away at their lettuce, and decided to give them a treat. Plucking the fresh buds off two of the stems, I gave each one a rose of their own. If tortoises could smile, they would have, and immediately abandoned their boring romaine for the tasty bright-red petals.

I put the remaining roses in a tall, clear glass vase and set a pack of gourmet red licorice next to it. Finally, I signed a mushy, romantic card with "Happy Anniversary!" and placed the card against the side of the flowers. I doubted I would even see my wife today, on our anniversary. As so often was the case, she would get home after I left for my animal hospital, and I would get home after she left for her hospital.

I worked until the wee hours of the morning on a project for Felix, the paralyzed tortoise. Bob and Michelle Queensbury were anxiously waiting for the old reptile in the exam room when I arrived. After exchanging greetings and shaking hands, Stacey stepped in behind me carrying a plastic bag that held a two-pound, off-white, spiculated, grapefruit-sized bladder stone.

"Oh my God!" Michelle covered her open mouth with her hand. "Did that really come out of his belly?"

"Yup." I nodded, smiling. "Go ahead, pick it up." Stacey handed her the clear bag.

"Wow. It's so heavy!" She repeatedly lifted it up and down.

"Now you can really understand how it must have wreaked havoc on Felix's insides."

"Fuck him." At this point Mr. Queensbury was playing with the bagged rock. He looked up at me. "That bastard's gonna pay!"

I sighed. I assumed he was referring to the other veterinarian, and I was getting a little tired of the expletives.

"Remember, as I told you before the surgery, Felix's obturator nerves have been damaged from the large stone. Nerves can regenerate, but that can take a *long* time." I emphasized the *long*. "And there's a chance that if there's permanent damage, he may never regain the use of his rear legs."

The mood of the duo turned momentarily somber.

"That said, he's still going to be much better off now that this rock is out of his gut. Even if he never returns to walking normally, the surgery will add years to his life."

"But what kind of life will he have if he can't walk?" Michelle Queensbury asked. She once again wiped a tear from her eye.

"Wait and see."

On cue, Stacey opened the exam room door and in walked—well, rolled—Felix, under his own power, pulling himself along with his front legs on his fancy new turtle cart.

"Oh my God!" Michelle said again, and this time she broke out in happy tears.

"I'll be a fucked monkey!" Mr. Queensbury responded.

Felix's rear legs were supported by a miniature skateboard that I'd made in my workshop the night before, attached using a Velcro patch under the shell. The limp, useless rear legs were supported with wide rubber wheels making it easy for him to navigate across the tile floor, turn corners, and even traverse the slight rise of the threshold as he entered. He steered and moved the cart forward using his normal front legs.

Felix booked his way directly across the room to the now crouching Bob Queensbury, who was also crying tears of joy. Stacey smiled and slipped out of the room. "How long will he need the skateboard?" Bob asked, carefully feeling Felix's rear legs.

"Don't know." I shrugged. "Possibly forever, perhaps less. Depends on how he responds to physical therapy."

I reviewed all of Felix's medications with the happy owners and reiterated many times that although he was doing well, he may never regain use of his rear legs. I had a feeling that Mr. Queensbury was no stranger to lawyers, courtrooms, and lawsuits. I wanted to make sure that my guarded prognosis was stated and noted, both verbally and in the written record, before they left.

I saw it in my own two tortoises when I fed them the roses yesterday morning. And, I saw it again when Felix came strolling into the room: tortoises really can smile.

• • •

I never thought I'd say this, but I spent the entire evening cruising the streets, up and down the Corridor, far past and deep into the danger zone, looking for a prostitute. When I arrived at work that morning I was greeted with sad news about Harriett the hooker's kitten, John. Harriett had brought John in as an emergency visit on Saturday night. For some reason Harriett's pimp had gone on a rampage and kicked the little kitten, sending it slamming against a wall. Although the staff made a heroic effort, Harriett's new love had died during the night. I asked how Harriett had handled it, and all my staff could say was that she was very sad. She paid her bill in cash, as usual, and left without saying much.

I wanted badly to talk with her, but after spending most of Saturday night on her normal corner outside our hospital, likely waiting anxiously for news of her kitten, she had not been seen by anyone since. I drove around the local neighborhoods, traversing side streets and even venturing down an alley where I knew hookers were known to frequent. I tried talking with a few ladies of the night, but none would give me any information on where Harriett might be. Finally, around midnight, I went home and took Wok to the park.

♦ ♦ ♦

"Please give your mother my best." I leaned past the handshake from Mr. Knight and gave the older gentleman a hug. He was by far one of my favorite clients. His little dog, Cindy, happily wagged her tail.

"I certainly will." The retired cobbler, hunched over his walker, was wearing one of his typical, infectious smiles. The receptionist staff members all waved goodbye as Mr. Knight headed out to his car.

Moments later, while I was consulting with another client, Lisa burst through the exam room door. "Dr. Mader, you need to come up front right now—it's an emergency!" Her tone of voice was sheer terror.

I followed her to the reception area and saw Mr. Knight there, alone, clutching the counter, no walker in sight, and Cindy nowhere to be seen. Worse, Mr. Knight's face, hair, and knuckles were covered with blood.

I raced over to the old man and caught him as he started to collapse. "Call 911!" I hollered out to no one in particular.

I gently set Mr. Knight down on the floor next to the fish tank, sliding him over and resting his back against the soft cushion of the bench. Stacey was instantly on scene with a cold towel and started wiping the blood from his face and hands.

"Mr. Knight, what happened? Where's Cindy?" I held him to my chest. Blood smeared over my shirt and tie.

"Please help me." The desperate man looked up at me, eyes red and watery. "She took Cindy!" he sobbed.

◆ ◆ ◆

Lisa rode with Mr. Knight in the back of the ambulance to the hospital. He did not have any family that we could call, with the exception of his mother, and given her Alzheimer's, she would not be of any help. On the way to Long Beach hospital's trauma center Mr. Knight told Lisa what had happened. After he left our office he had walked down the block to where he had parked his car. He had just finished placing Cindy in the front seat and turned to put his walker in the back when a woman came up behind him, hit him over his head, and threw him to the sidewalk, then stole his car—with Cindy inside.

According to Mr. Knight, the woman yelled, "I'm sorry!" as she drove off. Several people had walked by, he went on to say, but no one offered to help him. Finally, he got up, tears and blood in his eyes, and struggled back to our office.

I had Gene call the police. They went directly to Long Beach hospital and spoke with Lisa, and eventually, Mr. Knight once he was stable enough to talk. I also had Gene go over to Mr. Knight's house to check on his mother and arrange for someone to care for her, because it looked like the older gentleman would need to be kept overnight for observation. The ER doctors thought he might have suffered a concussion.

In the meantime, I had Fred call the animal shelter and all the vet hospitals within a ten-mile radius with a description of the little poodle. Peter and Leanne went driving around the neighborhood just in case the carjacker dumped Cindy out on the curb.

All we could do now was wait and pray.

Grant and Chloe Have "a Thing"

I couldn't believe it. It was already the first of July. Just *one month* until my veterinary specialty boards. The test was being administered in conjunction with the American Veterinary Medical Association's annual convention in Boston, on August 1 and 2. It was time to get my flights, hotel, and travel details organized.

It also meant that there was just one month left to study. I was decidedly not ready, and now there seemed to be so little time. How was I going to find the time to cram all the needed information into my tiny, slow brain in just *one month*?

Morning rounds were busy. I knew from Ellen, who had checked in on Mr. Knight the night before, that he was doing well, despite a concussion and several stitches in his head and elbow. He would likely be released that day. Meanwhile, Gene had called around again to the other veterinary hospitals in the area and made a couple of calls to the animal shelter. No one had seen little Cindy. The dog that never left its owner's side must have been petrified. We all continued to pray that it was still alive.

Dave's court appearance was scheduled for later in the morning.

It had been two days since Harriett's kitten died, and no one had seen or heard from Harriett either.

Since it was July, the beginning of summer, we had two student externs for the month. Chloe D'Amato, from my alma mater UC Davis, was staying upstairs in the apartment next to Alex. The two had already met and hit it off. In addition we had Grant Brooks, a true cowboy from Texas A&M. He came complete with a large rodeo belt buckle and shit-kickin' cowboy boots. He was staying with family friends who lived in the shore area.

I took charge of orienting the two new students, and I could sense that there was already some chemistry between them. Chloe was an attractive brunette, about five and a half feet tall, with a dancer's physique. Grant was an easy six feet tall with a V-shaped torso, chiseled jawline, and charming southern drawl. I had a feeling they would each have a summer experience to remember.

Just past noon, Dave stopped by the hospital after his court case had ended. It was the first time he'd been in since his arrest, and he was still sporting the stitches across his brow. His black eye was almost healed, but the scab over his temple was obvious.

"Dr. Mader, can we talk?" Dave came up behind me and gently pulled on my sleeve.

"Hey, Dave!" I turned and gave him a hug. "It's so good to see you." Everybody stopped what they were doing and came over to welcome him back. Dave gave an uncomfortable smile and exchanged pleasantries with the staff. After the last of the embraces he motioned for me to follow him back to the conference room. He pulled the door shut before sitting down.

"I am so sorry to have put you through all of this." He tried looking at me, but I could tell he was fighting back emotions as he looked down at the table. His stringy hair fell over his face, covering the injuries and tears.

"Hey, Dave." I reached across the table and touched his hand. "You are family. You have nothing to apologize about."

"I'll pay you back for Mr. Leonard," he sobbed. "It's gonna take some time, but I promise, I *will* pay you back."

"No," I said, shaking my head with emphasis. "No, you don't need to pay me back." I continued to hold his hand. "You'd have done the same thing for me."

"Yeah, but that's not right." He sat back, pulling away from my hand. "I don't even work here. You shouldn't have to pay for my mistakes."

"Of course you work here, and your only mistake was being in the wrong place at the wrong time!" I raised my voice and shook my head to make a point. "Now tell me, how did it go in court this morning?"

Dave sighed. "Okay, I guess. Mr. Leonard was able to plea-bargain me down from 'carrying a concealed weapon' to 'disturbing the peace.'"

"Wow." I was stunned. I thought for sure they would let him off with a warning, especially with the way the cops had brutalized him during the arrest. "What does that mean?"

"It means that I now have a criminal record, but since it was my first offense I won't have to do jail time, be on probation, pay a fine, or anything."

"So that sounds like a good thing?"

"I guess." He brushed his hair back away from his face. I noticed that the knuckles on his hand were also bruised. "Mr. Leonard was really hoping for a dismissal." He looked back at me. "Apparently after the Rodney King thing, the cops aren't taking any chances. They found a weapon on me, and to them that justified the force they used. They wanted it on the record."

That logic made no sense. The cops had no idea he was carrying the knife until after they tackled him. It was clearly a case of mistaken identity, but of all people, why Dave? He was the kindest, gentlest person on the planet.

"I will pay you back. Promise."

"Dave, you've already paid me back a million times. I'm honored to have you as a friend. You don't owe me anything. End of story. Okay?" I reached out and shook his hand.

Reluctantly, he reciprocated. A handshake. A hug. I was so glad he was back and not more seriously injured.

The rest of the day flew by. Dave spent the day in the wildlife ward catching up with the many cases that had come in while he was away. Robert had stepped up and cared for the wildlife during his absence.

◆ ◆ ◆

"Please help me!" Tina Scheelings screamed as she burst open the front door. Mai Tai immediately screamed as well, adding to the effect. "I need help!" Her voice cracked, petrified, pleading.

As with a "code blue" alarm in a human hospital, everybody in NAVH ran to the front lobby toward the commotion. Tina, standing in the door-way, was holding her crying baby in one arm, the open door with the other. Tina's face, arms, shirt, and baby were covered with blood.

"Max has been stabbed. He's in the car!" She pulled the door all the way open. "Please hurry!"

I was the first out the door. Grant was behind me, followed by Fred and Robert. A late-model black Ford Bronco, engine running, driver's door open, hastily parked in the wrong direction, was pulled up to and over our front curb. I noticed bloody handprints on the rear passenger door as I opened it. Max, the giant Rottweiler, covered with bright red blood, panting heavily between agonal, gurgling gasps, was on the floor wedged between the back and front seats.

I tried to lift him. He startled, jumped, yelping in pain, and whipped around, snapping his large, powerful jaws at me, missing my face by mere inches.

"Someone get me a large towel!" I commanded. Stacey tossed one over my shoulder. The next thing I knew Grant had gone around the other side of the car and was also in the back seat. I covered the struggling dog's head with the cloth to protect us from getting bitten, and we were able to lift the massive dog out, Grant pushing and me pulling.

We rushed the writhing, barking patient to the treatment area. Blood seemed to be pouring from his side, and the towel over his face was already soaked red. Stacey had raced ahead and was waiting at the treatment table with the oxygen cart at the ready. Within seconds of administering a sedative, the monstrous canine lay calm on the table, but with each breath bubbles percolated out the side of his ribcage.

"We need to plug the hole in his chest!" I pushed a large wad of white gauze sponges into the gaping wound. "Cover that with your palm!" I grabbed Grant's hand and placed it over the dressing. In the meantime Stacey inserted a breathing tube down Max's windpipe and started administering oxygen.

I grabbed a scalpel and sliced open Max's chest directly over the stab wound, then reached into his bloody, flailing chest and grasped the collapsed lung. To my horror, the knife had not just punctured the lung but actually shredded it.

I couldn't take the time to try to close all the lacerations, Max was bleeding excessively, so I made the decision to simply remove the entire affected lobe.

It worked immediately. The remaining portions of the lungs started to fill to capacity with each breath from the ventilator, and all the bloody bubbling ceased.

We all stood back and took let out a sigh.

"His gum color is coming back!" Stacey announced.

We looked at each other. The crisis was far from over. But at least for now, he was stable.

◆ ◆ ◆

Noah's Ark Veterinary Hospital was closed for the Fourth of July except for emergencies. I was taking emergency calls, like I usually did on holidays. Since Ellen was working, I took my books to work and decided to just sit in my office and study all day. I made rounds through the hospitalized patients before settling in upstairs to study. Max had made it through the night and was actually doing well considering he had lost a lot of blood, not to mention one of his lungs.

It turned out that Tina had gone for a walk in the park with her three-month-old daughter in a stroller, taking Max along. She had let Max off leash to wander about when out of nowhere this stranger, apparently unaware of Max, attacked her and attempted to steal her purse. Tina screamed for help, worried most about her baby. Max came from out of the bushes and jumped on the attacker. There was a struggle, but Max, being so large and powerful, had the mugger pinned down. Suddenly the man pulled out a large knife and stabbed Max in the chest several times.

Two men who saw what happened grabbed the attacker and held him down until the police arrived. A Good Samaritan helped Tina get Max into her car, and the rest was history.

Normally I hate being bothered while I'm studying, but there was an interruption that I would welcome anytime. Four and a half hours into my seven-hour Sunday studying intrinsic and extrinsic clotting pathways, clotting factors, and vascular response, Fred paged me with some unbelievable news. He had just received a call from Animal Control. One of their officers had found a little white dog wandering along the Corridor, about two miles north of our hospital, wearing one of our NAVH rabies tags. Fred looked up the number on the tag in our records for the officer. It was Cindy Knight! She was frightened and hungry from almost a week on the streets but unharmed.

◆ ◆ ◆

It was so satisfying to watch Tina walk out the door with an energetic, tail-wagging Max. Needless to say, he looked like he'd been through a war. His chest tube had been removed, but his entire left side had been shaved, reddish-purple bruising was everywhere, and he had stitches from top to bottom on his rib cage, making him look like some kind of dog Frankenstein.

Scars were cool though. I certainly had my share of them. They told a story, and Max's story was one of abject heroism. Who knows what would have happened to Tina and her baby if Max had not been with them in the park?

Equally satisfying as seeing them walk out the door was seeing Mr. Knight and Cindy walk in! Here he was for Cindy's regular Tuesday allergy shot. Just one week ago, a bloodied Mr. Knight had passed out from shock in our lobby. There were several bruises around Mr. Knight's head, the thin skin over his brow sported numerous stitches, and his elbow was wrapped in a padded bandage. Still, there he was, with his walker, carrying Cindy under his arm and a characteristic smile on his face. He could not stop thanking us for helping him the day he was carjacked and helping get Cindy back.

◆ ◆ ◆

Things seemed to be on a roll, both work and study. Sending Max home yesterday, seeing Mr. Knight on the mend, and more importantly, his getting Cindy back, plus actually getting the entire afternoon off to study—this was how life was supposed to work in a perfect world. I almost hated feeling so positive, as if I might jinx myself.

My first appointment of the afternoon was with the Queensburys for a recheck on Felix, the paralyzed, skateboarding tortoise. I was caught a bit off guard as I entered the conference room. "Hey, Dr. Mader!" All smiles, Mr. Queensbury immediately stood and extended his hand.

"Hi, Mr. Queensbury." I gave him a firm handshake. "How's Felix doing?"

"That's what I wanted to talk with you about. He's doing great." Again, nothing but smiles.

"That's good news." I was stumped. "I was really hoping to see him for a recheck. To check the shell patch and examine the nerves in his legs."

"Oh, you will." He waved off my statement. "First, I needed to talk with you about Dr. Fuckhead."

I knew he was talking about his previous veterinarian, but I hated to get into the middle of a situation like this. And I didn't like his language.

"I'm going to sue his ass, and I need your help."

"I'll make copies of Felix's records and X-rays." I tried to maintain a purely professional tone. "I can offer an objective second opinion. The medical records speak for themselves."

"I need to get you on the stand and tell the jury what a fuckup he was, and how you were able to make the diagnosis as soon as you touched him."

"I'll cooperate with a descriptive assessment, Mr. Queensbury. I'm required to do that per the Veterinary Practice Act, but I will not offer a subjective opinion."

That comment took the wind out of Queensbury's sails.

"My recommendation to you is to keep it objective." I tried to regain control of the conversation. "If you get sensational, you'll lose the respect of the judge." I held Felix's chart up and tipped it at the owner. "All you need to make your case is right here."

"Okay." He sighed. "I am just so pissed that I really want to nail his ass."

"That's your call."

"Whatever." He stood up and started to walk out of the room. As he got to the door, he turned back. "Wait here, would ya?"

That was odd. I looked out into the hall as Mr. Queensbury walked out the front door. Mai Tai screamed, and Lisa looked up at the door before turning and giving me a questioning what's-up-with-that shrug, which I returned.

No sooner had I then stepped across the hall and picked up the chart from the door slot for my next appointment than Mr. and Mrs. Queensbury came bounding back into the office. Felix was in Mrs. Queensbury's arms, and both Queensburys wore huge, happy smiles.

I put the chart back in the door slot, perplexed.

"Check it out!" Michelle Queensbury announced to the entire room. She bent over and placed the large desert tortoise on the tile floor. I instantly noticed that he was not wearing his skateboard. No sooner had the tortoise's feet hit the ground than he stood erect on all four legs and started walking toward me.

"Oh my God!" Lisa exclaimed.

Fred and Stacey were standing in the hall behind me, and both started clapping. "Woo hoo!"

Fantastic. I had really hoped that Felix would regain the use of his legs, but I had never expected it to be so soon.

◆ ◆ ◆

It was Tuesday, my half day. I had finished my surgeries and was about to head home and study when Tina and Max came in. Max was here to get his stitches out.

"Hey, Tina!" I walked over to her, Max, and the little baby in the stroller. Max sat steadfast next to the child, wagging his stump tail as I approached. The first thing I noticed was a forced smile from Tina.

"Hey, Dr. Mader." She wrapped her arms around me and gave me a hug that I thought was a bit more than just casual.

"Once again, I sense that something's rotten in Denmark." I had used that same line when I saw her back in November and she told me she was pregnant.

"You've got me figured out." She handed the leash to Stacey, who had stepped up behind me. I knelt down next to the muscular Max and took a quick look at my surgery site. It was completely healed, all eighteen inches of it.

"Stace, please take Max in the back and remove his sutures." With that I pointed to the conference room, figuring that Tina needed to talk in private.

"What's wrong?" I asked as Tina sat at the table, pulling her baby up next to her. She immediately buried her face in her hands and slowly shook her head side to side.

"You won't believe what's happening." Tina's eyes were red and moist from tears. "I can't believe it. These past ten days have been a nightmare!"

"What wrong?" I sat across from her and took her hand.

"The asshole," she said as she let go of my hand and wiped a tear from her face. I handed her a fresh hanky from my back pocket. "I'm sorry," she added, looking up at me, then down at her baby, "I shouldn't use that term." She stroked her baby on the top of his head. The child was happily sucking on a pink elephant-eared Binky pacifier, oblivious to the world's problems.

"That man who attacked me," she let out slowly as she wiped away another tear, "is suing me for his injuries and demanding that Max be euthanized because he's such an aggressive dog!"

Why didn't that surprise me?

"I'll do everything in my power to keep that from happening." I reached across the table and held her hand again. She looked up and gently put her other hand on top of mine.

"I don't know what to do."

"Do you have a lawyer?"

"No." She looked down. "I can't afford one, much less now after all of Max's medical bills."

"I'll get you the number of our attorney, Matt Leonard." I sat back and reached for the intercom. "He is amazing," I paged up front and asked Lisa to bring me Matt's number, adding, "and don't worry about Max's bill. Take all the time you need to get it paid off. I'm not in any hurry."

Tina looked up and I could see a forced but appreciative smile.

"I'll tell you something else. Not only will Matt get this a-hole off your back, I'll bet you anything that he will get the judge to mandate that this man will also have to pay you back for any and all of Max's veterinary bills."

After talking with Tina, I immediately called Matt. He said that he would take Tina's case pro bono and only accept payment if the judge mandated that the attacker pay restitution.

Feeling reasonably good about the morning yesterday, and seeing how well Max was doing, I went home and got in a solid six hours of studying. With only some two weeks to go and recognizing that I would never be totally ready, I was at least beginning to feel that I might have a chance to pass the specialty exam.

Shortly after morning rounds, just as I was starting to scrub in for surgery, Lisa came to get me.

"Dr. Mader." Her look was unsettled. "Harriett is here. She seems really upset. I put her in room three."

I could only assume that she was upset with us for not being able to save her adorable kitten. When I walked in I saw a different Harriett than the one I knew. No hooker regalia, but much more subdued clothes, including tattered jeans, a gray, long-sleeved sweatshirt, hood pulled up over her head, and large, dark sunglasses.

"Harriett . . ." She was looking down at the floor when I entered, and visibly shaking.

"Oh, Dr. Mader!" She spun in my direction and threw her arms around me, crying.

At that moment, Harriett was a client, a pet owner, somebody needing compassion, a friend. I held her and let her cry. She wept hard, her body jerking with each wail.

After what seemed like several minutes she calmed down and stepped back, again looking down at the floor. Tears ran from under the oversized shades.

I studied her for a moment. This was a very sad woman. The reaction and body language were not unexpected for a person who had lost a beloved pet. But I sensed something else going on.

I watched her for a moment more, then slowly reached over and touched her sunglasses. She jerked away at first, pushing my hand. But I reached again, even more gently, and removed her round, oversized shades.

Her face had been brutalized. Both eyes were blackened, and a multicolored, bruised, crescent-shaped cut rimmed her cheek.

"My God, Harriett! What happened?"

"I've had a bad time, Doc." She put her glasses back on gingerly, her face clearly still painful.

"I am so sorry to hear about John, Harriett." I wanted to hold her hand, but she had backed away. "I am sorry I was not there for you when you needed me."

"Dr. Doug!" I could see her jaw tighten. "I'm not upset with you. I know you can't be here all the time." She looked up and forced a partial smile. "Your people were solid. They did everything they could." The tears flowed again. I handed her a box of tissues from the pass-through window.

"Where have you been? I've been wanting to talk to you and haven't seen you." She looked up at me as in disbelief. "I even went driving around looking for you, to see if you had gone to another corner. I was afraid that you were mad at me."

She smiled—this time more naturally. "You went looking for me?" She pointed to herself and let out a sad chuckle.

"What happened, Harriett? Where have you been?"

"After your girl told me that John died, I didn't know what to do." She grabbed another tissue and blew hard into her hands. "I just started walking. Walking with nowhere to go. I tried to go home but my 'partment was just so empty without John waitin' for me. Next thing I know, I must've got into some bitch's territory, and she was beatin' my ass. I think she thought I was trying to cut in or somethin'."

I started to speak, but she cut me off by stepping close and placing her index finger over my lips.

"Dr. Doug," Harriett whispered, "I have to leave. I can't stay around here no more. Things have gotten real bad." She looked around for a garbage can for her tissue, then decided to put it in her pocket. "I just wanted to tell you . . . to thank you." As she got up close, I could see through the tinted shades. Harriett looked me in the eyes, "You have always treated me right. You've shown respect. You're real class."

She hugged me, held it for a few moments, her head pressed against my chest, then without saying anything further gave me a light kiss on the cheek, turned, and walked out.

◆ ◆ ◆

I took Wok to the park on Wednesday night and shared the saga of Harriett and her kitten. On the surface, she was such a harsh woman. She lived in a world where to survive she had to be tough, cold. Yet when kitten John entered her life, her true inner beauty came out. Now, her reason to live was gone. Her world had collapsed, and she felt that she had to leave.

I told Wok how young veterinary students always say that they go into veterinary medicine because they love animals and don't like people. In actuality, the animals are a small part of what veterinarians do—they are the excuse for people to come to see us. We often end up primarily caring for the owner. If all I had to do was treat sick animals, life would be simple. It's when you factor in the human component that the profession gets complicated.

Wok, as always, just sat there and listened.

◆ ◆ ◆

My mentor, Dr. Elliott Roberts, had given me a book titled *Self-Assessment: Internal Medicine*. The book was formatted like the specialty board exam and contained multiple questions. Some of the questions were simple, straightforward, like "How many bones are in the dog's carpus?" Others had images like X-rays, ultrasound photos, pictures of disease conditions, EKG strips, and the like. Each image had a question associated with it, and there were five possible answer choices.

The idea behind the book was to take the test cold and then check your score. The test was divided into sections, with each section broken down by subject, so you could tell by your scores which subject areas you needed to concentrate on.

I'm embarrassed to say that I scored just over 50 percent when I first took a practice test that December. That would not have been good enough to pass the specialty exam. Not only did it humble me, it directed me to the areas where I needed to focus my learning.

With just over a week to go before the big weekend, I had planned on retaking the test-book exam again. Granted, I'd already taken it once, and that certainly would give me an advantage this time, but that was seven months ago, and I had done a lot of studying in between.

I unplugged my phone so as not to be disturbed, set the timer on my watch, and grabbed my pencil and paper.

◆ ◆ ◆

"Judge Wapner wanted to film us for *The People's Court*." Bob Queensbury was laughing. "But Dr. Fuckhead wouldn't let him!"

"That's kinda funny," I acknowledged. I could see where a legal case involving a paralyzed tortoise would make for good TV. However, if I were the vet and I had made a big mistake like his, I too wouldn't want to air it on national television for everybody to see.

Felix wandered around the exam room floor, exploring the chairs, shoes, table, whatever he could reach. If you didn't know the old tortoise had been paralyzed a month ago and was still recovering from major surgery, you wouldn't think that anything was ever wrong.

"As it stands, the judge ruled that he was negligent and misdiagnosed Felix's problem. He ordered Dr. Fuckhead to refund all of my medical bills from my visits with him and to pay for all your fees."

"That's really great. I'm happy everything seems to have worked out." I writhed a bit about what I needed to say next. "But Mr. Queensbury, could you do me a favor and stop referring to the other doctor with an expletive?"

Mr. Queensbury looked at me like I just insulted his masculinity. Then after a momentary pause, he continued. "The ironic thing is that *The People's Court* would not only have paid us, and *him*, to be on the show, they would have paid all the veterinary bills, past and present, regardless of who won the case. Dr. Dickhead would have gotten off scot-free.

"I gave the judge a copy of your records and told him that Dr. Dickhead never even touched Felix and that you knew what was wrong the second you picked him up." Mr. Queensbury recounted. "Then I showed him the X-rays, and that sealed the deal!

"As soon as the judge saw Felix prancing around the courtroom he slammed the gavel down and proclaimed, 'Judgment for the plaintiff!'"

• • •

Sidney was curled up on my lap while I was sitting in my ugly chair reviewing cranial nerves when the phone rang.

"Hey, boss." Cliff's voice was quiet, reserved. "Just thought you'd want to know that Package came in."

My first reaction was irritation. Why, on my study day, was he calling to tell me this? News of a visit from our favorite drug dealer could wait until tomorrow.

"He was beaten up pretty bad." Cliff paused. "Seems that he must have crossed the wrong people. Some really nasty people."

"How's Powder?" I immediately thought about the little white guinea pig that Package always carried around with him.

"That's why I called." Again, a pause.

"After they beat Package, they threw Powder on the ground and stomped on him. He's dead."

• • •

That morning I made a quick stop by the hospital to grab some books for the final stretch of studying. It was my last Sunday before the big test. As I walked through the hospital I ran into Robert in the treatment area. He was standing quietly in the corner of the room, leaning against the counter, cuddling with Thor, Pat Peters's tegu.

"You're not scheduled to work today." Robert had taken it upon himself to personally care for the reptile. Still, he didn't need to come in on Sundays.

"Is everything okay?" I asked him. Although he always looked gaunt, today he seemed to have an inexplicable sadness in his eyes. His expression was hollow, distant.

"Yeah." He looked up at me. The black-and-white lizard was resting on his shoulder, its color pattern cryptic in the midst of Robert's neck tattoos. The pointy snout nestled into Robert's long hair, the same way a cat would snuggle with its owner.

"What brings you in?"

"I dunno." He didn't look at me as he spoke. He leaned his head over and rested his cheek on the back of the big lizard. The animal seemed so content on his warm shoulder. "I had a weird dream last night."

"Something you want to talk about?" I stepped over to him, but not so close as to invade his personal space.

He looked up and gave a tiny headshake in the negative.

Beyond his veneer of darkness, with all the tattoos of skulls and devil worship images, Robert had proven himself a sensitive, loyal, caring staff member.

"I've gotta go." I reached over and lightly stroked the back of the tegu, then placed my hand on Robert's free shoulder and gave a gentle squeeze. "If I haven't told you lately, you do a fantastic job. I'm so proud that you are part of our family."

He nodded.

I looked at Robert. Clearly something was troubling him. I thought I could see a real tear just above the black one tattooed on his cheek.

"Call me if you need anything, okay?" He looked up briefly. I was certain he was fighting something back. "Anything."

♦ ♦ ♦

"Where's Chloe?" I looked around the table. It was already past eight o'clock, and I was feeling the pressure of my personal time crunch. I wanted to get started, and I hated wasting time.

"She's running a bit behind," Cliff commented with a quiet chuckle.

Grant and Fred looked at each other, and Grant covered his mouth, clearly hiding a smile.

"What's up?" I was not in the mood for games today. Every minute wasted was a minute lost from preparing for my big test.

Dr. Nordic grabbed the stack of charts. "Mrs. Ingraham's Yorkie's bloody diarrhea—"

"Hematochezia!" I snapped. "It's hematochezia, not 'bloody diarrhea,' Cliff. Please use proper medical terminology." My stress was near redline right about now.

"As I was saying," Cliff, taken aback by my outburst, continued, "Mrs. Ingraham's Yorkie's hematochezia . . ."

Just then, in sashayed Chloe wearing full belly dancing regalia. Exposed cleavage, bare stomach with pierced belly button, and rings on her fingers. Her raiment was complete with all the ceremonial adornments.

What was going on here? I expected any minute to see an ensemble of Arab musicians come marching into the conference room playing the doumbek, riq, and rebab.

Once in the conference room, Chloe took her place at the table and opened her notebook, nonchalantly, as she would any other morning.

No one said a word. This was obviously some private joke, and any other time I would have been intrigued, maybe even found it funny, but today I had too much on my mind. So rather than encourage the theater, I ignored it. When we finished rounds and all the in-hospital cases had been discussed, I asked Stacey to stay behind while the group got up to attend to their assigned duties.

"What was that all about?" I knew she would tell me the truth.

"Chloe was pissed at Grant and Fred for going to a strip club last Saturday night."

I looked at Stacey, clearly clueless.

"You know that Grant and Chloe have been having a thing?" Stacey asked, as if it were common knowledge. I had suspected as much but was always the last to know.

"Chloe was pissed at Grant for going to the strip club. She told Grant that if he wanted to see a 'hot dancer,' all he had to do was ask."

"So that's why she showed up in her costume?"

"Apparently it's not just a costume. She really is a belly dancer. For a living. That's how she pays for school."

"Dr. Mader," Lisa interrupted. I was kind of glad she did.

"What?"

"Robert never showed up for work this morning." She had a look of true concern on her face. "He's never shown up late, much less missed a day."

I immediately thought about my encounter with him yesterday.

"Hopefully he just overslept. Can you call him?"

"He doesn't have a phone."

A chill shot through my body. I had a dreadful foreboding that this was not going to have a good outcome. "We must have his address. Take Fred and go over to his apartment. I have a bad feeling that something may have happened to him."

I couldn't stop replaying in my head the conversation I'd had with Robert yesterday morning. Clearly he was troubled. Did I miss something?

I was about to scrub in for my first surgery when my pager vibrated.

"9-1-1." Nothing else.

Immediately thereafter I received a second page from a phone number that I didn't recognize.

Lisa answered when I called back. "Robert's dead."

"What?" I was trying to process what she just told me.

"Robert," she paused, clearly sobbing, "is dead. He didn't answer his door, so we were able to get the landlord to open it for us." There was a long pause while she collected herself. "We found him in his coffin, where he always sleeps. Dead."

Oh my God. Why didn't I pick up the warning signs? Maybe I could have prevented this.

"Any idea what happened?" I took a few moments to respond.

"The police are here now." I could hear voices in the background. "They think it was an overdose. Possibly suicide." Another pause. More voices. "He looks so peaceful."

◆ ◆ ◆

Tuesday, my half day. Less than forty-eight hours until I had to leave for Boston and the most important two days of my life. I was not in the right mindset to be at work, much less study or take a test that would define my professional status among my peers for the rest of my career.

Ellen, as usual, was already at work when I got home the previous night after a very long day of patients and details dealing with Robert's senseless death. I so needed to talk with her.

Wok and I took an extra-long walk, and then we sat on our bench at the park for the rest of the night. I was in no mental state to study, so it would have been useless to even try. I told Wok all about Robert. I told him how I totally screwed up and didn't recognize that Robert was in trouble, and if I had only been more attentive, he would probably still be alive right now. I had told Robert how valuable he was to our team, but I did not react to his obvious cry for help. I failed him.

Wok leaned close against my shoulder.

◆ ◆ ◆

The drive into work the next morning was beautiful. The coastal fog had started to lift, blue sky teasing between drifting patches of white. Could the day continue so positively after what had happened? No.

The dark cloud of grief was palpable as soon as I entered the building. I tried my best to be cheerful, but it's impossible to pretend that everything is just fine when your friend was found dead less than twenty-four hours ago. As I passed each staffer I gave them a hug and told them how important they were to me.

I finally made it up to the receptionist's office. Lisa was sitting at the desk, her face buried in her hands.

"How are you holding up?" I walked up behind her and placed a hand on her shoulder.

"It just doesn't end." She started to sob.

"I know. I didn't sleep last night. I couldn't stop thinking about Robert and my conversation with him Sunday morning. I should have known that he needed help. If I had, he might still be alive."

Lisa stood up and gave me a big hug, burying her face in my chest. "It's not your fault, Dr. Mader." She stepped back.

After hugging Lisa one more time and telling her how much I appreciated everything she did, how important she was to us, I grabbed some charts and headed back to the conference room to start morning rounds.

We only had a few cases in the hospital, so patient review was quick. After, we all sat around the table talking about Robert, what we could have done differently, and how we could prevent anything like this from ever happening again.

Stacey had heard through the grapevine that Robert had recently been diagnosed with AIDS and there were suspicions that the diagnosis may have been why he decided to take his own life. He didn't leave a note, so we would never know.

♦ ♦ ♦

Less than one day before my flight to Boston, I still had a ton to do. I needed to put the horror of the past few days behind me and move forward, or I'd never get through this.

The day flew by. Between clients I gathered books and notes that I wanted to bring with me for the test. I had pretty much finished packing the previous afternoon, so I just needed to get home and organize my study material.

After finishing my last patient record, I made one final lap around the hospital and bade goodbye to the staff. They all wished me well with typical platitudes. "Good luck!" "You've got this!" and "Piece of cake!"

Ready or not, it was time.

I was glad to finally get out of the hospital. My plan was to get home, take Wok for his evening stroll, then spend some time getting my last bit of packing done and try to hit the sack early. My flight was scheduled to leave Los Angeles at 6:00 a.m. There would be no traffic on the 405 freeway at that time, but I still needed to leave my house no later than 4:00 in the morning.

I got home and opened the door. To my surprise Wok did not greet me with his leash like he usually did. I looked to see if Ellen's car was home, thinking that perhaps she had taken him out for a walk, but it was not in the driveway. "Wok!" I called out as I entered the hallway. I went to my office and put my books on the desk. "Wok!" I called out. No sound.

I went into the bedroom and there was Wok, lying in his dog bed. He didn't even lift his head when I entered the room. It seemed like it pained him just to look up in my direction.

I had an instant flashback to when he was a puppy and discovered he had bad hips. At least that time he had responded when I called his name.

I squatted down next to him and lifted his head. He was so weak. "What's going on, huh?" His eyes were sunken, his nose dry, and when I lifted his lips, his tongue and gums were pale.

I ran my hands over his body. Nothing. I felt for his pulse—it was weak and thready. I tried to get him to stand, but he resisted. When I tried to lift him up he immediately started to retch, and before I could react, he vomited foul-smelling, dark blood.

"Oh God, Wok. What did you get into?" I ran to the bathroom and grabbed a washcloth, wet it, and hurried back to my best friend. I cleaned his face and mouth and kept reassuring him that he was going to be all right.

Sidney came into the room and sat next to us, watching. He was concerned about his brother.

"I've gotta get you to the hospital!" I leaned over and kissed his forehead. I was just about to pick him up but decided that first I should check around the house for anything that he may have gotten into.

I ran out into the backyard and looked around the rose garden, storage shed, and woodpile. Along one of the fences I found a large puddle of what looked like dark, almost black diarrhea. I stuck my finger in it and sure enough, it was digested blood.

"He's got an ulcer," I said out loud.

I knew he looked bad. My dog was bleeding out internally.

I ran back inside and called Alex to let him know that I was on my way in with an emergency—Wok—and to please call Stacey and start preparing for a blood transfusion.

As I lifted Wok to carry him out to the car he grimaced in pain.

I grabbed a towel and placed him on the passenger seat, then raced across town to the hospital. I had already decided that I was not going to stop until I got to the hospital, even if a cop tried to pull me over. Alex, Stacey, Chloe, and Grant were all waiting for me as I pulled up. Grant picked up Wok and rushed him back to the treatment room, where Stacey and Alex had everything I needed ready.

As Stacey placed an IV catheter in Wok's leg, I got a blood sample. As expected, he was severely anemic. His packed cell volume was 18 percent. The value should be greater than 35 percent. He was in desperate need of a transfusion. The blood test confirmed the problem, and now I could treat the imminent threat, but I still did not know what had caused it.

While Alex and the rest of the team started Wok's transfusion, I raced back home to look around the yard and the house for clues. I also wanted to check Sidney, in case whatever made Wok sick had also affected him.

Nothing. Just nothing. I looked and looked. Sidney seemed fine, just concerned.

I needed to contact Ellen and tell her what was going on. I called her portable phone, but as expected, she did not have it turned on at work. I then called her work number, which was something generally frowned upon: the nurses were not allowed to take personal calls while on ER duty. But this was an emergency. I had to talk with her.

"Long Beach Trauma Center," the operator answered.

"This is Dr. Mader. I need to speak with Ellen Mader. It is an emergency."

"Okay, Doctor. Please hold while I page her." Then silence, interrupted every thirty seconds by a barely audible beeping tone.

It seemed like an eternity, but the operator finally was back on the line.

"I'm sorry, Doctor. She did not pick up her page. She must be with a patient. I can leave her a message." The woman was all business.

"Please do. It's critical," I pleaded, "and please keep trying until you reach her." I gave her both the home and NAVH numbers and then headed back to the hospital.

Cancer, foreign body, string, bacteria, amoeba, intussusception, toxin, bloat, autoimmune . . . the differential list went on and on.

Twelve months of intense studying to get myself ready to pass my specialty boards. To hell with the test! This was the real world. I was being tested with life or death right now, and the subject was my dog, my best friend in the world. I couldn't fail! I had to get 100 percent on this test. If something happened to Wok I didn't know how I could go on as a veterinarian.

My mind was spinning as I raced back to the hospital. My first thought was that I needed to pass the endoscope down into his stomach and see if I could identify the cause of the bleeding.

But why? I knew it was blood from the upper gastrointestinal tract. That's why it was black. If the bleeding was from the lower GI tract it would have been bright red—fresh, like blood from a bloody nose. That was basic GI medicine. Then again, the scope would tell me if the bleeding was caused by something he ate, like a nail or needle, or if it was from a tumor. Or was it just an ulcer?

Did it matter right now? At this moment, Wok was in no condition to be anesthetized and scoped. The most important thing was to fill his gas tank and get red blood cells back into his circulation. When he was stronger I could scope him and look around inside.

I had given myself an extra day in Boston to acclimate to the time change, so I could postpone my ticket for a day and scope him tomorrow morning if he was stable enough for the procedure.

He'd better be stable enough. He'd better not die. It was Wok. My soul mate.

Stacey met me at the front door.

"How is he?" I brushed past her.

"He's stable." She hurried to keep up. "Your wife just called," she announced as we headed back to the treatment area. "I didn't tell her what's going on."

I had been gone about forty-five minutes. In my mind, I expected Wok to jump up, tail wagging, happy to see me and ready to go for his evening walk. But that was the Hollywood movie world. It had been less than an hour, and the transfusion had barely started. Wok was lying in his cage, still depressed, still recumbent when I arrived.

I immediately went to him and opened the door, sitting as close as I could get in the floor-level cage. Leaning in, I hugged him and whispered in his ear, "I love you, Wok. Don't you dare die on me."

Transfusions are not without risk. Stacey had attached an EKG to Wok so we could monitor his heart rate, and every fifteen minutes we checked his body temperature to make sure that he was not having a negative reaction to the transfusion.

I called Ellen's trauma center again and again, each time getting a different operator with the same line: "She's with a patient and will have to call you back."

"It's urgent! Please have her call me right away!" was always my response.

Around 9:00 p.m. I thanked everybody for all their help and told them that they should head home.

"I'll stay with you, Dr. D." Stacey came over to where I was sitting with Wok and put her hand on my shoulder.

"Us too," Chloe and Grant both chimed in.

"We're not gonna let you go at this alone, boss man." Alex smiled.

"Don't you need to go get packed for tomorrow?" Stacey asked.

"If he's not any better, there won't be any tomorrow." I was talking to the group but didn't take my eyes off my buddy. He was still so obtunded that he didn't respond when I stroked his thick fur.

"If you are all going to stick around, why don't you order in some pizza. There's no reason why we have to starve while we wait this out."

Alex took it upon himself to call for delivery after taking everybody's requests.

Wok's vitals remained stable. His heart rate, breathing, and temperature were all within normal limits, meaning that the transfusion was being accepted by his body and the new red blood cells were doing their job.

Shortly after the pizza arrived the phone rang. It was Ellen.

"My God, I am so glad you called."

"What's the matter? I got a message that it was urgent, but I haven't had a chance to get to the phone for the past several hours."

"It's Wok. He's really sick." I told her the events of the evening. Because she was an ER nurse, she knew how dire the situation was. "Can you think of anything that he may have gotten into that could have caused him to bleed internally?"

There was a long pause. "No. I was with him all day." I could tell she was thinking it over. "I got home and was all amped up after a rough night and couldn't sleep. So I took him for a roller blade. After that, when we got back, I finally went to bed, and he went outside in the yard like he always does."

"And nothing happened on the roller blade?"

"No. Not on the run, but when I got up and was getting ready to leave he seemed a bit sore. That's all."

Because of his bad hips Wok didn't do much strenuous exercise. Just his regular evening walks in the park.

"Are you still planning on leaving in the morning?"

"Not if he's no better." I swallowed. I really couldn't imagine how I would react if he didn't improve. "I'll make that decision when the time comes."

"Keep me posted."

"It would be a lot easier if you could just call me whenever you get a chance. I can't ever seem to get through to you."

"Are you going to be home?"

"No. I'm staying right here with him." I paused. "I'm not leaving his side. Call me here."

She hung up. When I looked up from the phone, Stacey was looking at me in a way I'd never seen before.

"He's gonna be okay, Dr. D." She came over and gave me a hug. Stacey rarely ever showed any emotion. Once again, as during the past several days, I could not hold back my tears.

The ringing phone interrupted.

"Dr. Mader, it's your wife!" Alex announced over the intercom.

"There's no change," I told her. I had asked her to check in again when she could, but it had only been about ten minutes.

"I thought of something."

"What?"

"He seemed so sore when I got up that I gave him naproxen, the stuff you took for your knee. I figured it would be okay."

"You gave him *what*?" I was pretty sure I heard her right.

"Naproxen. Why?" Ellen was defensive.

"That's toxic in dogs!" My first emotion was anger. How could she give Wok something so dangerous! "Why would you do that?"

"He was sore. I was trying to help him!" I could tell she was starting to cry.

"It may be safe in people, but it's like battery acid in dogs. That's what gave him the ulcer!"

Oh God. What was I doing? I felt so stressed. It was wrong for me to chastise her. I knew Ellen didn't intend to harm Wok; she was just trying to ease his discomfort. At least now I knew what caused his internal bleeding. I've seen dogs take just one naproxen and develop such severe ulcers in less than twelve hours that they rupture their stomachs. Every case I'd seen had been diagnosed during necropsy—after the animal died.

"I'm sorry." I caught myself. "I'm not upset with you. I should not have snapped at you." I hesitated a moment, mad at myself. "Thank you for calling me back. I've got to get him on some medications to stop the bleeding."

"I'm *so* sorry." I could hear her voice tremble. I know she loved Wok as much as I did. "I thought I was helping him."

"I know, sweetie. I've gotta go." I paused. "I am just so stressed right now." I paused again, angry at myself on so many levels. "Love you."

"Love you too. I'll call as soon as I can."

Before I could say anything, Stacey had drawn up a syringe full of famotidine, a powerful histamine H2 receptor antagonist, also known as an antacid. Blocking Wok's natural production of stomach acid would help prevent additional injury to the already damaged gastric lining.

"Give it slowly by IV," I instructed, but I knew she already knew that.

"Do you want to give him sucralfate?" Chloe asked.

"Absolutely! Good thinking, Chloe." Sucralfate coats the lining of the esophagus, stomach, and duodenum, acting like a bandage, which also helps protect the damaged tissue. Finally, I added an intravenous antibiotic that would prevent any bacteria that might be in the stomach from entering Wok's bloodstream and potentially cause sepsis.

All the pieces of the medical puzzle had come together, and a sound treatment plan was in place. Now it was just a matter of time to give Mother Nature a chance to let Wok's damaged insides heal.

Just past midnight, I decided to run home and get my stuff for the trip. At this point there was no sense in trying to get any sleep, since if Wok was stable I'd have to leave for the airport in less than three hours.

I finally convinced Stacey to head home and the students to turn in. I made sure they all knew how appreciative I was for their help and support.

When I returned, I grabbed a book on gastrointestinal diseases and turned to the chapter on stomach ulcers. I put some blankets on the floor next to Wok's cage and reviewed the subject while my buddy slept.

Around 3:30 a.m. I put the book down, and Alex helped me get another blood sample. Wok's PCV had gone from 18 percent to 28 percent with the transfusion: still low, but out of the danger zone. The big thing was whether it would hold or he would keep bleeding. If that was the case, he'd need another transfusion.

I tried to call Ellen again but got put on hold. Since time was now a factor, I just hung up. I felt that Wok was stable for now, and there really was nothing more I could do. My team was good, and if Wok needed another transfusion I had total confidence that they would get it done.

I kissed my friend on his furry head and headed out to the airport.

◆ ◆ ◆

As soon as the plane touched down in Denver for my layover, I called my office. Stacey got on the phone and reported that Wok seemed much more alert that morning. He got up, went outside, and urinated and defecated. His stool was still loose and dark, but not pure blood like yesterday.

When he got back inside he ate some breakfast and even wagged his curly tail. Most importantly, his red cell count had seemed to stabilize at 26 percent. Even though it was down a little from the earlier result, this was to be expected after a transfusion. Not all of the donor cells survive, so a small percentage drop is generally of minimal concern. I hoped it was just a normal response and not a sign that he was still bleeding internally. He was not out of danger, but I was hopeful.

I had slept on the flight from LA to Denver, totally exhausted physically and emotionally. For the next leg to Boston I was hoping to do some more studying. I had packed a hematology book in my carry-on, figuring I'd review blood clotting again. Dr. Roberts had told me that questions about blood clotting pathways and clotting factors were common on the exam.

As soon as the plane lifted off I pulled out my book.

"That looks complicated," the elderly woman sitting next to me commented. Her voice was gravelly, as if she'd been a smoker her whole life. I heard her talking but had not at first realized that she was speaking to me.

"Young man, what is that you're reading?" She grabbed the top corner of my book and gave it a little shake to get my attention.

"Just a book to pass the time." I wasn't feeling conversational.

The lady appeared to be traveling by herself. She was sitting in the middle seat, and the aisle seat next to her was empty. I noticed that the skin on her hands was paper thin, covered with age spots; her knuckles were knurled and twisted. She clearly had a severe case of rheumatoid arthritis. The muscles in her arms were atrophied with age, and her flesh just hung in folds from her triceps. Every vein in her neck was visible. Her cheeks were prominent, lips thin and pale, eyes underscored with dark circles, no brows above. Her sparse gray hair suggested that she might be going through chemotherapy.

"It looks like some type of medical book to me," she continued. "I'm on my way to Boston General to get radiation therapy for a brain tumor." She pointed to her head as if to show me where it was.

"I'm so sorry to hear that." I sincerely was.

"They say I only have a couple of months to live."

I was dumbfounded, as she seemed to be smiling while she told me this horrible news.

"I'm eighty-four years old. I've seen it all. The development of air travel," she pointed around the plane, "two world wars, sixteen presidents, outlived two husbands, and traveled the globe three times around." Her tone became much more animated. "Two months may not seem like a long time, but for me, that's my lifetime and I still have a lot to do. I really don't have time for radiation. But as long as I'm strong enough to do it, by God, I'm going to."

Her lust for living was certainly impressive. Most people traveling on a plane will opt to leave an empty seat between themselves and the next passenger if available. It was obvious this woman had that choice and had not taken it. Clearly she wanted to talk. I closed my book and turned in my seat to engage her. For the next four hours I learned the story of Bernice.

When we landed, I helped my new friend with her carry-on bag as she exited the plane. After giving her a goodbye hug, I asked her to please stay in touch.

"Do let me know how your test goes. I know you'll pass it with flying colors!" And with that, Bernice was off to live the rest of her life.

• • •

I called the hospital from the airport in Boston as soon as I found a pay phone, and Stacey gave me another update. Although Wok's red cell count was still stable, he had developed a fever and his white cell count had gone up—a sign of sepsis. As I feared, he had developed an infection secondary to the ulcer. I gave her instructions to keep him on his IV fluids and to continue to monitor his red cell count every four hours. If it dropped below 20 percent I wanted him to get another transfusion. In the meantime, I told her to start him on a stronger antibiotic to try to stop the infection before it worsened.

I hung up, distraught. It was not the news I wanted to hear. The report from earlier in the morning had been so positive that I was hoping the worst was behind us. I had already made up my mind that if Wok started to decline I would blow off the test and head back to LA on the first flight out of Boston. Flights were leaving every hour, and I could be home and by Wok's side in less than eight hours if needed.

By the time I got my luggage, with all of my heavy books, it was almost 4:30 p.m., peak traffic time. The taxi took over an hour to get to Boston's Back Bay.

I had become so spoiled being treated to VIP rooms as a speaker that

I was aghast when I entered the room in the Sheraton. The $175-a-night room was smaller than my dorm room in college. Oh well, I wasn't there to party. I unpacked my suitcase and laid out the books on the windowsill (there was no desk). I struggled through the chapter on blood clotting, finding it difficult to concentrate due to lack of sleep and worries about Wok. Finally, I ordered some room service so I would not have to waste any more time by looking for a place to eat.

I continued to read as I made my way through the $28 hamburger and Diet Coke. After housekeeping picked up my dinner tray, I read for another four hours before finally falling asleep.

Between the jet lag and dreams and nightmares of brain tumors, bloody diarrhea, IV sets, clotting factors, and burying Wok, I think I may have gotten a rocky two to three hours of sleep when the wake-up call came in at 6:00 a.m. With the time change, that was 3:00 a.m. my time.

I felt like I had been beaten and dragged through salt. I took a cold shower to shock myself back to reality, then grabbed my overstuffed book pack and headed out of the hotel. I went to a nearby diner and downed some eggs and sausage, then made my way to the Boston Public Library, the largest library in the country outside of the Library of Congress. After finding a quiet table in one of the secluded, far-back recesses, I laid out my books, spreadsheets, and study guide.

For the next nine hours I left the table only to visit the facilities or to take a brief Diet Coke break on the outside steps. By six o'clock I was mentally fried. If I didn't know the material at this point, I was in a world of trouble.

I dropped my stuff off in my cubicle of a room at the Sheraton and then stepped out for a walk through the historic Back Bay to clear my head and get some feeling back in my sore butt.

I walked for what seemed like miles, taking in the history of the old city. It was a pleasant evening, and downtown was vivacious. Restaurants and bars were full of people milling about, music, and the smell of freshly baked goods. Just what the doctor ordered. In my meandering I passed by Fenway Park, where the Red Sox were losing the second half of a doubleheader to the Baltimore Orioles. Finally, around nine o'clock (six LA time), I started to get hungry, so I grabbed a small cup of clam chowder and crackers from a street vendor, which was absolutely delicious, then started back toward my hotel.

A few blocks from the Sheraton I passed a bustling cinema. Several blockbusters were playing, but for some reason *Buffy the Vampire Slayer* caught my eye. Why not? It was only 6:30 my time, I wasn't tired, and I was in no mood to do any more studying. So the night before the biggest test in my life, I watched a beautiful, blond teenage Valley girl save the world from evil vampires.

The Big Test

I don't think I slept much that night, but I did wake up feeling confident that I could recognize a vampire incognito and knew the best way to dispatch it if necessary.

I had brought an alarm clock with me. I set the alarm, set my watch, and scheduled a wake-up call. There was no way I was going to oversleep.

Before going to bed the previous night I had called the hospital and checked on Wok. Alex reported that his fever had broken, his red cell count was stable, his white cells were back to normal, and he was eating and acting like he wanted to go home.

What a relief!

I was as ready as I could be. It was game time.

I ate a light breakfast of protein. Carbohydrates give you a short boost, but it wears off quickly and you get tired. Also, the parasympathetic nervous system, the master of the "rest and digest" mode, does not need to be stimulated when you need your mind sharp and focused. A belly full of food is never a good idea prior to taking on any mental challenge.

The short walk from the hotel to the convention center was invigorating. It was a beautiful morning. The sun was out, and the rays felt warm on my face as I approached the testing hall.

A nervous buzz pervaded the foyer as candidates stood in line to sign in and get their testing materials. I was amazed at how many individuals were studying while waiting in line. The proctors at the registration table were carefully checking identification. Hard to believe, but people paying others to take their tests was not unheard of.

I had my good luck charm with me: a two-inch brown plastic horse named Montgomery, given to me when I was a freshman in college by my Secret Santa. Somewhere around my senior year he lost his left ear, but that never diminished his lucky powers. I've had that horse with me for every test I've ever taken, including my State and National Veterinary Boards.

I picked a seat adjacent to the outside aisle in the back row. It's an idiosyncrasy of mine, but I don't like having people behind me. I placed on the table my two #2 pencils, the limit we were allowed to bring to the test, then set Montgomery on the desk directly in front of me. No sooner had I done so than a proctor came over. "You can't have that on the table," he commanded tersely. "You have to put it away now."

I looked at him with an "Are you for real?" expression. I suppose I could have encrypted crib notes all over the tiny equine, but I didn't want to argue. "Okay, Monty," I whispered in his good ear, "into the stable you go," and slipped it into my pocket.

I sat there, looking around the room. You could feel the heightened anxiety all around. My mind was clear and totally focused on the task at hand. Things were in control back at home. Wok seemed to be on the mend. I was ready.

The proctors handed out the tests, face down. "Don't turn them over until instructed to do so," the executive director of the American Board of Veterinary Practitioners announced. "You should all be very proud. You've passed rigorous screening. You've completed extensive case reports. You are the cream of the veterinary crop."

The roomful of candidates was totally silent.

"You have four hours to complete the two hundred questions. When time is up, the proctors will collect your exam. If you finish early, you may turn in your exam to the proctor and leave. You will not be allowed back into the room once you've turned in your examination.

"There will be a one-hour lunch break. The afternoon session will start at exactly 1:00 p.m. If you are late, you will not be allowed in the room to sit for the next session. *No* exceptions." The director charged on like a drill sergeant. "Each question has five possible answers. This test is not designed to be easy, so read each question very carefully, and choose the *most correct* answer."

Really? There might be more than one correct answer for each question?

"If you have to go to the restroom, turn your test over and raise your hand. A proctor will accompany you to the restroom. Only one person can leave the testing room at a time."

If you didn't have to pee before, you probably did now.

"Any questions?" He looked around the room. I think I heard some candidates throw up in their throats. "There is to be *no* talking during the exam. If you talk, you will be asked to leave."

Silence.

"Begin!" He clicked a stopwatch.

I turned over my test booklet. It was thick like a novel. I flipped through the pages just to make sure that I had the complete test, all two hundred questions.

Taking a deep breath, I set it down in front of me and read the first question:

1. How many millimeters a day does an osteoclast move?

    A.   0.01 mm

    B.   0.02 mm

    C.   0.03 mm

    D.   0.04 mm

    E.   0.05 mm

I never studied that! I had no clue how many millimeters a day an osteoclast moves. Oh my God! It was only the first question, and I was already screwed. Should I just walk out now? Why was I even here? Who did I think I was, taking a veterinary specialty board exam?

Unbelievable. A year of studying and intense test preparation, and I felt as though I was done as soon as it started.

I closed my eyes and pushed on my forehead with my palm. Covertly, I slipped the other hand in my pocket and rubbed Montgomery's earless head.

Focus! In a moment of displaced reality I wondered if Buffy the Vampire Slayer knew the answer. That ridiculous thought brought my attention back to the situation at hand, and I silently chuckled. I thought about the choices, considered the question carefully, then picked an answer based on deduction.

Okay, I just needed to get over it and move on.

2. In a patient with hepatic pathology, which of the following clotting factors may be affected?

   A. Factor I
   B. Factor III
   C. Factor V
   D. Factor VII
   E. Factor VIII

Bam! Nailed that one. *Factor VII!* Thank you, Dr. Roberts, for warning me they would ask questions about blood clotting. Once again, I reached down and patted Montgomery on the head. Feeling a bit more confident, I trudged on.

And so it went for the next 198 questions. When I completed the last question, I flipped the test over and sat back to finally take a breath. I knew not to look around the room, so I just closed my eyes for a few minutes, then, when settled, flipped the booklet back over, and double-checked all of my answers.

I didn't change any of my first choices, so I felt reasonably good about my performance. I turned in my test booklet, and as I was leaving I passed several candidates in the foyer *either* discussing the questions and their answers with others or looking things up in books and journals. Dwelling on the uncertain questions at this juncture I think would have just rattled me, and discovering I had gotten an answer wrong would have unnerved me even more.

The conference center wasn't far from the street vendor where I got the clam chowder the previous night, so I headed over in that direction. It was close enough that I could grab a quick, tasty protein refill and still get back in time so as not to get locked out of the afternoon session.

Part two was just as mentally strenuous as the a.m. session. One candidate actually did return late from lunch and was not allowed back in. The woman was halted at the door by one of the proctors moments after 1:00 p.m. Refused entry, she went into a tirade and created quite a scene. Finally, security escorted her away. The drama left everybody inside a bit rattled, but the director was all business and got the examination back on track within minutes.

I left the afternoon session feeling moderately confident, but the osteo-clast question was really eating at me. As soon as I got back to the Sheraton I looked it up in my orthopedic textbook. Bingo! I had guessed right. At least I knew I got two of the two hundred questions correct.

Feeling good, I called NAVH and spoke with Cliff. Wok's red cell count was up to 29 percent, and his temperature had been normal since the change of antibiotics. I felt confident that he had turned the corner. Cliff even said that he was planning on sending Wok home with Ellen tomorrow morning when she got off work.

What great news! I ordered room service and spent the rest of the evening reviewing some subjects that I felt needed revisiting. Tomorrow's session was going to be all practical questions: case presentations with pictures, X-rays, EKGs, ultrasounds, blood smears, histology images, and more.

One last call to NAVH around 1:00 a.m. to check on Wok, and I was ready for the sack.

• • •

"I think there's something wrong with the image," I spoke out as soon as the proctor pointed at my raised hand, less than fifteen seconds into the first practical exam question of the morning.

We were allowed only sixty seconds per image before they automatically switched to the next question. Time was ticking, and something wasn't right.

All the edicts from yesterday applied this morning as well, which meant I was breaking the rules right out of the gate.

"I can't comment on any of the questions," the administrator replied abruptly.

My eyes darted around the room. From looking at the expressions on other examinees' faces, it seemed that almost everybody shared my confusion: the first written question did not appear to correspond to the image on the slide.

"With all due respect, sir." I was taking a chance of getting kicked out of the exam. I could blow off this question, but what if they had the sequence wrong? That could mean that every question was out of order.

"I am not allowed to discuss the test," he countered, more curtly.

"I'm not asking you to say anything about the question, but the image on the screen doesn't appear to match the first question on the written exam." There, I had said it.

Fortunately, almost the entire room nodded or mumbled in agreement. The mass response seemed to overwhelm the exam administrator.

"One second." He stepped from the podium and conferenced with the two other proctors working the room. Finally, the group of three walked back to the slide projector. After a minute of fussing with the gray slide carousel and flipping through the written test, the proctors succeeded in changing the image on the screen.

Ah, now it made sense! The first written question on the exam was about heart arrhythmias in a dog, but the image on the screen had been the X-ray of a cat. The new, clearly correct image was an EKG tracing.

"I apologize." The administrator resumed his place at the podium. "The carousel was not synchronized with the proper question number on the exam." He cleared his throat. "Let's continue."

He lifted the stopwatch and announced, "Start." As he went through the motions, several of the test takers thanked me for speaking up.

"*No talking!*" the commandant decreed.

◆ ◆ ◆

As I sat on the steps of the Bunker Hill Monument overlooking Boston Harbor later that afternoon, my spirits were more uplifted than they had been in months. The sun was high and bright in the midafternoon sky. Billowy white clouds floated across a light-blue background, so different from the Los Angeles brown smog to which I'd grown accustomed. Mindlessly, I watched plane after plane land or take off from Logan International Airport across the bay. At that moment I had nothing pressing, no one demanding my time, no books to cram, no phone calls to return, and no dying dog at home.

The first thing I did when I left the testing center was call work. Fred informed me that Ellen had picked up a happy, healthy Wok earlier in the morning. His fever was gone, and his red cell count was already back up to the mid-thirties. I called home but there was no answer, not surprising, as Ellen was probably sleeping. I wanted to talk to her about Wok and tell her about my exam. No worries, it could wait.

Next call was to Elliott Roberts to let him know that I was finished and to thank him profusely for all his help. Of course, he wanted to know how I did, and I had no idea. The examination was a bear. Unlike in college where tests are often graded on a curve, the specialty boards are a straight percentage. If you get enough answers correct, you pass and are a specialist. If not, you aren't. It was that simple. He was confident that I had done well. I wished I had his prescience.

I had walked to the monument from the convention center, but as I watched the busy airport off in the distance, I realized that time was running short, so I hailed a taxi to head out for my six o'clock flight. With the time change I'd be home shortly after ten. Ellen would be at work, but I couldn't wait to see Wok and the rest of my furry, scaly family.

What a year it had been. Trying to study for the exam while dancing with life's characters to a choreography totally out of my control. Managing the chaos created by a busy hospital, politics, teaching, personalities and egos, lawsuits, arrests, threats, life, death, and riots. It certainly had not been easy. Regardless of how I did on the exam, I knew that I was a better doctor for having made the effort. The executive director's final words to the group had been "Expect your scores in the next four to six weeks. Please don't call the ABVP office. We'll get the pass/fail letters out to you as soon as possible."

Epilogue

Dottie Shackleford from the West Coast Turtle and Tortoise Club waited patiently on the opposite side of the receptionist counter as Lisa processed her invoice. She had brought in two egg-bound female desert tortoises last week and come in today to pick them up. It was that time of year when female tortoises had their all-too-common reproductive problems.

"Here's your receipt." Lisa smiled and handed Dottie her paperwork. The Tortoise Club elder glanced down at the total on the bill, shaking her head.

I couldn't help but laugh to myself. Of all people to be critical of my prices, Dottie shouldn't be one of them. I charged the club only my actual costs on any procedures I did and never included a charge for my time.

Just then the front door opened, and in walked an enormous arrangement of flowers, bursting with a brilliant rainbow of colors and a silver Mylar balloon that read, "Congratulations!"

Mai Tai screamed, frightening the courier. After regaining his composure, he approached the reception area.

"For Dr. Mader." The deliveryman read from a small note.

"I'm Dr. Mader." I stepped up to the desk.

He placed the gigantic bouquet on the counter. "Here you go!"

I took the small card from the stick in the front of the basket and opened it while Lisa and Dottie watched.

> *Congratulations, Dr. Doug Mader!*
> *Diplomate, American Board of Veterinary Practitioners*
> *(Companion Animal Practice)*
> *I am so proud of your accomplishments. I knew you could do it!*
> *Love,*
> *Kristin*

Wow. How nice. Kristin Sullivan, my *human doctor* friend. She was a boarded specialist in human medicine, so she knew what it took.

"Congratulations for what?" Dottie's smoker voice disrupted my musings.

"Dr. Mader just passed his Veterinary Specialty Boards!" Stacey answered with a huge smile, her pride in my accomplishment evident. She had heard the commotion from Mai Tai and come up front to see what was happening.

"Oh?" Dottie did not seem at all impressed. "I suppose that means you're going to raise your prices?"

Acknowledgments

My greatest appreciation goes out to my agent, the late Peter Miller of Global Lion Intellectual Property Management. There is a reason he was known as the Literary Lion. Sadly, Peter passed away and never got to see this book in print. I know he would have been proud. Carl Hiaasen has been a great friend and mentor over the years. Elizabeth Green of Brief Media told me to quit my day job and keep writing. Nanette LeFevre and Kelly Martin gave me the motivation to see this project through. Paul DeAngelis is a consummate professional and helped shape this story into the work of art it is. Adam O'Brien and Julia Abramoff have been wonderful editors to work with at Apollo. Finally, I want to thank my nonhuman family: Aragon, Atigun, Bali, Dalton, Simon, Traci, Kevin, Rinca, London, Stella, and Astro. Most importantly, much forever love to Swatch, who encouraged me to pursue my dream of writing about the most wonderful career in the world.

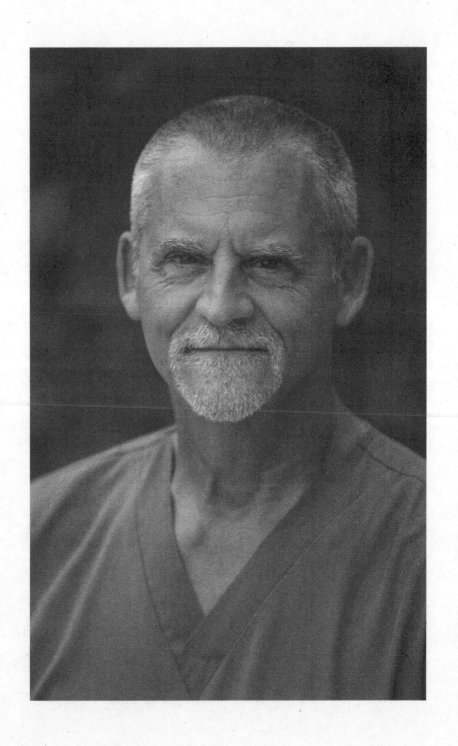

About the Author

DR. DOUG MADER is a triple board-certified veterinary specialist and has been a veterinarian for over three decades. He is an internationally recognized speaker, has written four best-selling medical textbooks and numerous book chapters and scientific publications, and has had long-standing pet columns in the *Long Beach Press Telegram*, *Reptiles* magazine, and the *Key West Citizen*. Dr. Mader is the recipient of the U.S. Fish & Wildlife Service Award, the UC Davis School of Veterinary Medicine Alumni Achievement Award, and the Fred L. Frye Lifetime Achievement Award for Veterinary Medicine, and is a six-time winner of the North American Veterinary Community Speaker of the Year award and a four-time winner of the Western Veterinary Conference Educator of the Year award. He is also a fellow of the Royal Society of Medicine in the UK. Dr. Mader practiced in California for many years, but today lives and works in the Florida Keys.